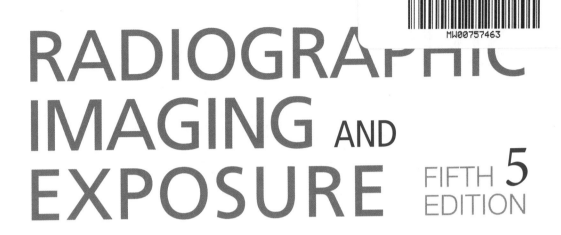

RADIOGRAPHIC IMAGING AND EXPOSURE

FIFTH 5 EDITION

TERRI L. FAUBER, EdD, RT(R)(M)

Associate Professor and Radiography Program Director
Department of Radiation Sciences
School of Allied Health Professions
Virginia Commonwealth University
Richmond, Virginia

with 207 illustrations

ELSEVIER

ELSEVIER

3251 Riverport Lane
St. Louis, Missouri 63043

RADIOGRAPHIC IMAGING & EXPOSURE, FIFTH EDITION   ISBN: 978-0-323-35624-4
Copyright © 2017 by Elsevier, Inc. All rights reserved.

Notices

Previous editions copyrighted 2013, 2009, 2004, and 2000.

Library of Congress Cataloging-in-Publication Data

Names: Fauber, Terri L., author.
Title: Radiographic imaging & exposure / Terri L. Fauber.
Other titles: Radiographic imaging and exposure
Description: Fifth edition. | St. Louis, Missouri : Elsevier, [2017] |
    Includes bibliographical references and index.
Identifiers: LCCN 2016009225 | ISBN 9780323356244 (pbk. : alk. paper)
Subjects: | MESH: Radiography | Radiographic Image Enhancement
Classification: LCC RC78 | NLM WN 200 | DDC 616.07/572--dc23 LC record available at
http://lccn.loc.gov/2016009225

Content Strategist: Sonya Seigafuse
Content Development Manager: Billie Sharp
Associate Content Development Specialist: Samantha Dalton
Publishing Services Manager: Jeff Patterson
Book Production Specialist: Bill Drone
Design Direction: Paula Catalano

Printed in the United States of America

Last digit is the print number: 9   8   7   6   5   4   3

CONTRIBUTORS

James N. Johnston, PhD, RT(R)(CV)
Professor Radiologic Sciences
Dean of the Robert D. & Carol Gunn College of
 Health Sciences and Human Services
Midwestern State University
Wichita Falls, Texas

Rebecca Harris Keith, MS, RT(R)(CT)
Assistant Professor & Director of Admissions
Department of Radiation Sciences
School of Allied Health Professions
Virginia Commonwealth University
Richmond, Virginia

Andrew Woodward, MA, RT(R)(CT)(QM)
Assistant Professor
Division of Radiologic Science
School of Medicine
University of North Carolina at Chapel Hill
Chapel Hill, North Carolina

REVIEWERS

Dean Ann Brake, MEd, RT(R)
Associate Professor
St. Louis Community College
St. Louis, Missouri

**Mary Doucette, MS RRA, RT(R)(M)(MR)
(CT)(QM)**
Program Director, AAS Radiology Technology
Great Basin College
Elko, Nevada

Pamela L. Harmon, MA, RT(R)
Radiologic Technology Program Coordinator
Triton College
River Grove, Illinois

Deborah R. Leighty, MEd, RT(R)(BD)
Clinical Coordinator, Radiography Program
Hillsborough Community College
Tampa, Florida

Radiographic Imaging & Exposure takes a unique and more effective approach to teaching imaging and exposure by focusing on the practical fundamentals. With a topic such as radiographic imaging, it is impossible to entirely depart from theoretic information, and we do not want to do so. A concerted effort was made to present the most important and relevant information on radiographic imaging and exposure. This book highlights the practical application of theoretical information to make it more immediately useful to students and practicing radiographers alike. Our ultimate goal is to provide the knowledge to effectively solve problems for consistently producing quality radiographic images in a clinical environment.

WHO WILL BENEFIT FROM THIS BOOK?

Radiographic Imaging & Exposure provides a fundamental presentation of topics that are vital for students to master to be competent radiographers. Moreover, radiographers will benefit from the practical approach to the topics of imaging and exposure presented here.

ORGANIZATION

Radiographic Imaging & Exposure begins with a description of Wilhelm Conrad Roentgen's discovery of x-rays in 1895 and the excitement it first caused among the members of the nineteenth-century society, who feared that private anatomy would be exposed for all to see! The introductory chapter moves into the realm of radiologic science with discussions of x-rays as energy, the unique characteristics of x-rays, and the fundamentals of radiation protection. Chapter 2 provides a more detailed discussion of the x-ray beam. The subsequent chapters describe image formation and radiographic quality (Chapter 3), digital imaging (Chapter 4), film-screen imaging (Chapter 5), exposure technique factors (Chapter 6), and scatter control (Chapter 7). Chapter 8 focuses on the tools available to assist the radiographer in selecting appropriate exposure techniques, such as automatic exposure control devices, anatomically programmed techniques, and exposure technique charts. Chapter 9 helps the reader apply previously gained knowledge to evaluate image quality and to identify factors contributing to poor-quality images and strategies for improvement. Chapter 10 discusses the components of fluoroscopic units, viewing and recording systems, and finally, the digital fluoroscopy technology in use today.

Radiation exposure and imaging continues to be a complex subject even in the digital age. This text provides a thorough yet practical level of imaging and exposure to equip radiographers with the knowledge they need to produce high-quality images on the first attempt.

DISTINCTIVE FEATURES

Radiographic imaging and exposure is a complex topic, and a mastery of the fundamentals is necessary to become competent, whether you are a student or a practicing radiographer. Three special features have been integrated within each chapter to facilitate the understanding and retention of the concepts discussed and to underscore their applicability in a clinical setting. In addition, these special features give the practicing radiographer quick visual access to fundamental information that they need every day. Each feature is distinguished by its own icon for easy recognition.

Important Relationships summarize the relationships being discussed in the text, as each one occurs, for immediate summary and review. The topic of radiographic imaging and exposure is replete with fundamental, important relationships, and they are emphasized in short, meaningful ways at every opportunity.

 Mathematical Applications demonstrate the importance of mathematical formulas. Radiographic imaging also has a strong quantitative component, and this feature helps accustom the reader to the necessity of mastering mathematical formulas. Because the formulas are presented with clinical scenarios, an immediate application and explanation of the formulas is provided.

 Radiation Protection Alerts emphasize the imaging and exposure variables that can have an impact on radiation exposure to patients and others. Because computer processing can mask exposure errors, it is even more important for radiographers to comprehend how their exposure technique choices can affect the patient.

NEW TO THIS EDITION

Digital imaging and film-screen imaging content have been separated into two chapters in this edition of *Radiographic Imaging & Exposure*. The digital imaging content has been expanded to include the most current concepts. Providing a chapter exclusively for film-screen imaging and adding more content will assist educators who still teach film-screen imaging. Educators who limit the amount of film-screen imaging taught can choose to skip Chapter 5. As in previous editions, emphasis is placed on the responsibilities radiographers have in limiting the radiation exposure to the patient.

The fifth edition of *Radiographic Imaging & Exposure* includes the following:

- Expanded and in-depth coverage of digital and film-screen imaging and an increased coverage of fluoroscopy, including digital fluoroscopy, that meets the ARRT examination content specifications.
- Emphasis on radiographers' responsibilities in minimizing radiation exposure to patients and themselves.
- Chapter 9, *"Image Evaluation,"* gives students the opportunity to apply the knowledge they have gained from earlier chapters by evaluating image quality and practicing problem-solving skills related to exposure technique factors. This practical application enhances learning and builds on the knowledge students have already acquired.

LEARNING AIDS

One of the primary goals of *Radiographic Imaging & Exposure* is to be a practical textbook that prepares student radiographers for the responsibilities of radiographic imaging in a clinical setting. Every effort has been made to make the material easily accessible and understandable while remaining thorough.

- The writing style is straightforward and concise, and the textbook includes numerous features to aid in the mastery of its content, including *Important Relationships, Mathematical Applications,* and *Radiation Protection Alerts.*
- All the *Important Relationships, Mathematical Applications,* and *Radiation Protection Alerts* are also collected in separate appendices for quick reference and review, and are organized by chapter.
- *Radiographic Imaging & Exposure* also includes traditional learning aids. Each chapter begins with a list of objectives and key terms and concludes with a set of multiple-choice review questions, which help readers to evaluate whether they have achieved the chapter's objectives. An answer key is provided in the back of the book.

ANCILLARIES

For the Instructor

Evolve Resources is an interactive learning environment designed to work in coordination with *Radiographic Imaging & Exposure,* 5th edition. It includes laboratory activities, PowerPoint slides, mathematical worksheets, an image collection of approximately 207 images, two practice tests with 60 questions each, and a Test Bank in Exam View with more than 620 questions.

The ancillary material on Evolve is useful for both the practiced and the novice educator. The laboratory exercises accommodate different resources and instructor preferences with recommended laboratory activities. Additional mathematical worksheets are included for educators to provide more practice for students if required.

Instructors may also use Evolve to provide an Internet-based course component that reinforces and expands the concepts presented in class. Evolve may be used to publish the class syllabus, outlines, and lecture notes; set up "virtual office hours" and e-mail communication; share important dates and information through the online class calendar; and encourage student participation through chat rooms and discussion boards. Evolve allows instructors to post exams and manage their grade books online. For more information, visit *http://evolve.elsevier.com*, or contact an Elsevier sales representative.

ACKNOWLEDGMENTS

The opportunity to publish a 5th edition has far exceeded my expectations for this textbook, and I continue to be amazed by its reception within the radiography community. It takes many dedicated and knowledgeable people to revise and improve a textbook on radiographic imaging and exposure. Sonya Seigafuse has been extraordinarily supportive throughout this journey to publication. Samantha Dalton and William Drone have worked diligently to ensure the quality and accuracy of the chapters.

Educators, students, and radiographers have challenged me to pursue excellence in producing an imaging textbook that is comprehensible, accurate, and relevant to radiographic imaging. I am also indebted to the many authors before me who have explored complex physics concepts in an effort to explain the theory and practice of radiographic imaging. Comprehending the intricacies of digital imaging continues to be a challenge, and I am grateful for the knowledge and expertise of Andrew Woodward in helping me explain complex digital imaging concepts. His contributions have been invaluable. My admiration continues for all the educators, students, and imaging professionals who desire to achieve excellence in radiographic imaging.

Terri L. Fauber

CONTENTS

1 **Radiation and Its Discovery,** 1

2 **The X-ray Beam,** 15

3 **Image Formation and Radiographic Quality,** 42

4 **Digital Imaging,** 67

5 **Film-Screen Imaging,** 110

6 **Exposure Technique Factors,** 147

7 **Scatter Control,** 178

8 **Exposure Technique Selection,** 208

9 **Image Evaluation,** 237

10 **Dynamic Imaging: Fluoroscopy,** 262

Appendix A: Summary of Important Relationships, 285

Appendix B: Summary of Mathematical Applications, 295

Appendix C: Summary of Radiation Protection Alerts, 299

Appendix D: Answer Key for Chapter 9: Image Evaluation, 302

Chapter Review Questions Answer Key, 314

Illustration Credits, 316

Glossary, 318

Index, 324

Radiation and Its Discovery

CHAPTER OUTLINE

Discovery
X-rays as Energy
   Radiation Units of
     Measurement

Properties of X-rays
The Fundamentals of Radiation
    Protection

OBJECTIVES

After completing this chapter, the reader will be able to perform the following:

1. Define all the key terms in this chapter.
2. State all the important relationships in this chapter.
3. Describe the events surrounding the discovery of x-rays.
4. Describe the dual nature of x-ray energy.
5. State the characteristics of electromagnetic radiation.
6. Differentiate among the units of measurement for radiation.
7. List the properties of x-rays.
8. Recognize the fundamentals of radiation protection.

KEY TERMS

absorbed dose
air kerma
ALARA
dose equivalent

electromagnetic radiation
exposure
fluorescence
frequency

photon
quantum
radioactivity
wavelength

X-rays were discovered in Europe in the late nineteenth century by German scientist Dr. Wilhelm Conrad Roentgen. Although Roentgen discovered x-rays by accident, he proceeded to study them so thoroughly that within a very short time, he identified all the properties of x-rays that are recognized today. Roentgen was more interested in the characteristics of x-rays as a form of energy than their practical application. X-rays are classified as a specific type of energy termed *electromagnetic radiation*, and like all other types of electromagnetic energy, x-rays act like both waves and particles.

DISCOVERY

X-rays were discovered on November 8, 1895, by Dr. Wilhelm Conrad Roentgen (Figure 1-1), a German physicist and mathematician. Roentgen studied at the Polytechnic Institute in Zurich. He was appointed to the faculty of the University of Würzburg and was the director of the Physical

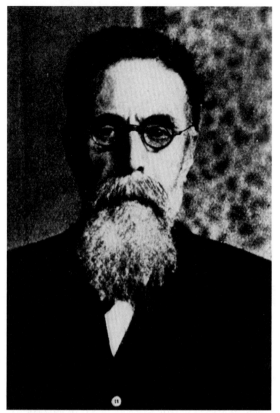

FIGURE 1-1 Dr. Wilhelm Conrad Roentgen.

Institute at the time of his discovery. As a teacher and researcher, his academic interest was the conduction of high-voltage electricity through a low-vacuum tubes. A low-vacuum tube is simply a glass tube from which a certain amount of air is evacuated. The specific type of tube that Roentgen was working with was called a *Crookes tube* (Figure 1-2).

At the end of his workday on November 8, Roentgen prepared his research apparatus for the next experimental session to be conducted when he would return to his workplace. He darkened his laboratory to observe the electrical glow (cathode rays) that occurred when the tube was energized. This glow from the tube would indicate that the tube was receiving electricity and was ready for the next experiment. That day, Roentgen covered his tube with black cardboard and again electrified it. By chance, he noticed a faint glow coming from a certain material located several feet from his electrified tube. The source was a piece of paper coated with barium platino-cyanide. Not believing that the cathode rays could reach that far from the tube, Roentgen repeated the experiment. Each time Roentgen energized his tube, he observed this glow coming from the barium platinocyanide-coated paper. He concluded that the energy emanating from his tube was causing this paper to produce light, or fluoresce. **Fluorescence** refers to the instantaneous production of light resulting from the interaction of some type of energy (in this case x-rays) and some element or compound (in this case barium platinocyanide).

Roentgen was understandably excited about this apparent discovery; however, at the same time, he was cautious not to make any early assumptions about what he had observed. Before sharing information about his discovery with colleagues, Roentgen spent time meticulously investigating

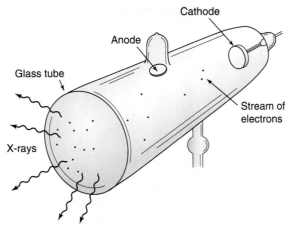

FIGURE 1-2 A Crookes tube as used by Roentgen to discover x-rays.

the properties of this new type of energy. Of course, this new type of energy was not new at all; it had always existed and had likely been produced unknowingly by Roentgen and his contemporaries who were also involved in experiments with electricity and low-vacuum tubes. Knowing that others were doing similar research, Roentgen worked in earnest to exactly determine what this energy was.

Roentgen spent the next several weeks working feverishly in his laboratory to investigate as many properties of this energy as he could. He noticed that when he placed his hand between his energized tube and the barium platinocyanide-coated paper, he could see the bones of his hand glow on the paper, with this fluoroscopic image moving as he moved his hand. Curious about this, he produced a static image of his wife Anna Bertha's hand using a 15-min exposure. This became the world's first radiograph (Figure 1-3). Roentgen gathered other materials and interposed them between his energized tube and the fluorescent paper. Some materials, such as wood, allowed this energy to pass through and caused the paper to fluoresce, whereas some materials, such as platinum, did not.

In December 1895, Roentgen decided that his investigations of this energy were sufficient to inform his physicist colleagues of what he now believed to be a discovery of a new form of energy. He called this energy *x-rays*, with *x* representing the mathematical symbol for the unknown. On December 28, 1895, Roentgen submitted a scholarly paper on his research activities to his local professional society, the Würzburg Physico-Medical Society. Written in his native language, German, his article was titled "On a new kind of rays," and it caused a buzz of excitement in the medical and scientific communities. Within a short time, an English translation of this article appeared in the journal *Nature*, dated January 23, 1896.

While Roentgen deemed his discovery important, he also considered it to have primarily academic value. His concern was in the x-ray itself as a form of energy and not in its possible practical applications. Others quickly began assembling their own x-ray-producing devices and exposed inanimate objects as well as tissue, both animal and human and both living and dead, to determine the range of use of these x-rays. Their efforts were driven largely by skepticism, rather than belief that x-rays could do what had been claimed. Skepticism eventually gave way to productive curiosity as investigations concentrated on ways of imaging living human bodies for medical benefits.

As investigations into legitimate medical applications of the use of x-rays continued, the non-medical and non-scientific communities began taking a different view of Roentgen's discovery. X-ray-proof underwear was offered as protection from these rays, which were known to penetrate solid materials, and a New Jersey legislator attempted to enact legislation that would ban the use of x-ray-producing devices in opera glasses. Both these efforts were presumably aimed at

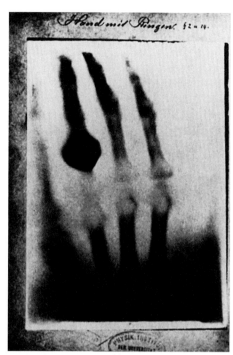

FIGURE 1-3 The first radiograph that demonstrates the bones of the hand of Roentgen's wife, Anna Bertha, with a ring on one finger.

protecting an individual's private anatomy from unscrupulous users of x-rays. The public furor reached such a height that a London newspaper, the *Pall Mall Gazette*, offered the following editorial in 1896: "We are sick of Roentgen rays. Perhaps the best thing would be for all civilized nations to combine to burn all the Roentgen rays, to execute all the discoverers, and to corner all the equipment in the world and to whelm it in the middle of the ocean. Let the fish contemplate each other's bones if they like, but not us."

In a similar vein, but in a more creative fashion, another London periodical, *Photography*, in 1896 offered the following:

"Roentgen Rays, Roentgen Rays?
What is this craze?
The town's ablaze
With this new phase
Of x-ray ways.
I'm full of daze, shock and amaze,
For nowadays
I hear they'll gaze
Through cloak and gown and even stays!
The naughty, naughty Roentgen rays!"

Fortunately, despite these public distractions, the scientific applications of x-rays continued to be investigated for the benefit of society. Roentgen's discovery was lauded as one of great significance to science and medicine, and Roentgen received the first Nobel Prize presented for physics in 1901. The branch of medicine that was concerned with the use of x-rays was called *roentgenology*. A unit of radiation exposure was called the *roentgen*. X-rays were, at one time at least, called *roentgen rays*.

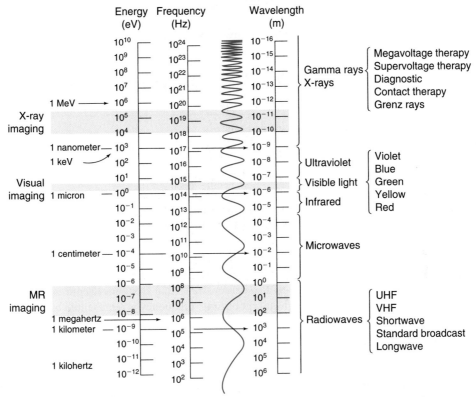

FIGURE 1-4 Electromagnetic spectrum. Radiowaves are the least energetic on the spectrum, and gamma rays are the most energetic.

Excitement over this previously undiscovered type of energy was tempered by the realization in 1898 that x-rays could cause biological damage. This damage was first noticed as a reddening and burning of the skins (called *erythema*) of individuals who were exposed to large doses of x-rays required at that time. More serious effects, such as the growth of malignant tumors and chromosomal changes, were attributed in later decades to x-ray exposure. However, despite these disturbing findings, it was realized that x-rays could be used safely. When radiation-protection procedures to safeguard both the radiographer and the patient are followed, x-rays can assist medical diagnosis by imaging virtually every part of the human body.

X-RAYS AS ENERGY

Energy is the ability to do work and it can exist in different forms, such as electrical energy, kinetic energy, thermal energy, and electromagnetic energy. Energy can also be transformed from one form to another; for instance, the electrical energy applied to a stove is changed into heat. Similarly, the electrical energy applied to an x-ray tube is transformed into heat and x-rays.

X-radiations, or x-rays, are a type of electromagnetic radiation. **Electromagnetic radiation** refers to radiation that has both electrical and magnetic properties. All radiations that are electromagnetic make up a spectrum (Figure 1-4).

In the academic discipline of physics, energy can generally be described as behaving according to the wave or the particle concept of physics. X-rays have a dual nature: they behave like both waves and particles. Higher-energy electromagnetic radiation, such as x-rays, tends to exhibit more particle-like characteristics and lower-energy electromagnetic radiation, such as radiowaves, tend to exhibit more wave-like characteristics.

 IMPORTANT RELATIONSHIP

The Dual Nature of X-ray Energy

X-rays act like both waves and particles.

X-rays can be described as waves because they move in waves that have wavelength and frequency. Looking at a sine wave (Figure 1-5), one can see that the **wavelength** represents the distance between two successive crests or troughs. Wavelength is represented by the Greek letter lambda (λ), and its values are given in units of angstroms (Å). An angstrom is a metric unit of length equal to one ten-billionth of a meter, or 10^{-10} m. X-rays used in radiography range in wavelength from approximately 0.1 to 1.0 Å. Another unit of measurement for wavelength is nanometer (nm); 1 Å equals 0.1 nm.

The sine wave (Figure 1-5) also demonstrates that **frequency** represents the number of waves passing a given point per given unit of time. Frequency is represented by a lowercase f or by the Greek letter nu (ν), and its values are given in units of Hertz (Hz). X-rays used in radiography range in frequency from approximately 3×10^{19} to 3×10^{18} Hz. Wavelength and frequency are inversely related—that is, as one increases, the other decreases.

 IMPORTANT RELATIONSHIP

Wavelength and Frequency

Wavelength and frequency are inversely related. Higher-energy x-rays have decreased wavelength and increased frequency. Lower-energy x-rays have increased wavelength and decreased frequency.

This relationship can be observed in Figure 1-6 and is demonstrated by the expression $c = \lambda\nu$, where c represents the speed of light. In this expression, if wavelength increases, frequency must decrease because the speed of light is a constant velocity (3×10^8 m/s or 186,000 miles/s). Conversely, if wavelength decreases, frequency must increase, again because the speed of light is constant. Mathematically, the formulas are $\lambda = c/\nu$ to solve for wavelength and $\nu = c/\lambda$ to solve for frequency.

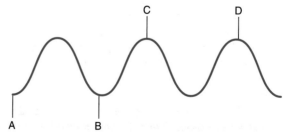

FIGURE 1-5 Sine wave demonstrating wavelength and frequency. One wavelength is equal to the distance between two successive troughs (points *A* to *B*) or the distance between two successive crests (points *C* to *D*).

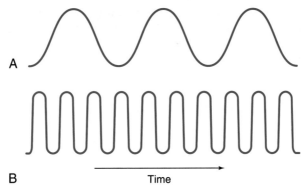

FIGURE 1-6 A, Sine wave demonstrating long wavelength and low frequency. **B,** Sine wave demonstrating short wavelength and high frequency; Comparison of sine waves. **A** and **B** demonstrates the inverse relationship between wavelength and frequency.

X-rays also behave like particles and move as photons or quanta (plural). A **photon** or **quantum** (singular) is a small, discrete bundle of energy. For most applications in radiography, x-rays are referred to as *photons*. When x-rays interact with matter, they behave more like particles than waves. The energy of an individual photon is measured in units of electron volts (eV) and the energy of diagnostic x-rays is approximately between 10^4 and 10^5 eV. Decreasing the wavelength and/or increasing the frequency of the x-ray will increase its energy.

Radiation Units of Measurement

It is important to recognize the units of radiation quantity to obtain an accurate understanding of radiation exposure and dose. There are two systems for quantifying radiation exposure: the conventional one and the International System (SI). SI has become the more widely adopted of the two. Radiation exposure can be measured in the following units:

Unit of Measure	Conventional	International System (SI)
Exposure	roentgen (R)	air kerma (Gy)
Absorbed Dose	radiation absorbed dose (rad)	gray (Gy)
Dose Equivalent	radiation equivalent in man (rem)	sievert (Sv)
Radioactivity	curie (Ci)	becquerel (Bq)

Exposure

The quantity of radiation **exposure** expressed in roentgens (R) measures the amount of ionization or electrical charge in a specified amount of air; this is a measure of the *intensity* of radiation exposure. **Air kerma** is the amount of energy deposited in a unit mass of air and expressed in units of gray (Gy). Radiation exposure is typically expressed in smaller units by adding the prefix "milli," where 1 R = 1000 mR and 1 Gy = 1000 mGy.

Absorbed Dose

The rad and gray are units measuring the transfer of radiation energy into matter (e.g., tissue), known as the **absorbed dose**. One rad equals a transfer of 100 ergs per gram of any absorbing matter. One gray (Gy) is defined as 1 joule of energy absorbed in each kilogram of absorbing material. One gray equals 100 rads. A conversion factor of 0.01 is used to convert rads into grays. For example, an absorbed dose of 5 rads = 0.05 Gy.

Absorbed dose is typically used in referring to patient exposure and is expressed as millirads or mGy because of the low level of radiation-absorbed dose that occurs during medical procedures. The amount of absorbed dose is dependent on the energy of the ionizing radiation and the type of interacting tissues.

Dose Equivalent

The units used in measuring occupational radiation exposure (**dose equivalent**) are radiation equivalents in man (rem) and sieverts (Sv). One sievert equals 100 rem. These units are derived by multiplying a quality factor by the units of absorbed exposure, rads or grays. The quality factor takes into consideration the biological effects of different types of ionizing radiation. X- and gamma rays have a quality factor of 1 and therefore are equal in their biological effect on tissues. Consequently, 1 rad or 0.01 Gy is equal to 1 rem or 0.01 Sv. Differing particulate radiations have associated quality factors, resulting in changes in the biologic effects following exposure.

Radioactivity

Unstable atoms will spontaneously emit particles and energy from the nucleus in an effort to reach stability (**radioactivity**). This process is called radioactive disintegration or decay. Radioisotopes are the radioactive elements used in nuclear medicine and radiation therapy.

The curie and the becquerel measure the rate of nuclear disintegration or decay of a material. Radioactive disintegration or decay refers to the decrease in the activity of a radiation source. Half-life is a term that describes the time it takes for the radiation activity to reduce to 50% of its original activity.

PROPERTIES OF X-RAYS

X-rays are known to have several characteristics or properties. These characteristics are briefly explained here and presented in Box 1-1.

- *X-rays are invisible.* In addition to being unable to see x-rays, one cannot feel, smell, or hear them.
- *X-rays are electrically neutral.* X-rays have neither a positive nor a negative charge; they cannot be accelerated or made to change direction by a magnet or electrical field.
- *X-rays have no mass.* X-rays create no resistance to being put into motion and cannot produce force.
- *X-rays travel at the speed of light in a vacuum.* X-rays move at a constant velocity of 3×10^8 m/s or 186,000 miles/s in a vacuum.
- *X-rays cannot be optically focused.* Optical lenses have no ability to focus or refract x-ray photons.
- *X-rays form polyenergetic or heterogeneous beams.* The x-ray beam that is used in diagnostic radiography is composed of photons that have many different energies. The maximum energy that a photon in any beam may have is expressed by the kilovoltage peak (kVp), which is set on the control panel of the radiographic unit by the radiographer.
- *X-rays can be produced in a range of energies.* These are useful for different purposes in diagnostic radiography. The medically useful diagnostic range of x-ray energies is 30–150 kVp.
- *X-rays travel in straight lines.* X-rays used in diagnostic radiography form a divergent beam in which each individual photon travels in a straight line.
- *X-rays can cause certain substances to fluoresce.* When x-rays strike certain substances, those substances produce light. These substances are used in diagnostic radiography, such as image receptors.
- *X-rays cause chemical changes to occur in radiographic and photographic films.* X-rays are capable of causing images to appear on radiographic film and are capable of fogging photographic film.

BOX 1-1   Characteristics of X-rays
Are invisible
Are electrically neutral
Have no mass
Travel at the speed of light in a vacuum
Cannot be optically focused
Form a polyenergetic or heterogeneous beam
Can be produced in a range of energies
Travel in straight lines
Can cause some substances to fluoresce
Cause chemical changes in radiographic and photographic film
Can penetrate the human body
Can be absorbed or scattered in the human body
Can produce secondary radiation
Can cause damage to living tissue

- *X-rays can penetrate the human body.* X-rays have the ability to pass through the body based on the energy of the x-rays and on the compositions and thicknesses of the tissues being exposed.
- *X-rays can be absorbed or scattered by tissues in the human body.* Depending on the energy of an individual x-ray photon, that photon may be absorbed in the body or made to scatter, moving in another direction.
- *X-rays can produce secondary radiation.* When x-rays are absorbed as a result of a specific type of interaction with matter (photoelectric effect), a secondary or characteristic photon is produced.
- *X-rays can cause chemical and biologic damage to living tissue.* Through excitation and ionization (removal of electrons) of atoms comprising cells, damage to the cells can occur.

THE FUNDAMENTALS OF RADIATION PROTECTION

A central message throughout this textbook is that it is the radiographer's responsibility to minimize the radiation dose to the patient, to themselves, and to others in accordance with the **As Low As Reasonably Achievable (ALARA) Principle.**

! **Radiation Protection Alert**
ALARA Principle
It is the radiographer's responsibility to minimize the radiation dose to the patient, to themselves, and to others in accordance with the **As Low As Reasonably Achievable (ALARA) Principle.**

Central to minimizing the radiation dose to oneself and to others are the cardinal principles of shielding, time, and distance. Shielding broadly refers to the use of radiopaque materials (i.e., materials through which x-rays do NOT pass easily) to greatly reduce radiation exposure to areas of the patient not essential for the exam being performed, to radiographers during exams, and to others. Lead-impregnated materials are a common example. Leaded/rubber sheets of varying sizes may be directly laid on the patient to shield radiosensitive areas. One example of this is gonadal shielding; these are specifically shaped lead materials that are placed directly over the gonadal area to minimize radiation dose to these radiosensitive areas. They must be carefully and precisely placed to prevent interference with the image and the anatomic area of interest. They should be used on all patients within reproductive age and when it will not interfere with the primary imaging objective of the examination being performed. Lead aprons may be worn by the radiographer or other health care workers when it is necessary to be in close proximity to the patient during an exposure. In addition, thyroid shields are commonly used in conjunction with lead aprons during fluoroscopic exams by those personnel that remain in the room. This collar wraps around the neck and fastens in the back to shield the entire front portion of the neck. Leaded curtains may be draped from the fluoroscopy tower to provide a barrier between the fluoroscopist and the x-ray beam during fluoroscopic exams. The walls of the radiographic suite provide lead or lead equivalent (thicknesses of other materials that provide equivalent radiopaque properties as lead) to limit exposure beyond that intended for the radiological exam. The primary barriers are those to which the x-ray beam is routinely directed, such as the floor beneath the x-ray table and the wall behind the upright Bucky. Secondary barriers are the others, such as the wall separating the control panel from the room and the ceiling. The general rule of thumb is to always maximize shielding (use as much as possible).

Time broadly refers to the duration of exposure to ionizing radiation and the time spent in a health care environment where exposure to ionizing radiation is accumulated. This may include the length exposure and number of times the patient is exposed for a radiological exam or the time a radiographer spends in a fluoroscopy suite (or any procedure involving fluoroscopy). Whether one is referring to the patient, to the radiographer, or to other health care workers, the general rule of thumb is always minimize time (limit duration of exposure to ionizing radiation).

Distance refers to the space between oneself and the source of ionizing radiation. This is an effective means of limiting exposure simply because the intensity (quantity) of radiation diminishes over distance. This is an application of the inverse-square law discussed in detail in Chapter 6. Suffice it to say here that as one increases the distance from an ionizing radiation source, the intensity of that source significantly decreases. This principle is applied mostly to radiographers and others to maintain a safe distance from the source of radiation during exposure. The general rule of thumb is always to maximize distance (maintain a safe distance from the radiation source during exposure).

> **! Radiation Protection Alert**
>
> *Cardinal Principles for Minimizing Radiation Dose*
>
> *Time*- Limit the amount of time exposed to ionizing radiation
> *Distance*- Maintain a safe distance from source of ionizing radiation exposure
> *Shielding*- Maximize the use of shielding from ionizing radiation exposure

Another important tool in radiation protection is the limiting of the field of x-ray exposure, essentially beam restriction, through the use of a collimator. By limiting the area of exposure, this device limits the radiation dose to the patient; that is, the smaller the area of x-ray exposure, the lower the total dose to the patient. When we discuss radiation interactions in the body, we are talking about x-ray photons interacting with atoms of tissue. The greater the volume of tissue we expose, the greater the opportunity for such interactions to occur. With these interactions, the photon's energy will either be totally absorbed (which contributes to patient dose) or scattered (which may contribute to the dose to radiographers or others if in the immediate area). See Chapter 3 for a full discussion of x-ray interactions with matter.

Radiation Protection Alert

Beam Restriction

Limiting the size of the x-ray exposure field reduces the volume of tissue irradiated and limits the radiation dose to the patient.

Next among our "tools" of radiation protection are the primary controls of the x-ray beam's kilovoltage peak (kVp), milliamperage (mA), and duration (s), mAs = mA × s. These are the factors selected by the radiographer to produce an x-ray beam of a given quality (penetrating power), controlled by kVp, and quantity (number of photons), ultimately controlled by mAs. The combination of kVp and mAs is selected on the basis of a number of considerations including the anatomic part being examined, patient age, condition, pathology, etc. and should be ideally suited to the circumstance to minimize radiation dose while producing a quality image. See Chapter 6 for a complete discussion of these factors.

Radiation Protection Alert

Primary Exposure Factors

The combination of kVp and mAs is selected based on a number of considerations, including the anatomic part being examined, patient age, condition, and pathology, and should be ideally suited to the circumstance to minimize radiation dose while producing a quality image.

Finally, there are a number of daily "work flow" tasks and processes that address radiation protection. A major one, for which the radiographer serves as a front line advocate for the patient, is the avoidance of duplication of exams. This means preventing the patient from having the same exam performed twice owing to an error. With so much computerization, automation, and team approach to patient care, it is easy to duplicate an order (accidentally order the same radiographic exam more than once) or for two different physicians involved in a patient's care to unknowingly order the same thing. There are instances where a patient's condition rapidly changes and it is necessary to perform the same exam a number of times in succession; but it is okay to double-check an order or to stop and question. The radiographer must recognize and accept his/her role as a patient advocate and do what is necessary to avoid unnecessary duplication of exams. Think of each duplicate exam as a doubling of the radiation dose that is otherwise needed (the first exam was a normal dose, and the unnecessary one doubles that dose). Thus, this radiation protection measure alone significantly impacts the radiation dose administered to the patient and to others.

Radiation Protection Alert

Avoid Duplicate Exams

The radiographer must recognize and accept his/her role as a patient advocate and do what is necessary to avoid duplication of exams.

Screening for pregnancy is another important task for minimizing unnecessary exposure to a developing fetus. Departmental protocols for pregnancy screening may vary and should be consistently employed. When it is necessary to perform a radiographic exam on a pregnant patient, shielding materials and precise collimation, as discussed previously, should be used to minimize radiation dose administered to the fetus. Be sure to follow the clinical site policy for pregnancy screening.

> **⚠ Radiation Protection Alert**
>
> ### Screening for Pregnancy
>
> Screening for pregnancy is another important task for minimizing unnecessary exposure to a developing fetus. When it is necessary to perform a radiographic exam on a pregnant patient, shielding materials and precise collimation should be used to minimize the radiation dose administered to the fetus.

Lastly, as a developing radiographer, good work habits and skills have not yet been developed. Use sufficient time and concentration to "get it right the first time." Develop a mental checklist for radiographic procedures and perform them the same way every time. By doing so, mistakes involving the details of a task can be minimized along with unnecessary radiation dose administered to the patient and to others. See Box 1-2 for a summary of radiation protection fundamentals.

Since the publication of Roentgen's scientific paper, no other properties of x-rays have been discovered. However, the discussion of x-rays has expanded far beyond the early concerns about modesty or even danger. Today, x-rays are accepted as an important diagnostic tool in medicine, and the radiographer is an important member of the health care team. The radiographic imaging professional is responsible for the care of the patient in the radiology department, the production and control of x-rays, and the formation of the radiographic image. Figure 1-7 shows a standard

---

BOX 1-2   Summary of Radiation Protection Fundamentals

- Minimize the radiation dose to the patient, to themselves, and to others in accordance with the **A**s **L**ow **A**S **R**easonably **A**chievable (**ALARA**) Principle
- Limit the amount of *time* exposed to ionizing radiation
- Maintain a safe *distance* from source of ionizing radiation exposure
- Maximize the use of *shielding* from ionizing radiation exposure
- Limit the size of the x-ray exposure field to the area of interest
- Select a combination of kVp and mAs to produce a diagnostic image while minimizing patient radiation exposure
- Avoid unnecessary duplicate exams
- Screen for pregnancy
- Develop a mental checklist for radiographic procedures and perform consistently

---

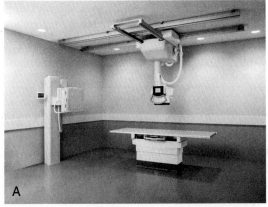
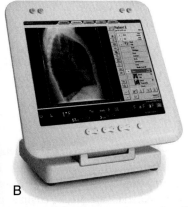

FIGURE 1-7   A, Typical radiographic unit showing the x-ray table, overhead x-ray tube, and collimator. **B,** Control panel.

radiographic room that includes an x-ray table, overhead x-ray tube and collimator, and a control panel for the selection of exposure technique factors. The subsequent chapters of this book uncover the intricate and fascinating details of the art and science of medical radiography.

CHAPTER SUMMARY

- X-rays were discovered on November 8, 1895, by Dr. Wilhelm Conrad Roentgen, a German physicist, mathematician, and recipient of the first Nobel Prize for physics.
- The discovery of x-rays was met with skepticism and curiosity and subsequently by acceptance of its medical benefit.
- X-rays are a type of electromagnetic radiation with both electrical and magnetic properties.
- Electromagnetic radiation is a form of energy that moves in waves with wavelength and frequency.
- Wavelength and frequency are inversely related. Higher-energy x-rays have decreased wavelength and increased frequency.
- X-rays act like both waves and particles and have a higher energy than other types of electromagnetic radiation, such as visible light.
- There are two systems of quantifying radiation exposure: the conventional system and the International System (SI). Exposure in air - roentgen (R) and air kerma; Absorbed Dose - radiation absorbed dose (rad) and gray (Gy); Dose Equivalent - radiation equivalent in man (rem) and sievert (Sv); Radioactivity - curie (Ci) and becquerel (Bq).
- X-rays have several important characteristics: they are invisible and electrically neutral, have no mass, travel at the speed of light, penetrate matter, and can cause chemical and biologic changes.
- The fundamentals of radiation protection include adhering to the ALARA principle, time, distance, shielding, beam restriction, careful selection of exposure technique factors, avoidance of duplicate exams, and screening for pregnancy.

REVIEW QUESTIONS

1. In what year were x-rays discovered?
   A. 1892
   B. 1895
   C. 1898
   D. 1901
2. In what year were some of the biologically damaging effects of x-rays discovered?
   A. 1892
   B. 1895
   C. 1898
   D. 1901
3. X-rays were discovered in experiments dealing with electricity and _____.
   A. ionization
   B. magnetism
   C. atomic structure
   D. vacuum tubes
4. X-rays were discovered when they caused a barium platinocyanide-coated plate to _____.
   A. fluoresce
   B. phosphoresce
   C. vibrate
   D. burn and redden

5. X-radiation is classified in which spectrum?
   A. Radiation
   B. Energy
   C. Atomic
   D. Electromagnetic

6. X-rays have a dual nature, which means that they behave like both _____.
   A. atoms and molecules
   B. photons and quanta
   C. waves and particles
   D. charged and uncharged particles

7. The wavelength and frequency of x-rays are _____ related.
   A. directly
   B. inversely
   C. partially
   D. not

8. X-rays have _____ electrical charge.
   A. a positive
   B. a negative
   C. an alternately positive and negative
   D. no

9. X-rays have _____.
   A. no mass
   B. the same mass as electrons
   C. the same mass as protons
   D. the same mass as neutrons

10. The x-ray beam used in diagnostic radiography can be described as being _____.
    A. homogeneous
    B. monoenergetic
    C. polyenergetic
    D. scattered

11. The unit that measures the transfer of radiation energy into tissues is known as the _____.
    A. roentgen
    B. REM
    C. gray
    D. sievert

12. Which of the following will minimize radiation exposure to the patient?
    A. Beam restriction
    B. Gonadal shielding
    C. Screening for pregnancy
    D. All of the above

The X-ray Beam

CHAPTER OUTLINE

X-ray Production
Cathode
Anode
X-ray Tube Housing
Target Interactions
Bremsstrahlung Interactions
Characteristic Interactions

X-ray Emission Spectrum
X-ray Exposure
X-ray Quality and Quantity
Kilovoltage
Milliamperage
Exposure Time
Milliamperage and Time

Line-focus Principle
Anode Heel Effect
Beam Filtration
Compensating Filters
Heat Units
Extending X-ray Tube Life

OBJECTIVES

After completing this chapter, the reader will be able to perform the following:

1. Define all the key terms in this chapter.
2. State all the important relationships in this chapter.
3. Describe the construction of an x-ray tube.
4. State the function of each component of an x-ray tube.
5. Describe how x-rays are produced.
6. Explain the role of the primary exposure factors in determining the quality and quantity of x-rays.
7. Explain the line-focus principle.
8. State how the anode heel effect can be used in radiography.
9. Differentiate among the types of filtration and explain their purpose.
10. Calculate heat units.
11. Recognize how changing generator output, kVp, mA, and filtration affect the x-ray emission spectrum.
12. List the guidelines followed to extend the life of an x-ray tube.

KEY TERMS

actual focal spot size
added filtration
anode
anode heel effect
bremsstrahlung interactions
cathode
characteristic interactions
compensating filter
dosimeter
effective focal spot size
exposure time
filament

filament current
focusing cup
half-value layer (HVL)
heat unit (HU)
inherent filtration
kilovoltage
leakage radiation
line-focus principle
milliamperage
off-focus radiation
rotor
space charge

space charge effect
stator
target
thermionic emission
total filtration
trough filter
tube current
voltage ripple
wedge filter
x-ray emission spectrum

The x-ray tube is the most important part of the x-ray machine because the tube is where the x-rays are produced. Radiographers must understand the construction and operation of an x-ray tube. The radiographer controls many actions that occur within the tube. Kilovoltage peak (kVp), milliamperage (mA), and exposure time all are factors that the radiographer adjusts on the control panel to produce a quality image. The radiographer also needs to be aware of the amount of heat produced during x-ray production because excessive heat can damage the tube.

X-RAY PRODUCTION

The production of x-rays requires a rapidly moving stream of electrons that are suddenly decelerated or stopped. The source of electrons is a cathode, or negative electrode. The negative electrode is heated and electrons are emitted. The electrons are attracted to the positively charged anode (positive electrode) and move rapidly toward the anode where they are stopped or decelerated. When the kinetic energy of the electrons is transferred to the anode, x-rays and heat are produced.

Cathode

The **cathode** of an x-ray tube is a negatively charged electrode. It comprises a **filament** and a **focusing cup**. Figure 2-1 shows a double-filament cathode surrounded by a focusing cup. The **filament** is a coiled tungsten wire, which is the source of electrons during x-ray production.

 IMPORTANT RELATIONSHIP

Filament

The filament is the source of electrons during x-ray production.

Most x-ray tubes are referred to as *dual-focus tubes* because they have two filaments: one large and one small. Only one filament is energized at any one time during x-ray production. If the radiographer selects a large focal spot when setting the control panel, the large filament is energized. If a small focal spot is chosen, the small filament is energized. The **focusing cup** is made of nickel and nearly surrounds the filament. It is open at one end to allow electrons to flow freely across the tube from cathode to anode. It has a negative charge, which keeps the cloud of electrons emitted from the filament from spreading apart. Its purpose is to focus the stream of electrons.

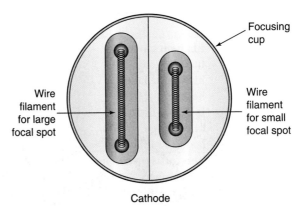

FIGURE 2-1 Most x-ray tubes use a small filament and a large filament, corresponding to a small focal spot size and a large focal spot size.

Anode

The **anode** of an x-ray tube is a positively charged electrode composed of molybdenum, copper, tungsten, and graphite. These materials are used for their thermal and electrical conductive properties. The anode consists of a **target** and, in rotating anode tubes, a **stator** and **rotor**. The **target** is a metal that abruptly decelerates and stops electrons in the tube current, allowing the production of x-rays. The target can be either rotating or stationary. Tubes with rotating targets are more common than tubes with stationary ones. Rotating anodes are manufactured to rotate at a set speed ranging from 3000 to 10,000 revolutions per minute (rpm). Figure 2-2 shows how a rotating anode and stationary anode differ in appearance.

 IMPORTANT RELATIONSHIP

Target

The target is the part of the anode that is struck by the focused stream of electrons coming from the cathode. The target stops the electrons and creates the opportunity for the production of x-rays.

The target of the rotating anode tubes is made of a tungsten and rhenium alloy. This layer, or track, is embedded in a base of molybdenum and graphite (Figure 2-3). Tungsten generally constitutes 90% of the composition of the rotating target, with rhenium constituting the other 10%. The face of the anode is angled to help the x-ray photons exit the tube. Rotating targets generally have a target angle ranging from 5° to 20°. Tungsten is used for both rotating and stationary targets because it has a high atomic number of 74 for efficient x-ray production and a high melting point of 3400°C (6152°F). Most of the energy produced by an x-ray tube is heat; thus, melting of the target can sometimes become a problem, especially with high exposures.

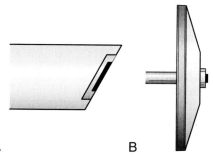

A   B

FIGURE 2-2 Side views of a stationary anode (**A**) and a rotating anode (**B**).

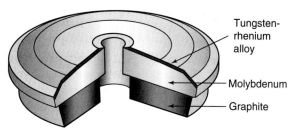

Tungsten-rhenium alloy

Molybdenum

Graphite

FIGURE 2-3 Typical construction of a rotating anode.

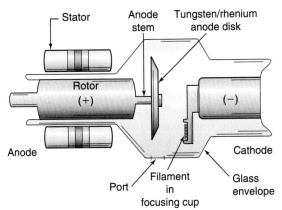

FIGURE 2-4 Structure of a typical x-ray tube, including the major operational parts.

 IMPORTANT RELATIONSHIP

Tungsten

Because tungsten has a high atomic number (74) and a high melting point (3,400°C [6,152°F]), it efficiently produces x-rays.

In order to turn the anode during x-ray production, a rotating anode tube requires a stator and rotor (Figure 2-4). The **stator** is an electric motor that turns the rotor at very high speed. The **rotor** (made of copper) is rigidly connected to the target through the anode stem (made of molybdenum), causing the target to rapidly rotate during x-ray production. High-strength ball bearings in the rotor allow it to smoothly rotate at high speeds.

During x-ray production, most of the energy produced at the anode is heat, with a very small percentage being x-ray energy. Heat can pose a problem if allowed to build up; hence, it is transferred to the envelope and then to the insulating oil surrounding the tube. Moreover, many tube assemblies have a fan that blows air over the tube to help dissipate heat.

 IMPORTANT RELATIONSHIP

Dissipating Heat

The heat produced when the x-ray exposure is activated is transferred to the insulating oil that surrounds the x-ray tube.

Rotating anodes can withstand high heat loads; this ability relates to the actual focal spot, which is the physical area of the target that is bombarded by electrons during x-ray production. With stationary targets, the focal spot is a fixed area on the surface of the target. With rotating targets, this area is represented by a focal track. Figure 2-5 shows the stationary anode's focal spot and the rotating anode with its focal track. The size of the focal spot is not altered with a rotating anode, but the actual physical area of the target bombarded by electrons is constantly changing, causing a greater area—a focal track—to be exposed to electrons. Because of the larger area of the target being bombarded during an exposure, the rotating anode is able to withstand higher heat loads produced by greater exposure factors. Rotating anode x-ray tubes are used in all applications in radiography, whereas stationary anode tubes are limited to studies of small anatomic structures such as teeth.

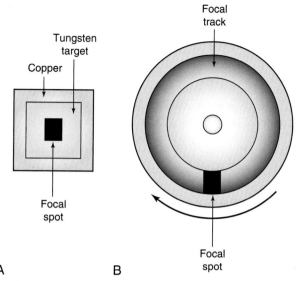

FIGURE 2-5 A, Front view of a stationary anode. **B,** The target area of the rotating anode turns during exposure along with an increased physical area—a focal track—that is exposed to electrons.

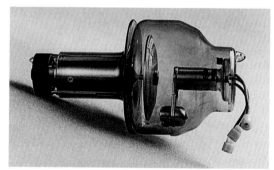

FIGURE 2-6 A glass envelope x-ray tube as it appears before installation in a tube housing.

IMPORTANT RELATIONSHIP

Rotating Anodes

Rotating anodes can withstand higher heat loads than stationary anodes because the rotation causes a greater physical area, or focal track, to be exposed to electrons.

X-ray Tube Housing

The components necessary for x-ray production are housed in a glass or metal envelope. Figure 2-6 shows the appearance of a glass x-ray tube. Metal envelopes are more commonly used because of their superior electrical properties.

A disadvantage of a glass envelope x-ray tube is that tungsten evaporated from the filament during exposure can be deposited upon the inside of the glass, especially in the middle portion of the envelope. This evaporation can affect the flow of electrons and cause the tube to fail. Replacing this section of glass with metal prevents these problems and extends the tube life. An additional advantage of a metal envelope is the reduction of **off-focus radiation.** Off-focus radiation occurs when projectile electrons are reflected and x-rays are produced from outside the focal spot. The metal tube envelope can collect these electrons and conduct them away from the anode.

The envelope allows air to be completely evacuated from the x-ray tube, which in turn allows an efficient flow of electrons from cathode to anode. The envelope serves two additional functions: it provides some insulation from electrical shock that may occur because the cathode and anode contain electrical charges and it dissipates heat in the tube by conducting it to the insulating oil surrounding the envelope. The purpose of insulating oil is to provide more insulation from electrical shock and to help dissipate heat away from the tube. All of these components are surrounded by metal tube housing on all sides except for a port, or window, which allows the primary beam to exit the tube. It is the metal tube housing that the radiographer observes and handles when moving the x-ray tube. The tube housing is lined with lead to provide additional shielding from **leakage radiation.** Leakage radiation refers to any x-rays, other than the primary beam, that escape the tube housing. The tube housing is required to allow a leakage radiation of no more than 100 mR/hr to escape when measured at a distance of 1 m from the source while the tube operates at maximum output. Electrical current is supplied to the x-ray tube using two high-voltage cables that enter the top of the tube assembly.

TARGET INTERACTIONS

The electrons that move from the cathode to the anode travel extremely fast, approximately at half the speed of light. The moving electrons, which have kinetic energy, strike the target and interact with the tungsten atoms in the anode to produce x-rays.

IMPORTANT RELATIONSHIP
Production of X-rays

As electrons strike the target, their kinetic energy is transferred to the tungsten atoms in the anode to produce x-rays.

These interactions occur within the top 0.5 mm of the anode surface. Two types of interactions produce x-ray photons: **bremsstrahlung interactions** and **characteristic interactions.**

IMPORTANT RELATIONSHIP
Interactions that Produce X-ray Photons

Bremsstrahlung interactions and characteristic interactions both produce x-ray photons.

Bremsstrahlung Interactions

Bremsstrahlung is a German word meaning "braking" or "slowing down radiation." **Bremsstrahlung interactions** occur when a projectile electron completely avoids the orbital electrons of a tungsten atom and travels very close to its nucleus. The very strong electrostatic force of the nucleus causes the electron to suddenly "slow down." As the electron loses energy, it suddenly changes its direction, and the energy loss then reappears as an x-ray photon (Figure 2-7).

In the diagnostic energy range from 30 to 150 kVp, most x-ray interactions are bremsstrahlung. Below 70 kVp (with a tungsten target), 100% of the x-ray beam results from bremsstrahlung interactions. Above 70 kVp, approximately 85% of the beam results from bremsstrahlung interactions.

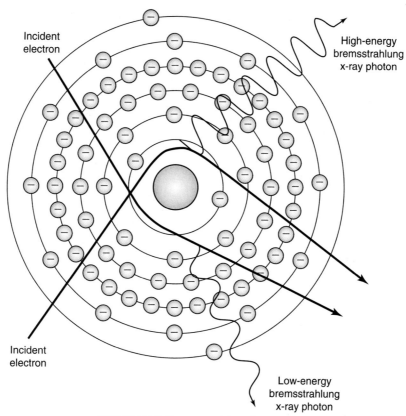

Incident electron

High-energy bremsstrahlung x-ray photon

Incident electron

Low-energy bremsstrahlung x-ray photon

FIGURE 2-7 Bremsstrahlung interaction.

 IMPORTANT RELATIONSHIP

Bremsstrahlung Interactions

Most x-ray interactions in the diagnostic energy range are bremsstrahlung.

Characteristic Interactions

Characteristic interactions are produced when a projectile electron interacts with an electron from the inner shell (K-shell) of a tungsten atom. The electron must have enough energy to eject the K-shell electron from its orbit. K-shell electrons in tungsten have the strongest binding energy at 69.5 keV. For a projectile electron to remove this orbital electron, it must possess energy equal to or greater than 69.5 keV. When the K-shell electron is ejected from its orbit, an outer-shell electron drops into the open position and creates an energy difference. The energy difference is emitted as an x-ray photon (Figure 2-8). Electrons from the L-, M-, O-, and P-shells of the tungsten atom are also ejected from their orbits. However, the photons created from these interactions have very low energy and, depending on filtration, may not even reach the patient. K-shell characteristic x-rays have an average energy of approximately 69 keV; therefore, they significantly contribute to the useful x-ray beams. Below 70 kVp (with a tungsten target), no characteristic x-rays are present in the beam; above 70 kVp, approximately 15% of the beam consists of characteristic x-rays. X-rays produced through these interactions are termed *characteristic x-rays* because their energies are characteristic of the tungsten target element.

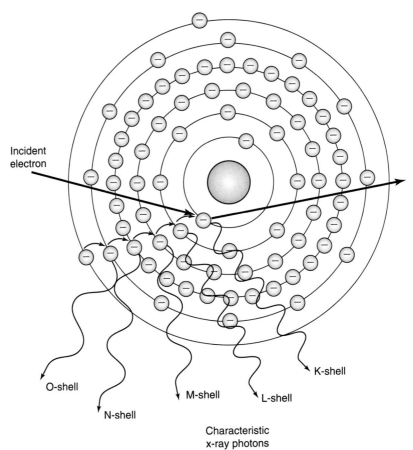

Incident
electron

O-shell

N-shell

M-shell

L-shell

K-shell

Characteristic
x-ray photons

FIGURE 2-8 Characteristic interaction.

> ### IMPORTANT RELATIONSHIP
>
> #### *Characteristic Interactions*
>
> Characteristic x-rays can be produced in a tungsten target only when the kVp is set at 70 or greater because the binding energy of the K-shell electron is 69.5 keV.

To summarize, when comparing bremsstrahlung and characteristic interactions, most x-ray interactions produced in diagnostic radiology result from bremsstrahlung interactions. There is no difference between a bremsstrahlung x-ray and a characteristic x-ray at the same energy level; they are simply produced by different processes.

X-RAY EMISSION SPECTRUM

X-ray energy is measured in kiloelectron volts (keV) (1 keV = 1000 electron volts). The x-ray beam is polyenergetic (has many energies) and consists of a wide range of energies known as the **x-ray emission spectrum**. The lowest energies are always approximately 15 to 20 keV, and the highest energies are always equal to the kVp set on the control panel. For example, an 80 kVp x-ray exposure technique produces x-ray energies ranging from 15 to 80 keV (Figure 2-9). The

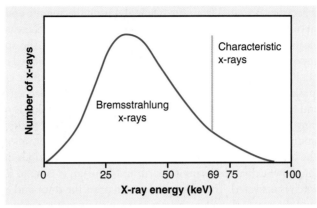

FIGURE 2-9 An 80 kVp x-ray emission spectrum from a tungsten target. Most x-rays occur between 30 and 40 keV. Characteristic x-ray energies are discrete and are represented by the line at 69 keV.

smallest number of x-rays occurs at the extreme low and high ends of the spectrum. The greatest number of x-ray energies occurs between 30 keV and 40 keV for an 80 kVp exposure. The x-ray emission spectrum, or the range and intensity of x-rays emitted, changes with different exposure technique settings on the control panel.

X-RAY EXPOSURE

A radiographic exposure is produced by a radiographer using two switches located on the control panel of the x-ray unit. These are sometimes combined into a single switching device that has two levels of operation corresponding to rotor preparation and x-ray exposure. In either case, the switches that are used to make an x-ray exposure are called *deadman switches*. Deadman switches require positive pressure to be applied during the entire x-ray exposure process. If the radiographer lets off either switch, thus releasing positive pressure, the exposure process is immediately terminated.

The first switch is usually called the *rotor*, or *prep button*, and the second switch is usually called the *exposure*, or *x-ray button*. The activation of the exposure switch by the radiographer produces specific reactions inside the x-ray tube. The rotor must be activated before the x-ray exposure to properly produce an x-ray exposure.

Pushing the rotor, or prep button, causes an electrical current to be induced across the filament in the cathode. This **filament current** is approximately 3 to 5 A and operates at approximately 10 V. The amount of current flowing through the filament depends on the mA set at the control panel. The **filament current** heats the tungsten filament. This heating of the filament causes thermionic emission to occur. **Thermionic emission** refers to the boiling off of electrons from the filament.

IMPORTANT RELATIONSHIP

Thermionic Emission

When the tungsten filament gains enough heat (therm), the outer-shell electrons (ions) of the filament atoms are boiled off, or emitted, from the filament.

The electrons liberated from the filament during thermionic emission form a cloud around the filament called **space charge**. This term is descriptive because there is an actual negative charge from these electrons that exists in the space around the filament. The **space charge effect** refers to the tendency of the space charge to prevent more electrons to be boiled off of the filament. The focusing cup, with its own negative charge, forces the electrons in the space charge to remain together.

By pushing the rotor, or prep button, the radiographer also activates the stator that drives the rotor and rotating target (Box 2-1). While thermionic emission is occurring and the space charge is forming, the stator starts to turn the anode, accelerating it to top speed in preparation for x-ray production. If an exposure were to be made before the target was up to speed, the heat produced would be too great for the slowly rotating target, causing serious damage. The machine therefore does not allow such an exposure to occur until the target is up to full speed, even when the exposure switch is activated. The radiographer can press the rotor and exposure switches one after the other, and the machine makes the exposure as soon as it is ready, with no damage to the tube. It takes only a few seconds for the space charge to be produced and for the rotating target to reach its top speed (Figure 2-10).

When the radiographer pushes the exposure, or x-ray button, the x-ray exposure begins (Box 2-2). The kVp level, which depends on the actual kVp value set on the control panel by the radiographer, is applied across the tube from cathode to anode. This creates potential difference and the cathode becomes highly negatively charged, strongly repelling the thus created negatively charged electrons. The anode becomes positively charged, strongly attracting the electrons.

Electrons that comprised the space charge now flow quickly from the cathode to the anode in a current. **Tube current** refers to the flow of electrons from cathode to anode and is measured in units called *milliamperes* (mA). It is important to note that electrons flow only in one direction in the x-ray tube—from cathode to anode.

 IMPORTANT RELATIONSHIP

Tube Current

Electrons flow only in one direction in the x-ray tube—from cathode to anode. This flow of electrons is called the *tube current* and is measured in milliamperes (mA).

As these electrons strike the anode target, their kinetic energy is converted into either electromagnetic energy (x-rays) or thermal energy (heat); in other words, an energy conversion occurs. Most of the electron kinetic energy in the tube current (greater than 99%) is converted to heat, whereas less than 1% of it is converted to x-rays. These events are illustrated in Figure 2-11.

BOX 2-1   Preparing the Tube for Exposure

When the rotor, or prep button, is activated:

On the Cathode Side of the X-ray Tube
1. The filament current heats up the filament.
2. This heat boils electrons off of the filament (thermionic emission).
3. These electrons gather in a cloud around the filament (space charge).
4. The negatively charged focusing cup keeps the electron cloud focused together.
5. The number of electrons in the space charge is limited (space charge effect).

On the Anode Side of the X-ray Tube
1. The rotating target begins to turn rapidly, quickly reaching top speed.

IMPORTANT RELATIONSHIP

Energy Conversion in the X-ray Tube

As electrons strike the anode target, more than 99% of their kinetic energy is converted to heat, whereas less than 1% of their energy is converted to x-rays.

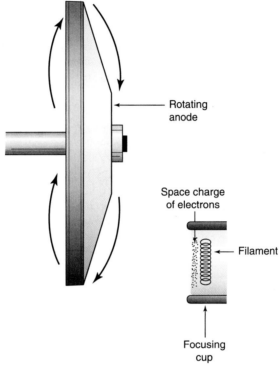

FIGURE 2-10 When the radiographer activates the rotor, or prep button, a filament current is induced across the filament, causing electrons to be burned off and gather in a cloud around the filament. Simultaneously, the rotating anode begins to turn.

BOX 2-2   Making an X-ray Exposure

After activation of the rotor and the exposure is initiated:

On the Cathode Side of the X-ray Tube
1. High negative charge strongly repels electrons.
2. These electrons stream away from the cathode and toward the anode (tube current).

On the Anode Side of the X-ray Tube
1. High positive charge strongly attracts electrons in the tube current.
2. These electrons strike the anode.
3. X-rays and heat are produced.

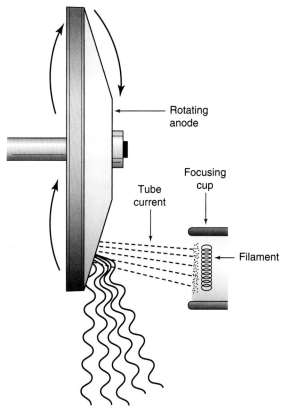

FIGURE 2-11 After activation of the rotor and initiation of the exposure, a high voltage, or kilovoltage, is applied across the tube, making the cathode highly negative and the anode highly positive. Electrons are repelled from the cathode side and attracted to the anode side. The negatively charged focusing cup focuses the electrons into a stream, and they quickly cross the tube gap in a tube current. The kinetic energy of electrons interacting with the target is converted into x-rays and heat.

X-RAY QUALITY AND QUANTITY

The radiographer initiates and controls the production of x-rays. Manipulating the prime exposure factors on the control panel (kVp, mA, and exposure time) allows both the quantity and the quality of the x-ray beam to be altered. The quantity of the x-ray beam indicates the number of x-ray photons in the primary beam, and the quality of the x-ray beam indicates its penetrating power. Knowledge of the prime exposure factors and their effect on the production of x-rays assists the radiographer in producing quality radiographs.

Kilovoltage

The **kilovoltage** (kVp) that is set by the radiographer and applied across the x-ray tube at the time the exposure is initiated determines the speed at which the electrons in the tube current move.

 IMPORTANT RELATIONSHIP

Kilovoltage and the Speed of Electrons

The speed of the electrons traveling from the cathode to the anode increases as the kilovoltage applied across the x-ray tube increases.

Selecting a higher voltage results in greater repulsion of electrons from the cathode and greater attraction of electrons toward the anode. The speed at which the electrons in the tube current move determines the quality or energy of the x-rays that are produced. The higher the energy of the x-ray photons, the greater their penetrability, or ease with which they move through tissue. Whether addressing the x-ray photons themselves or the primary beam, *quality* refers to the energy level of the radiation (Box 2-3).

 IMPORTANT RELATIONSHIP

Speed of Electrons and Quality of X-rays

The speed of the electrons in the tube current determines the quality or energy of the x-rays that are produced. The quality or energy of the x-rays in turn determines the penetrability of the primary beam.

 IMPORTANT RELATIONSHIP

kVp and Beam Penetrability

As kVp increases, beam penetrability increases; as kVp decreases, beam penetrability decreases.

In addition to kVp affecting the quality of x-ray photons produced, it affects the quantity or number of x-ray photons produced (Figure 2-12). Increased kVp results in more x-rays being produced because it increases the efficiency of x-ray production (Box 2-4 describes quality-control methods for evaluating kilovoltage accuracy).

BOX 2-3   **kVp and X-ray Quality**
1. Higher kVp results in electrons that move faster in the tube current from the cathode to the anode.
2. The faster the movement of the electrons in the tube current, the greater the energy of the x-rays produced.
3. The greater the energy of the x-rays produced, the greater the penetrability of the primary beam.
4. The quality of the x-ray beam refers to its energy level; hence, adjusting kVp affects the quality of the x-ray beam.

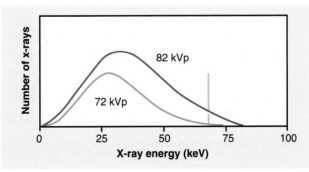

FIGURE 2-12 Increasing the kVp from 72 to 82 shows an increase in the quantity of x-rays (amplitude), and the x-ray emission shifts toward the right, indicating an increase in the energy or quality of the beam.

In order to provide a sufficient potential difference (kVp) to allow x-ray production, a generator is required to convert low voltage (volts) to high voltage (kilovolts). Three basic types of x-ray generators are available: single phase, three phase, and high frequency. Each generator produces a different voltage waveform (Figure 2-13). These waveforms are a reflection of the consistency of the voltage supplied to the x-ray tube during an x-ray exposure. The term **voltage ripple** describes voltage waveforms in terms of how much the voltage varies during x-ray production. Figure 2-13 shows that for single-phase generation, voltage varies from the peak to a value of zero. The voltage ripple for single-phase generators is said to be 100% because there is total variation in the voltage waveform, from peak voltage to zero voltage. For three-phase generators, the voltage ripple is 13% for the 6-pulse mode and 4% for the 12-pulse mode. High-frequency generators produce a voltage ripple of less than 1%. Voltage used in the x-ray tube is most consistent with high-frequency generators. The more consistent the voltage applied to the x-ray tube throughout the exposure, the greater the quantity and energy level (quality) of the x-ray beam. Figure 2-14 shows x-ray emission for different types of generators.

Milliamperage

Milliamperage (mA) is the unit used to measure tube current. Tube current is the number of electrons flowing per unit time between the cathode and the anode. For example, at 200 mA, there is a specific amount of current applied to the filament, causing a certain amount of thermionic emission. Based on the amount of thermionic emission, there is a space charge consisting of a certain number of electrons; 200 mA indicates the number of electrons (based on the space charge) flowing in the tube per second. Generally, changing to the 400 mA station on the control

---

BOX 2-4   Quality-Control Check: Kilovoltage Accuracy

- X-ray quality can be affected if the actual kilovoltage used is inaccurate.
- A digital kVp meter measures the actual kilovoltage, and a Wisconsin Test Cassette estimates the kilovoltage by measuring densities (blackness) produced on a film.
- The maximum variability of the kilovoltage is ±5%.

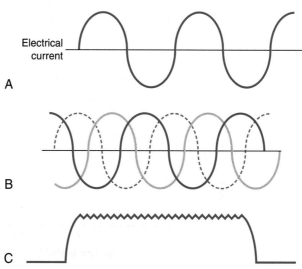

FIGURE 2-13 Voltage waveforms produced by various x-ray generators. **A,** Single phase. **B,** Three phase. **C,** High frequency.

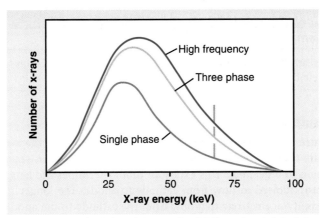

FIGURE 2-14 The quantity (amplitude) and the quality (shift to the right) of the x-ray beam are increased when using high-frequency and three-phase generators because they are more efficient in x-ray production.

panel causes twice as much thermionic emission, twice as big a space charge and twice as many electrons to flow per second. The milliamperage set by the radiographer determines the number of electrons flowing in the tube and the quantity of x-rays produced (Box 2-5). The quantity of electrons in the tube current is directly proportional to the milliamperage; if milliamperage increases, the quantity of electrons and x-rays proportionally increase, and if it decreases, the quantity of electrons and the x-rays proportionally decrease. Milliamperage does not affect the quality or energy of the x-rays produced (Figure 2-15).

BOX 2-5   mA and X-ray Quantity

1. Higher mA results in more electrons moving in the tube current from the cathode to the anode.
2. The more electrons in the tube current, the more x-rays produced.
3. The number of x-rays produced is directly proportional to mA.

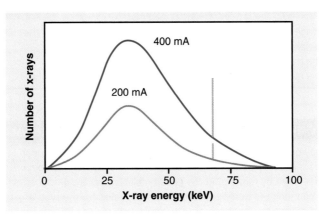

FIGURE 2-15 Changing the mA results in a proportional change in the quantity (amplitude) of x-rays produced.

IMPORTANT RELATIONSHIP

Milliamperage, Tube Current, and X-ray Quantity

The quantity of electrons in the tube current and quantity of x-rays produced are directly proportional to the milliamperage.

Exposure Time

Exposure time determines the length of time over which the x-ray tube produces x-rays. The exposure time set by the radiographer can be expressed in seconds or milliseconds as either a fraction or a decimal. This exposure time determines the length of time for which the tube current is allowed to flow from cathode to anode. The longer the exposure time, the greater the quantity of electrons that flow from the cathode to the anode and the greater the quantity of x-rays produced (Box 2-6). For example, if an exposure time of 0.25 s at 400 mA produces 5000 x-rays, then doubling the exposure time to 0.50 s at 400 mA would produce 10,000 x-rays. Changes in exposure time produce the same effect on the number of x-rays produced as do changes in milliamperage (Box 2-7 describes quality-control methods for evaluating exposure timer accuracy).

 IMPORTANT RELATIONSHIP

Exposure Time, Tube Current, and X-ray Quantity

The quantity of electrons flowing from the cathode to the anode and the quantity of x-rays produced are directly proportional to the exposure time.

Milliamperage and Time

When milliamperage is multiplied by exposure time, the result is known as *mAs*, which the radiographer can set at the control panel. Mathematically, mAs is simply expressed as follows: $mA \times s = mAs$, where *s* represents the exposure time in fractions of a second (as actual fractions or in decimal form) or in seconds.

BOX 2-6   Exposure Time and X-ray Quantity

1. Longer exposure time results in more electrons moving in the tube current from the cathode to the anode.
2. The more electrons in the tube current, the more x-rays produced.
3. The number of x-rays produced is directly proportional to the exposure time.

BOX 2-7°   Quality-Control Check: Exposure Timer Accuracy

- X-ray quantity can be affected if the actual exposure time used is inaccurate. A digital timer device measures the actual exposure time. A synchronous spinning top test device estimates the actual time by measuring the density (blackness) arc produced on film with a timer protractor or by counting the number of black dots expected for the type of x-ray generator.
- The maximum variability of the exposure timer is ±5% for times >10 ms and ±10% for times <10 ms.

MATHEMATICAL APPLICATION

Calculating mAs

$$mAs = mA \times seconds$$

Examples:

$$200 \, mA \times 0.25 \, s = 50 \, mAs$$

$$500 \, mA \times 2/5 \, s = 200 \, mAs$$

$$800 \, mA \times 100 \, ms \, (milliseconds \, or \, 0.1 \, s) = 80 \, mAs$$

The quantity of electrons flowing from the cathode to the anode is directly proportional to mAs (Box 2-8). The quantity of x-ray photons produced is directly proportional to this quantity of electrons. An increase or decrease in mA, exposure time, or mAs directly affects the quantity of x-rays produced; mAs has no effect on the quality of the x-rays produced (Box 2-9 describes quality-control methods for evaluating radiation output).

 IMPORTANT RELATIONSHIP

Quantity of Electrons, X-rays, and mAs

The quantity of electrons flowing from the cathode to the anode and the quantity of x-rays produced are directly proportional to mAs.

BOX 2-8   mAs and X-ray Quantity

1. Higher mAs results in more electrons moving within the tube current from the cathode to the anode.
2. The more electrons in the tube current, the more x-rays produced.
3. The number of x-rays produced is directly proportional to the mAs.
4. mAs affects only the quantity of x-rays produced; it has no effect on the quality of the x-rays.

BOX 2-9   Quality-Control Check: Radiation Output

- Variations in the generator or x-ray tube performance may cause inconsistent exposures and affect the x-ray quantity. Three quality-control tests are typically performed with a **dosimeter** (a device that measures x-ray exposure) to evaluate the radiation output by measuring the radiation intensity: reproducibility of exposure, mAs reciprocity, and milliamperage and exposure time linearity.
- **Reproducibility of exposure** verifies the consistency of the radiation output for a given set of exposure factors. The maximum variability of the reproducibility of radiation exposures is ±5%.
- **mAs reciprocity** verifies the consistency of radiation intensity for changes in mA and exposure time with constant mAs. The maximum variability of reciprocity is ±10%.
- **Milliamperage and exposure time linearity** verifies that proportional changes in mA or exposure time or both likewise change the radiation intensity. Doubling the mA or exposure time should double the radiation intensity. The maximum variability of linearity is ±10%.

LINE-FOCUS PRINCIPLE

The **line-focus principle** describes the relationship between the actual and the effective focal spots in an x-ray tube.

 IMPORTANT RELATIONSHIP

Line-focus Principle

> The line-focus principle describes the relationship between the actual focal spot, where the electrons in the tube current bombard the target, and the effective focal spot, which is the same area as seen from directly below the tube.

The **actual focal spot size** refers to the size of the area on the anode target that is exposed to electrons from the tube current. It depends on the size of the filament producing the electron stream. The **effective focal spot size** refers to focal spot size as measured directly under the anode target (Figure 2-16).

A tube's focal spot is an important factor because a large focal spot can withstand the heat produced by large exposures, whereas a small one produces better image quality. The line-focus principle demonstrates how, by angling the face of the anode target, the actual focal spot can remain relatively large while the effective focal spot is reduced in size. Greater heat capacity can be achieved while maintaining a good image quality.

When manufactured, every tube has a specific anode target angle, typically ranging from 5° to 20°. Based on the line-focus principle, the amount of the target angle determines the size of the effective focal spot. It should be noted that the anode target angle is determined on the basis of the intended use of the tube and is not something the radiographer "selects" at the operating console.

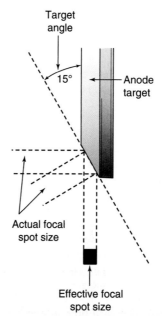

FIGURE 2-16 The line-focus principle addresses the relationship between the size of the actual focal spot (where the electrons actually bombard the target) and the effective focal spot (the same area as viewed and measured directly below the target).

A larger target angle produces a larger effective focal spot and a smaller target angle produces a smaller one. The relationship among target angle, effective focal spot size, and actual focal spot size is illustrated in Figure 2-17.

 IMPORTANT RELATIONSHIP

Anode Angle and Effective Focal Spot Size

Based on the line-focus principle, the smaller the anode target angle, the smaller the effective focal spot size.

ANODE HEEL EFFECT

A phenomenon known as the **anode heel effect** occurs because of the angle of the target. The heel effect describes how the x-ray beam has greater intensity (number of x-rays) on the cathode side of the tube but a lower intensity toward the anode side (Figure 2-18).

 IMPORTANT RELATIONSHIP

Anode Heel Effect

X-rays are more intense on the cathode side of the tube; their intensity decreases toward the anode side.

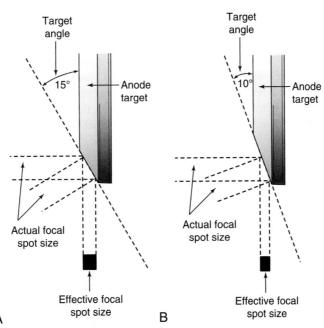

FIGURE 2-17 Based on the line-focus principle, a large target angle produces a large effective focal spot size **(A)** and a small target angle produces a small one **(B)**. Both actual focal spot sizes are the same, meaning that they can withstand the same heat loading. The smaller effective focal spot results in improved image quality.

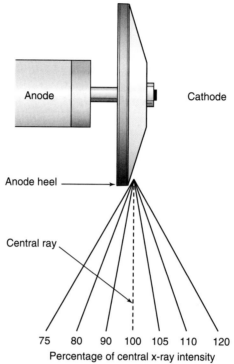

75   80   90   100   105   110   120
Percentage of central x-ray intensity
FIGURE 2-18 Anode heel effect.

As x-rays are produced, they leave the anode in all directions. The x-rays that are emitted toward the anode side of the tube have farther to travel, and some are absorbed by the anode itself (anode heel), reducing them in number compared with the photons that are emitted in the direction of the cathode. The difference in the intensities between the two ends can be as much as 45%. The heel effect can be used to advantage in radiography because the cathode end of the tube can be placed over a thicker body part, resulting in a more even exposure to the image receptor.

The anode heel effect can be used in imaging the thoracic spine, which has small vertebrae at the top and large vertebrae at the bottom. By placing the patient's head under the anode end of the tube, more intense radiation is directed toward the lower, larger portion of the spine, and the upper, smaller vertebrae are exposed to less intense radiation exposure.

BEAM FILTRATION

The x-ray beam produced at the anode exits the tube housing to become the primary beam. The primary beam is the x-ray beam that eventually records the body part onto the image receptor. The x-rays that exit the tube are polyenergetic; they consist of low-energy, medium-energy, and high-energy photons. The low-energy photons cannot penetrate parts of the anatomy and do not contribute to image formation. They contribute only to patient dose.

  IMPORTANT RELATIONSHIP

Low-Energy Photons, Patient Dose, and Image Formation

Low-energy photons serve only to increase patient dose and do not contribute to image formation.

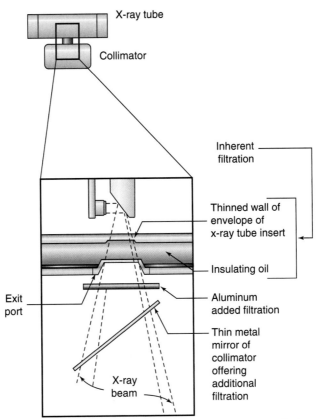

X-ray tube

Collimator

Inherent filtration

Thinned wall of envelope of x-ray tube insert

Insulating oil

Exit port

Aluminum added filtration

Thin metal mirror of collimator offering additional filtration

X-ray beam

FIGURE 2-19 Aluminum (Al)-added filtration is shown at the port, or window, of the x-ray tube and the collimator mirror. The inherent filtration of the envelope and the oil are shown.

Reduction of the low-energy photons requires that filtration be added to the x-ray beam to attenuate or absorb these photons. **Added filtration** describes the filtration that is added to the port of the x-ray tube. Aluminum is the material primarily used for this purpose because it absorbs more low-energy photons while the useful higher-energy photons can exit (Figure 2-19).

Various components within the x-ray tube assembly also contribute to the attenuation of low-energy x-rays. **Inherent filtration** refers to the filtration that is permanently in the path of the x-ray beam. Three components contribute to inherent filtration: (1) the envelope of the tube, (2) the oil that surrounds the tube, and (3) the window in the tube housing. The mirror inside the collimator (beam restrictor located just below the x-ray tube) adds additional filtration (see Figure 2-19). The **total filtration** in the x-ray beam is the sum of the added and inherent filtration. The U.S. government sets standards for total filtration to ensure that patients receive minimal doses of radiation. The current guidelines state that x-ray tubes operating at above 70 kVp must have a minimum total filtration of 2.5 mm of aluminum or its equivalent. Increasing the amount of tube filtration increases the x-ray beam quality because there is a greater percentage of x-rays that have high energy rather than low energy. In addition, increasing tube filtration decreases the quantity of x-rays or x-ray emission (Figure 2-20) (Box 2-10 describes quality-control methods for evaluating filtration).

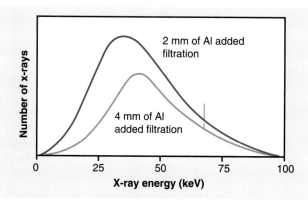

FIGURE 2-20 Increasing beam filtration decreases the quantity (amplitude) and increases the quality (shift to the right) of the x-ray beam.

BOX 2-10   Quality-Control Check: Beam Filtration

- **Half-value layer (HVL)**, the amount of filtration that reduces the intensity of the x-ray beam to one-half of its original value, is considered the best method for describing x-ray quality.
- The HVL can be used as an indirect measure of the total filtration in the path of the x-ray beam. It is expressed in millimeters of aluminum (mm-Al).
- During the HVL test, a radiation-measuring device, such as a dosimeter, is used to measure both the radiation intensity of the original exposure and that following the addition of increasing millimeters of aluminum filtration in the path of the primary beam. The radiation intensity can be graphed for the increasing levels of aluminum filtration to determine the HVL.
- According to the NCRP Report #102, for equipment operated at or above 70 kVp, the required minimum total filtration should be at least 2.5 mm, which indicates the total filtration in the x-ray tube is adequate to protect patients from unnecessary low-energy radiation.
- Normal HVL of general diagnostic beams is 3–5 mm aluminum.

⚠ Radiation Protection Alert

Beam Filtration

Low-energy photons, created during x-ray production, are unable to penetrate the patient. Patients are protected from unnecessary exposure to this low-energy radiation by the placement of inherent and added filtration in the path of the x-ray beam.

COMPENSATING FILTERS

Compensating filters can be added to the primary beam to alter its intensity. These types of filters are used to image anatomic areas that are non-uniform in makeup and assist in producing more consistent exposure to the image receptor.

The most common type of compensating filter is a simple **wedge filter** (Figure 2-21A). The thicker part of the wedge filter is lined up with the thinner portion of the anatomic part being imaged, allowing fewer x-ray photons to reach that end of the part. A wedge filter may be used for an anteroposterior (AP) projection of the femur, where the hip end is considerably larger than the knee end. A **trough filter** performs a function similar to a wedge filter; however, it is differently designed (Figure 2-21B). In particular, the trough filter has a double wedge. A trough filter may be used for an AP projection of the thorax to compensate for the easily penetrated air-filled lungs.

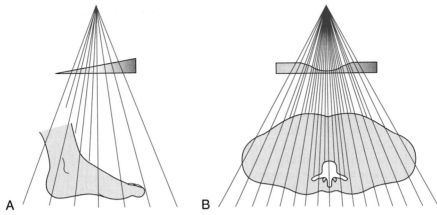

FIGURE 2-21 A, Wedge filter. **B,** Trough filter.

TABLE 2-1	Generator Factor
Generator Type	**Factor**
Single phase	1.00
Three phase	1.35
High frequency	1.40

HEAT UNITS

During x-ray production, most of the kinetic energy of the electrons is converted to heat. This heat can damage the x-ray tube and the anode target. The amount of heat produced from any given exposure is expressed by the **heat unit (HU)**. The number of HUs produced depends on the type of x-ray generator being used and the exposure factors selected for a particular exposure and can be mathematically expressed as follows:

$$HU = mA \times time \times kVp \times generator\ factor.$$

The generator factor (Table 2-1) accounts for the fact that the use of more consistent x-ray generators results in more heat.

 MATHEMATICAL APPLICATION

Calculating Heat Units

An exposure is made with a three-phase x-ray unit at 600 mA and 75 kVp over 0.05 s. How many heat units are produced from this exposure?

$$HU = mA \times time \times kVp \times generator\ factor$$
$$HU = 600 \times 0.05 \times 75 \times 1.35$$
$$= 3037.5\ HU$$

Different models of x-ray tubes vary in their ability to withstand the heat produced by x-ray exposures. Prior to modern x-ray tubes, radiographers were responsible for evaluating their exposure technique selection to avoid excessive heat load. Box 2-11 explains the use of tube-rating charts to avoid heat damage. Manufacturers of current x-ray units build their equipment so that tube-damaging exposures cannot be made. In general, if an inappropriate technique is set, the radiographer sees a message such as "Technique Overload," or the machine may simply not expose after the button is activated. The routine use of high-exposure techniques, although within the x-ray tube's limit, can potentially damage the x-ray tube.

BOX 2-11   Tube-Rating Charts

Prior to today's x-ray tubes, manufacturers used instantaneous-load tube-rating charts, also called *single-exposure rating charts*, to describe the exposure limits of x-ray tubes. An instantaneous-load tube-rating chart is used to determine whether a particular exposure would be safe to make and to determine what limits on kVp, mA, and exposure time must be made for safe exposure. Violation of these limits, as indicated by the tube-rating chart, would almost certainly result in permanent and irreparable damage to the x-ray tube. Figure 2-22 shows a typical instantaneous-load tube-rating chart. For example, the maximum kVp that can be used with 700 mA and 0.3 s exposure time is 90 kVp. The maximum mA that can be used with 105 kVp and 0.2 s exposure time is 600 mA. The maximum exposure time that can be used with 85 kVp and 900 mA is 0.05 s. Although 130 kVp, 500 mA, and 0.1 s would produce a safe exposure, 130 kVp, 500 mA, and 0.2 s would not.

In addition to tube-rating charts, manufacturers provided anode and housing cooling charts. Based on the quantity of heat units, these charts provided radiographers with information regarding the amount of time that must elapse before initiating another exposure.

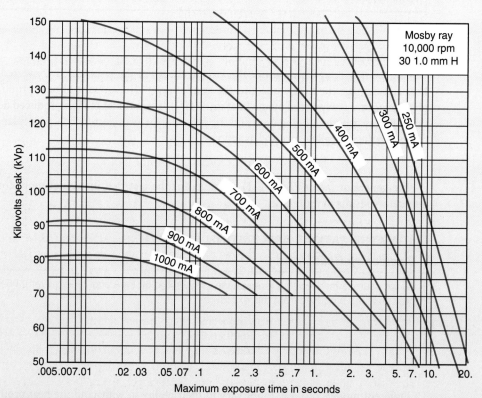

FIGURE 2-22 Typical instantaneous-load tube-rating chart that can be used to determine safe and unsafe exposures.

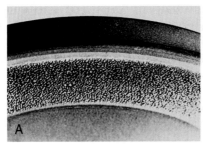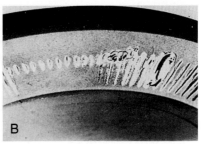

FIGURE 2-23 Two heat-damaged anode targets. **A,** Target shows pitting of the anode track caused by consistent overloading of exposure factors. **B,** Target shows melting of the focal track caused by failure of the rotor to rotate the anode. This failure is usually due to heat damage to the rotor bearings from overloading the exposure factors.

EXTENDING X-RAY TUBE LIFE

X-ray tubes are expensive devices that can fail because of radiographer errors or carelessness. Not only do failed tubes result in an expense for purchasing a new tube but there is also a down time for a radiographic room when a failed tube is being replaced, thus decreasing the room's productivity. A few simple but important guidelines for x-ray tube operation should be consistently adhered to by the radiographer to extend tube life:

- If applicable, warm up the tube according to the manufacturer's specifications, especially if it has not been energized for 2 h or more.
- Avoid excessive heat unit generation. Repeatedly using exposure techniques near an x-ray tube's limit increases the total number of heat units. Figure 2-23 shows anode targets that have been damaged as a result of excessive heat loading.
- Do not hold down the rotor button without making an exposure. Unnecessarily holding down the rotor button causes excessive wear on both the filament and the rotor.
- Use lower tube currents with longer exposure times when possible to minimize wear on the filament.
- Do not move the tube while it is energized. This movement can cause damage to the anode and anode stem as a result of torque, the angular analog of force that acts to produce rotation.
- If the rotor makes noticeable noise, stop using the tube until it has been inspected by a qualified service personnel. Noises can be indicative of a potentially serious problem.

Radiographers create diagnostic images by producing an x-ray beam that visualizes anatomic structures. The x-rays produced by the radiographer affect not only the quality of the image but also the life of the x-ray tube. Understanding the prime exposure factors and their effect on the x-ray beam and knowing what happens inside the x-ray tube are important considerations in radiography.

CHAPTER SUMMARY

- X-rays are produced when electrons are boiled off (thermionic emission) the cathode filament, accelerated across to the anode target and suddenly stopped. Heat is also produced.
- The anode, containing a tungsten–rhenium alloy target, typically rotates, allowing for larger exposures.
- X-rays are produced by bremsstrahlung (primarily) and characteristic interactions that occur as the electrons interact with the tungsten atoms in the target.

- Manipulation of the primary factors affects the quality and quantity of radiation. kVp affects both the quality (energy and penetrability) and the quantity of x-rays, whereas mA and exposure time (or mAs when combined) affect only quantity.
- The line-focus principle describes the relationship between the anode angle and the effective focal spot. The anode heel effect results in more intense radiation exiting the tube toward the cathode side.
- Added and inherent beam filtration ensures that a minimal amount of low-energy x-ray photons reach the patient. The half value layer (HVL) is an indirect measure of total filtration and is used to describe x-ray quality.
- There are numerous methods for extending tube life, including attending to the amount of heat produced during x-ray production. Heat units are the measure of the amount of heat produced using specific exposure factors.

REVIEW QUESTIONS

1. Which x-ray tube component serves as a source of electrons for x-ray production?
   A. Focusing cup
   B. Filament
   C. Stator
   D. Target
2. Electrons interact with the _____ to produce x-rays and heat.
   A. focusing cup
   B. filament
   C. stator
   D. target
3. The cloud of electrons that forms before x-ray production is referred to as _____.
   A. thermionic emission
   B. space charge
   C. space charge effect
   D. tube current
4. The burning or boiling-off of electrons at the cathode is referred to as _____.
   A. thermionic emission
   B. space charge
   C. space charge effect
   D. tube current
5. Which primary exposure factor influences both the quantity and the quality of x-ray photons?
   A. mA
   B. mAs
   C. kVp
   D. Exposure time
6. The unit used to express tube current is _____.
   A. mA
   B. mAs
   C. kVp
   D. s
7. What percentage of the kinetic energy is converted to heat when moving electrons strike the anode target?
   A. 1%
   B. 25%

C. 59%

D. 99%

8. The intensity of the x-ray beam is greater on the _____.
   A. cathode side of the tube
   B. anode side of the tube
   C. short axis of the beam
   D. long axis of the beam

9. According to the line-focus principle, as the target angle decreases, the _____.
   A. actual focal spot size decreases
   B. actual focal spot size increases
   C. effective focal spot size decreases
   D. effective focal spot size increases

10. _____ extends x-ray tube life.
   A. Selecting higher tube currents
   B. Using small focal spots when possible
   C. Producing exposures with a wide range of kVp values
   D. Warming up the tube after 2 h of non-use

11. Which type of target interaction is responsible for most of the x-rays in the diagnostic beam?
   A. Characteristic interaction
   B. Thermionic emission
   C. Bremsstrahlung interaction
   D. None of the above

12. What value of mAs is produced when the radiographer sets a kilovoltage peak of 70 kVp, a milliamperage of 600 mA, and an exposure time of 50 ms?
   A. 3.5 mAs
   B. 30 mAs
   C. 300 mAs
   D. 350 mAs

13. Increasing the kVp results in _____.
   A. x-rays with higher energy
   B. x-rays with lower energy
   C. more x-rays
   D. A and C
   E. B and C

14. Total filtration in the x-ray beam includes _____.
   A. compensating filters
   B. inherent filtration
   C. added filtration
   D. B and C
   E. all of the above

15. How many heat units result from an exposure made on a single-phase x-ray unit using a beam current of 400 mA, an exposure time of 0.2 s, and a kilovoltage peak of 70 kVp?
   A. 5600 HU
   B. 7560 HU
   C. 7896 HU
   D. 8120 HU

3

Image Formation and Radiographic Quality

CHAPTER OUTLINE

Image Formation
  Differential Absorption
Radiographic Quality
  Image Brightness

Image Contrast
Spatial Resolution
Distortion
Scatter

Quantum Noise
Image Artifacts
Digital versus Film-Screen
  Imaging

OBJECTIVES

After completing this chapter, the reader will be able to perform the following:

1. Define all the key terms in this chapter.
2. State all the important relationships in this chapter.
3. Describe the process of radiographic image formation.
4. Explain the process of beam attenuation.
5. Identify the factors that affect beam attenuation.
6. Describe the x-ray interactions termed *photoelectric effect* and *Compton effect*.
7. Define the term *ionization*.
8. State the composition of exit radiation.
9. Explain the process of creating the various shades of image brightness.
10. Describe the necessary components of radiographic quality.
11. Explain the importance of brightness and contrast to image quality.
12. Differentiate between high-contrast and low-contrast images.
13. Explain the importance of spatial resolution and both size and shape distortion to image quality.
14. State the effects of quantum noise, scatter, and image artifacts on image quality.
15. Recognize the advantages of digital imaging and the limitations of film-screen imaging.

KEY TERMS

absorption
artifact
attenuation
brightness
coherent scattering
Compton effect
Compton electron
contrast resolution
density
differential absorption
distortion

dynamic range
elongation
exit radiation
fog
foreshortening
gray scale
high contrast
image receptor
invisible image
ionization
latent image

long-scale contrast
low contrast
magnification
manifest image
photoelectric effect
photoelectron
quantum noise
remnant radiation
scale of contrast
scattering
secondary electron

KEY TERMS—cont'd

shape distortion	spatial resolution	transmission
short-scale contrast	subject contrast	visible image
size distortion	tissue density	

To produce a radiographic image, x-ray photons must pass through tissue and interact with an **image receptor (IR)**, a device that receives the radiation leaving the patient. Both the quantity and the quality of the primary x-ray beam affects its interactions within the various tissues that make up anatomic parts. In addition, the composition of the anatomic tissues affects the x-ray beam interaction. The absorption characteristics of the anatomic part are determined by its thickness, atomic number of the atoms contained within it, and tissue density or compactness of the cellular structures. Finally, the radiation that exits the patient is composed of varying energies and interacts with the image receptor to form a latent or invisible image and must be processed.

A visible radiographic image is produced following the processing of the latent or invisible image. Depending on the type of imaging system, the acquiring, processing, and displaying of images can vary significantly. However, the attributes of a quality radiographic image are similar regardless of the type of imaging system. This chapter will focus on how images are formed and their quality after processing.

IMAGE FORMATION

Differential Absorption

The process of image formation is a result of **differential absorption** of the x-ray beam as it interacts with anatomic tissue. Differential absorption is a process whereby some amount of the x-ray beam is absorbed in the tissue and some passes through (transmits) the anatomic part. The term *differential* is used because varying anatomic parts do not *absorb* the primary beam to the same degree. Anatomic parts composed of bone absorb more x-ray photons than parts filled with air. Differential absorption of the primary x-ray beam creates an image that structurally represents the anatomic area of interest (Figure 3-1).

 IMPORTANT RELATIONSHIP

Differential Absorption and Image Formation

A radiographic image is created when an x-ray beam passes through a patient and then interacts with an image receptor, such as a digital-imaging system. The variations in the absorption and transmission of the exiting x-ray beam structurally represent the anatomic area of interest.

Creating a radiographic image by differential absorption requires several processes to occur: beam attenuation, absorption, and transmission.

Beam Attenuation

As the primary x-ray beam passes through anatomic tissue, it loses some of its energy (intensity). Fewer x-ray photons remain in the beam after it interacts with anatomic tissue. This reduction in the intensity or number of photons in the primary x-ray beam is known as **attenuation**. Beam attenuation occurs as a result of the photon interactions with the atomic structures that comprise the tissues. Two distinct processes occur during beam attenuation: absorption and scattering.

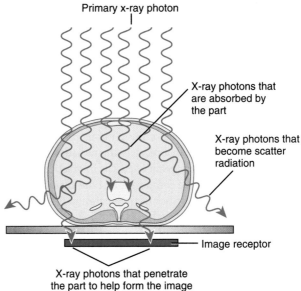

Primary x-ray photon

X-ray photons that are absorbed by the part

X-ray photons that become scatter radiation

Image receptor

X-ray photons that penetrate the part to help form the image

FIGURE 3-1 As the primary x-ray beam interacts with an anatomic part, photons are absorbed, scattered, and transmitted. The differences in the absorption characteristics of the anatomic part create an image that structurally represents the part.

Absorption. As the energy of the primary x-ray beam is deposited within the atoms comprising the tissue, some x-ray photons are completely absorbed. Complete **absorption** of the incoming x-ray photon occurs when it has enough energy to remove (eject) an inner-shell electron. The ejected electron is called a **photoelectron**, and it quickly loses energy by interacting with nearby tissues. The ability to remove (eject) electrons, known as **ionization**, is a characteristic of x-rays. In the diagnostic range, this x-ray interaction with matter is known as the **photoelectric effect**.

With the photoelectric effect, an ionized atom has a vacancy, or electron hole, in its inner shell. An electron from an outer shell drops down to fill this vacancy. Because of the difference in binding energies between the two electron shells, a secondary x-ray photon is emitted (Figure 3-2). This secondary x-ray photon typically has a very low energy and is unlikely to exit the patient.

IMPORTANT RELATIONSHIP

X-ray Photon Absorption

During attenuation of the x-ray beam, the photoelectric effect is responsible for the total absorption of the incoming x-ray photon.

The probability of total photon absorption by the photoelectric effect depends on the energy of the incoming x-ray photon and the atomic number of the anatomic tissue. The energy of the incoming x-ray photon must be at least equal to the binding energy of the inner-shell electron. After absorption of a certain amount of x-ray photons, the overall energy or quantity of the primary beam decreases as it passes through the anatomic part.

Scattering. Some incoming photons are not absorbed but instead lose energy during interactions with the atoms comprising the tissue. This process is called **scattering**. It results from an interaction

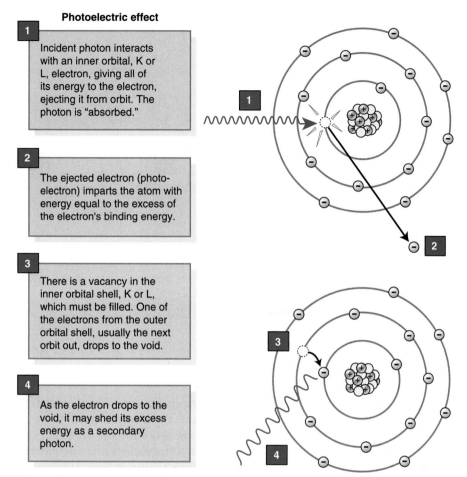

Photoelectric effect

1 Incident photon interacts with an inner orbital, K or L, electron, giving all of its energy to the electron, ejecting it from orbit. The photon is "absorbed."

2 The ejected electron (photo-electron) imparts the atom with energy equal to the excess of the electron's binding energy.

3 There is a vacancy in the inner orbital shell, K or L, which must be filled. One of the electrons from the outer orbital shell, usually the next orbit out, drops to the void.

4 As the electron drops to the void, it may shed its excess energy as a secondary photon.

FIGURE 3-2 The photoelectric effect is responsible for total absorption of the incoming x-ray photon.

between diagnostic x-rays and matter, known as the **Compton effect**. The loss of energy of the incoming photon occurs when it ejects an outer-shell electron from a tissue atom. The ejected electron is called a **Compton electron** or **secondary electron**. The remaining lower-energy x-ray photon changes direction and may leave the anatomic part to interact with the image receptor (Figure 3-3).

 IMPORTANT RELATIONSHIP

X-ray Beam Scattering

During attenuation of the x-ray beam, the incoming x-ray photon may lose energy and change direction as a result of the Compton effect.

Compton interactions can occur at any diagnostic x-ray energy and are an important interaction in radiography. The probability of a Compton interaction occurring depends on the energy of the incoming photon. It does not depend on the atomic number of the anatomic tissue. For example, a Compton interaction is just as likely to occur in soft tissue as in tissue composed of bone;

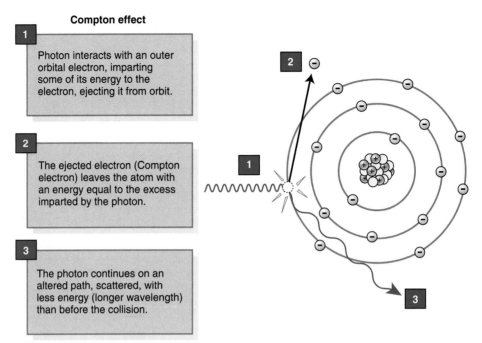

Compton effect

1 Photon interacts with an outer orbital electron, imparting some of its energy to the electron, ejecting it from orbit.

2 The ejected electron (Compton electron) leaves the atom with an energy equal to the excess imparted by the photon.

3 The photon continues on an altered path, scattered, with less energy (longer wavelength) than before the collision.

FIGURE 3-3 During the Compton effect, the incoming photon loses energy and changes its direction.

however, if the tissue has more complex atoms, there are more opportunities for interaction. With higher atomic number particles, such as bone, if the energy of the incoming photon is sufficiently high, more scatter will occur; otherwise, more absorption will occur. For Compton interactions to occur, the energy of the photon is more important, whereas the atomic number of elements in the tissue is only related to the opportunity for x-ray interactions. When a higher kVp within the diagnostic range is used, the overall number of x-ray interactions within matter decrease because of increased photon transmission; however, the percentage of photoelectric interactions generally decreases at higher kilovoltages within the diagnostic range, whereas the percentage of Compton interactions is likely to increase at higher kilovoltages within the diagnostic range. Box 3-1 compares photoelectric and Compton interactions. Scattered and secondary radiations provide no useful information and must be controlled during radiographic imaging.

Coherent scattering is an interaction that occurs with low-energy x-rays, typically below the diagnostic range. The incoming photon interacts with the atom, causing it to become excited. The x-ray does not lose energy, but it changes direction. Coherent scattering could occur within the diagnostic range of the x-rays and may interact with the image receptor, but it is not considered an important interaction in radiography.

If a scattered photon strikes the image receptor, it does not contribute any useful information about the anatomic area of interest. If scattered photons are absorbed within the anatomic tissue, they contribute to radiation exposure to the patient. In addition, if the scattered photon leaves the patient and does not strike the image receptor, it could contribute to radiation exposure of anyone near the patient.

The preceding discussion focused on photon interactions that occur in radiography when using x-ray energies within the moderate range. X-rays with energies above the diagnostic range result in other interactions, namely, pair production and photodisintegration. X-ray interactions above the diagnostic range are important in radiation therapy.

BOX 3-1 Comparing the Photoelectric and Compton Effects

Photoelectric Effect
- An incoming photon has sufficient energy to eject an inner-shell electron and be completely absorbed.
- An electron from an upper-level shell fills the electron hole or vacancy.
- A secondary photon is created because of the difference in the electrons' binding energies.
- The probability of this effect depends on the energy of the incoming x-ray photon and the composition of the anatomic tissue.
- Fewer photon interactions occur at a higher kVp, but of those interactions, a smaller percentage are photoelectric interactions.

Compton Effect
- An incoming photon loses energy when it ejects an outer shell electron and changes direction.
- The scattered photon may be absorbed within the patient tissues, leave the anatomic part, interact with the image receptor, or expose anyone near the patient.
- Scattered photons that strike the image receptor provide no useful information.
- The probability of this effect depends on the energy of the incoming x-ray photon but not on the composition of the anatomic tissue.
- Fewer photon interactions occur at a higher kVp, but a greater percentage of those interactions are Compton interactions.

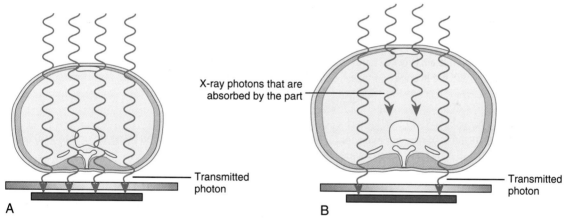

X-ray photons that are absorbed by the part

Transmitted photon

Transmitted photon

A

B

FIGURE 3-4 A, a thinner patient transmits more radiation than a thicker patient. **B,** a thicker patient absorbs more radiation than a thinner patient.

Factors Affecting Beam Attenuation

The amount of x-ray beam attenuation is affected by the thickness of the anatomic part, the atomic number of the atoms contained within it, its tissue density, and the energy of the x-ray beam.

Tissue Thickness. Increasing the thickness of a given anatomic tissue increases beam attenuation by either absorption or scattering (Figure 3-4). X-rays are exponentially attenuated and are generally reduced by approximately 50% for each 4–5 cm (1.6–2 in) of tissue thickness (Figure 3-5). More x-rays are needed to produce a radiographic image for a thicker anatomic part. Fewer x-rays are needed to produce a radiographic image for a thinner anatomic part.

Type of Tissue. Tissues composed of elements with a higher atomic number, such as bone (which has an effective atomic number of 13.8), attenuates the x-ray beam more than tissue composed of elements with a lower atomic number, such as fat (which has an effective atomic number of 6.3). The higher atomic number indicates there are more atomic particles for interactions with x-ray photons. X-ray absorption is more likely to occur in tissues with a higher effective atomic number than in those with a lower effective atomic number (Figure 3-6).

Tissue density (matter per unit volume), or the compactness of atomic particles comprising the anatomic part, also affects the amount of beam attenuation. For example, muscle (effective atomic number 7.4) and fat (effective atomic number 6.3) tissue are similar in effective atomic number; however, their atomic particles differ in compactness and their tissue densities vary. Muscle tissue has atomic particles that are more densely packed or compact and therefore attenuate the x-ray beam more than fat cells. Bone is composed of tissue with a higher atomic number, and the atomic particles are more compacted or densely packed. Anatomic tissues are typically ranked on the basis of their attenuation properties. Four substances account for most of the beam attenuation in the human body: bone, muscle, fat, and air. Bone attenuates the x-ray beam more than muscle, muscle

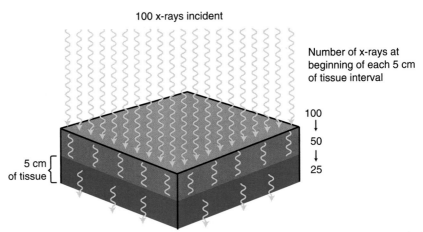

FIGURE 3-5 X-rays are exponentially attenuated and generally reduced by approximately 50% for each 4–5 cm (1.6–2 in) of tissue thickness.

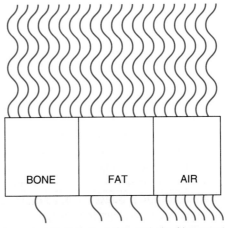

FIGURE 3-6 Bone absorbs more radiation than fat and air. Air transmits more radiation than fat and bone.

attenuates the x-ray beam more than fat, and fat attenuates the x-ray beam more than air. The atomic number of the anatomic part and its tissue density affect x-ray beam attenuation.

X-ray Beam Quality. The quality of the x-ray beam or its penetrating ability affects its interaction with anatomic tissue. Higher-penetrating x-rays (shorter wavelength with higher frequency) are more likely to be transmitted through anatomic tissue without interacting with the tissues' atomic structures. Lower-penetrating x-rays (longer wavelength with lower frequency) are more likely to interact with the atomic structures and be absorbed. The kilovoltage selected during x-ray production determines the energy or penetrability of the x-ray photon, and this affects its attenuation in anatomic tissue (Figure 3-7). Beam attenuation decreases with a higher-energy x-ray beam and increases with a lower-energy x-ray beam (Table 3-1).

 IMPORTANT RELATIONSHIP

Factors Affecting Beam Attenuation

Increasing tissue thickness, atomic number, and tissue density increases x-ray beam attenuation because more x-rays are absorbed by the tissue. Increasing the quality of the x-ray beam decreases beam attenuation because the higher-energy x-rays penetrate the tissue.

Transmission. If the incoming x-ray photon passes through the anatomic part without any interaction with the atomic structures, it is called **transmission** (Figure 3-8). The combination of absorption and transmission of the x-ray beam provides an image that structurally represents the anatomic part. Because scatter radiation is also a process that occurs during interaction of the x-ray beam and the anatomic part, the quality of the image created is compromised if the scattered photon strikes the image receptor.

Exit Radiation

When the attenuated x-ray beam leaves the patient, the remaining x-ray beam, referred to as **exit radiation** or **remnant radiation**, is composed of both transmitted and scattered radiation (Figure 3-9). The varying amounts of transmitted and absorbed radiation (differential absorption) create an image that structurally represents the anatomic area of interest. Scatter exit radiation (Compton

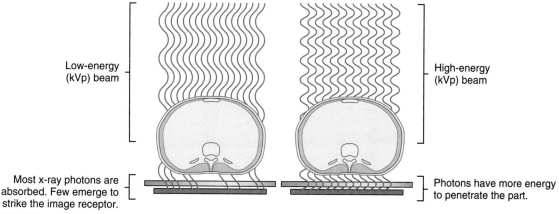

Low-energy (kVp) beam

High-energy (kVp) beam

Most x-ray photons are absorbed. Few emerge to strike the image receptor.

Photons have more energy to penetrate the part.

FIGURE 3-7 The energy of the x-ray beam affects its interaction within anatomic tissues. Lower kVp results in more absorption in the tissue; higher kVp results in more transmission through the tissue.

interactions) that reach the image receptor do not provide any diagnostic information about the anatomic area. Scatter radiation creates unwanted exposure on the image called **fog**. Methods used to decrease the amount of scatter radiation reaching the image receptor are discussed in Chapter 7.

 IMPORTANT RELATIONSHIP

X-ray Interaction with Matter

When the diagnostic primary x-ray beam interacts with anatomic tissues, three processes occur: absorption, scattering, and transmission.

The areas within the anatomic tissue that absorb incoming x-ray photons (photoelectric effect) create the white or clear areas (increased brightness) on the displayed image. The incoming x-ray photons that are transmitted create black areas (decreased brightness) on the displayed image.

Factor	Beam Attenuation	Absorption	Transmission
TABLE 3-1 Factors Affecting Attenuation			
Tissue Thickness			
• Increasing thickness	↑	↑	↓
• Decreasing thickness	↓	↓	↑
Tissue Atomic Number			
• Increasing atomic #	↑	↑	↓
• Decreasing atomic #	↓	↓	↑
Tissue Density			
• Increasing tissue density	↑	↑	↓
• Decreasing tissue density	↓	↓	↑
X-ray Beam Quality			
• Increasing beam quality	↓	↓	↑
• Decreasing beam quality	↑	↑	↓

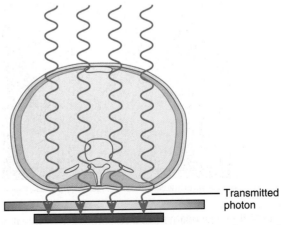

Transmitted photon

FIGURE 3-8 Some incoming x-ray photons pass through the anatomic part without any interactions.

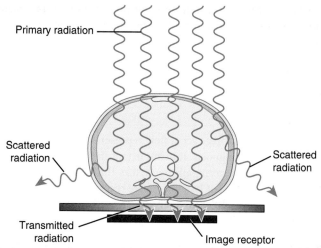

FIGURE 3-9 Radiation that exits the anatomic part comprises transmitted and scattered radiation.

Anatomic tissues that vary in absorption and transmission create a range of dark and light areas (shades of gray) (Figure 3-10). The various shades of gray recorded in the radiographic image make anatomic tissues visible. Skeletal bones are differentiated from the air-filled lungs because of their differences in absorption and transmission.

Less than 5% of the primary x-ray beam interacting with the anatomic part actually reaches the image receptor, and an even lower percentage is used to create the radiographic image. The exit radiation interacting with an image receptor creates the **latent image**, or **invisible image**. This latent image is not visible until it is processed to produce the **manifest image**, or **visible image**.

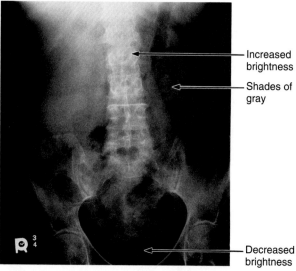

FIGURE 3-10 Anatomic tissues vary in their absorption and transmission of x-ray photons to create the range of brightness or gray levels that structurally represent the anatomic area of interest. Increased brightness represents absorbed radiation, whereas decreased brightness represents transmitted radiation.

IMPORTANT RELATIONSHIP

Image Brightness

The range of image brightness levels visible after processing is a result of the variation in x-ray absorption and transmission as the x-ray beam passes through anatomic tissues.

RADIOGRAPHIC QUALITY

A quality radiographic image accurately represents the anatomic area of interest, and information is well visualized for diagnosis. It is important to identify the attributes of a quality radiographic image before comprehending all the factors that affect its quality. Radiographic images can be acquired from two different types of image receptors: digital and film-screen. The process of creating a latent image by differential absorption is the same for both digital and film image receptors; however, the acquisition, processing, and display vary greatly.

 IMPORTANT RELATIONSHIP

Creating the Latent Image

The process of differential absorption for image formation is the same for digital and film-screen imaging. The varying x-ray intensities exiting the anatomic area of interest form the latent image.

The *visibility* of the anatomic structures and the *accuracy* of their recorded structural lines (sharpness) determine the overall quality of the radiographic image. The visibility of the recorded detail refers to the *brightness* and *contrast* of the image, and the accuracy of the structural lines is achieved by maximizing the amount of *spatial resolution* and minimizing the amount of *distortion* (Figure 3-11). Visibility of the recorded detail is achieved by the proper balance of image brightness and contrast.

Image Brightness

How the radiograph is displayed determines whether the image is evaluated in terms of brightness or density. Digital images are typically displayed on a computer monitor, whereas film-screen images are displayed on film. Digital images can also be printed on specialized film. Brightness and density refer to the same image quality attribute but are differently defined. **Brightness** is the amount of luminance (light emission) of a display monitor. **Density** is the amount of overall blackness on the processed film image. An area of increased brightness viewed on a computer monitor shows decreased density on a film image, whereas an area of decreased brightness visualized on a computer monitor has increased density on a film image.

Radiographic Quality

Visibility

Sharpness

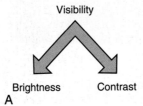

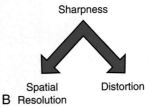

Brightness   Contrast

A

Spatial   Distortion

B   Resolution

FIGURE 3-11 Factors affecting radiographic image quality. **A**, Visibility factors. **B**, Sharpness factors.

A radiograph must have sufficient brightness to visualize the anatomic structures of interest (Figure 3-12). A radiograph that is too light has too much brightness to visualize the structures of the anatomic part (Figure 3-13). Conversely, a radiograph that is too dark has insufficient brightness and the anatomic part cannot be well visualized (Figure 3-14). The radiographer must evaluate the overall brightness in the image to determine whether it is sufficient to visualize the anatomic area of interest. He/she then decides whether the radiograph is diagnostic or unacceptable.

IMPORTANT RELATIONSHIP
Brightness and Radiographic Quality

A radiographic image must have sufficient brightness to visualize the anatomic structures of interest.

The primary factor that affects the amount of density produced in a film-screen image is the amount or quantity of radiation reaching the image receptor. However, the quantity of radiation reaching the image receptor has less of an effect on the brightness of a digital image because of computer processing. To evaluate other attributes of radiographic quality, such as contrast and sharpness, the image must have sufficient brightness or density to visualize the anatomic area of interest.

Image Contrast

In addition to sufficient brightness or density, the radiograph must exhibit differences in the brightness levels or densities (image contrast) to differentiate among anatomic tissues. The range of brightness levels is a result of the tissues' differential absorption of the x-ray photons. An image that has sufficient brightness but no differences appears as a homogeneous object (Figure 3-15). This appearance indicates that the absorption characteristics of the object are equal. When the absorption characteristics of an object differ, the image has varying levels of

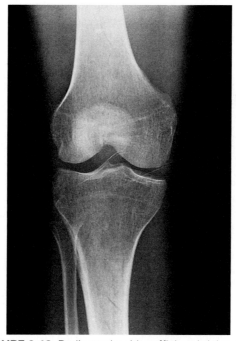

FIGURE 3-12 Radiograph with sufficient brightness.

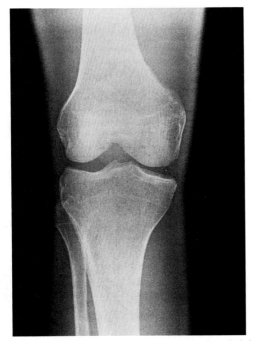

FIGURE 3-13 Radiograph with excessive brightness.

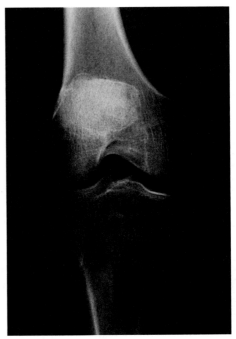

FIGURE 3-14 Radiograph with insufficient brightness.

brightness (Figure 3-16). The anatomic tissues are easily differentiated because of these differences in brightness levels (i.e., contrast). Tissues that attenuate the x-ray beam equally are more difficult to visualize because the brightness levels are too similar to differentiate.

Radiographic contrast is the combined result of multiple factors associated with the anatomic structure, radiation quality, image-receptor capabilities, and, in digital imaging, computer processing and display. **Subject contrast** refers to the absorption characteristics of the anatomic tissue imaged and the quality of the x-ray beam. Differences in tissue thickness, density, and effective atomic number contribute to subject contrast (Figure 3-17). For example, the chest is composed of tissues that vary greatly in x-ray lucency, such as the air-filled lungs, the heart, and the bony thorax. This anatomic region creates high subject contrast because the tissues attenuate the x-ray beam very differently compared with the abdomen for the same beam quality. When the thorax is imaged, great differences in brightness levels are recorded for the varying tissues (Figure 3-18). The abdomen is composed of tissues that attenuate the x-ray beam similarly and is considered to be a region of low subject contrast. The brightness levels representing the organs in the abdomen are more similar (Figure 3-19). Therefore, it is difficult to distinguish the stomach from the kidneys. As previously discussed, the quality of the x-ray beam also affects its attenuation in tissues, which alters subject contrast. Increasing the penetrating power of the x-ray beam decreases attenuation, reduces absorption, and increases x-ray transmission, resulting in fewer differences in the brightness levels recorded in the radiographic image.

IMPORTANT RELATIONSHIP
Differentiating Among Anatomic Tissues

The ability to distinguish among types of tissues is determined by the differences in brightness levels in the image, or contrast. Anatomic tissues that attenuate the beam similarly have low subject contrast. Anatomic tissues that attenuate the beam very differently have high subject contrast.

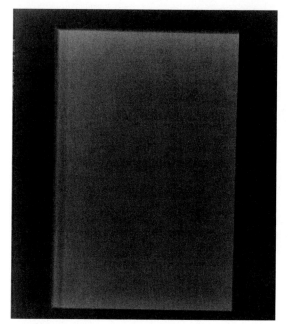

FIGURE 3-15 Radiograph of a homogeneous object having no differences in brightness levels.

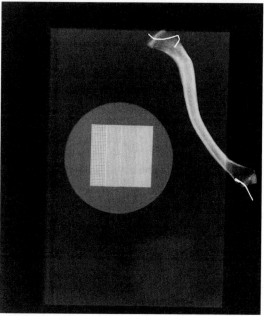

FIGURE 3-16 An object with different absorption characteristics produces an image with varying brightness levels.

Brightness or density is easily measurable; however, contrast is a more complex attribute. Evaluating radiographic quality in terms of contrast is more subjective (it is affected by individual preferences). The level of radiographic contrast desired in an image is determined by the composition of the anatomic tissue to be imaged and the amount of information needed to visualize the tissue for an accurate diagnosis. For example, the level of contrast desired in a chest radiograph is different from that required in a radiograph of an extremity.

Radiographic or *image contrast* is a term used in both digital and film-screen imaging to describe variations in brightness and density. In digital imaging, the number of different shades of gray that can be stored and displayed by a computer system is termed **gray scale**. Because the digital image is processed and reconstructed in the computer as digital data, its gray scale or contrast can be altered. Digital images can be displayed to show a range of gray levels from high to low contrast. High-contrast images display fewer shades of gray but greater differences among them (Figure 3-20). Low-contrast images display a greater number of gray shades but smaller differences among them (Figure 3-21).

The term **contrast resolution** is used to describe the ability of an imaging receptor to distinguish between objects having similar subject contrast. Digital image receptors have improved contrast resolution compared with film-screen image receptors.

Radiographic film images are typically described by their **scale of contrast**, or the range of visible densities. A film image with a few visible densities but great differences among them is said to have **high contrast**; this is also described as **short-scale contrast**. A radiograph with a large number of densities but few differences among them is said to have **low contrast**; this is also described as **long-scale contrast**.

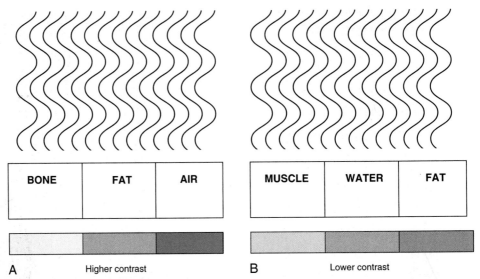

FIGURE 3-17 A, Higher contrast resulting from great differences in radiation absorption between tissues that vary greatly in composition. **B,** Lower contrast resulting from fewer differences in the radiation absorption for tissues that are more similarly composed.

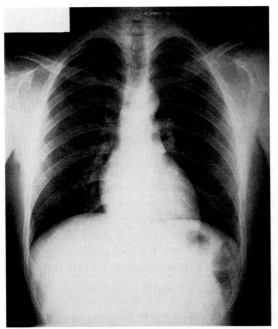

FIGURE 3-18 The thorax is an anatomic area of high subject contrast because there is great variation in tissue composition.

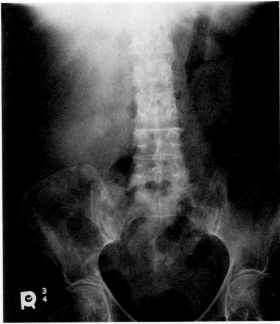

FIGURE 3-19 The abdomen is an anatomic area of low subject contrast because it is composed of similar tissue types.

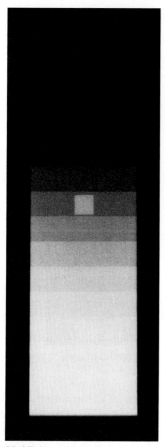

FIGURE 3-20 High-contrast image showing fewer gray levels and greater differences among them.

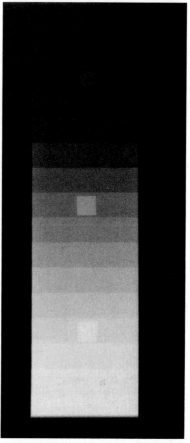

FIGURE 3-21 Low-contrast image showing many gray levels and few differences among them.

Spatial Resolution

The quality of a radiographic image depends on both the visibility and the accuracy of the recorded anatomic structural lines (sharpness). Adequate visualization of the anatomic area of interest (brightness and contrast) is just one component of radiographic quality. To produce a quality radiograph, the anatomic details must be accurately recorded and with the greatest amount of sharpness. Spatial resolution is a term used to evaluate the accuracy of the recorded anatomic structural lines. **Spatial resolution** refers to the smallest object that can be detected in an image.

The ability of a radiographic image to demonstrate sharp lines determines the quality of the spatial resolution. The imaging process makes it impossible to produce a radiographic image without a certain degree of unsharpness. A radiographic image that has greater spatial resolution minimizes the unsharpness of the anatomic structural lines.

 IMPORTANT RELATIONSHIP

Sharpness of Anatomic Detail

The accuracy of the anatomic structural lines recorded in the radiographic image is determined by its spatial resolution.

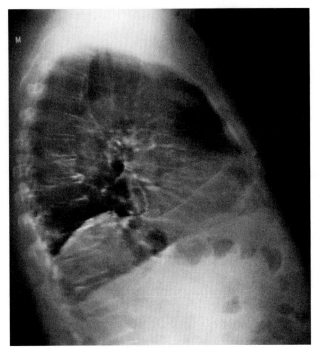

FIGURE 3-22 Image showing motion unsharpness.

A radiographic image cannot be an exact reconstruction of the anatomic structure. Some information is always lost during the process of image formation. In addition, factors such as patient motion increase the amount of unsharpness recorded in the image (Figure 3-22). It is the radiographer's responsibility to minimize the amount of information lost by manipulating the factors that affect the sharpness of the recorded image. Diagnostic quality is achieved by maximizing the amount of spatial resolution and minimizing the amount of image distortion.

The sharpness and visibility of recorded detail have typically been discussed as two separate qualities of a radiographic image. Generally, this separation remains true except when imaging small anatomic structures. A small anatomic structure is best visualized when its brightness varies significantly from the background. If unsharpness is increased, the visibility of small anatomic details is compromised. An increase in the amount of unsharpness recorded on the image decreases the contrast of small anatomic structures, reducing the overall visibility of the structural lines. The spreading of the structural lines with increased unsharpness decreases the differences in brightness levels between the structural lines of the area of interest and the background. As a result, the difference in brightness levels between the area of interest and the background lessens (low contrast) and the visibility of the anatomic structure is reduced (Figure 3-23).

Distortion

Distortion results from the radiographic misrepresentation of either the size (magnification) or the shape of the anatomic part. When an image is distorted, spatial resolution is also reduced.

Size Distortion (Magnification)

The term **size distortion** (or **magnification**) refers to an increase in the image size of an object compared with its true or actual size. Radiographic images of objects are always magnified in

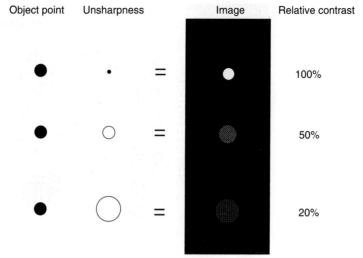

Object point   Unsharpness   Image   Relative contrast

100%

50%

20%

FIGURE 3-23 Unsharpness and image contrast. Increasing the amount of unsharpness decreases the brightness between the area of interest and its surrounding background.

terms of the true object size. The source-to-image-receptor distance (SID) and object-to-image-receptor distance (OID) play important roles in minimizing the amount of size distortion of the radiographic image.

Because radiographers produce radiographs of three-dimensional objects, some size distortion always occurs as a result of OID. The parts of the object that are farther away from the image receptor are radiographically represented with greater size distortion than the parts of the object that are closer to the image receptor. Even if the object is in close contact with the image receptor, some part of the object is farther away than other parts of the object. SID also influences the total amount of magnification of the image. As SID increases, size distortion (magnification) decreases; as SID decreases, size distortion (magnification) increases.

IMPORTANT RELATIONSHIP

Size Distortion

Radiographic images of objects are always magnified in terms of the true object size. The SID and OID play important roles in minimizing the amount of size distortion or magnification created.

Shape Distortion

In addition to size distortion, objects that are being imaged can be radiographically misrepresented by distortion of their shape. **Shape distortion** can radiographically appear in two different ways: elongation or foreshortening. **Elongation** refers to images of objects that appear longer than the true objects. **Foreshortening** refers to images that appear shorter than the true objects. Examples of elongation and foreshortening can be seen in Figure 3-24.

Shape distortion can arise from inaccurate central ray (CR) alignment of the tube, the part being radiographed, or the image receptor. Any misalignment of the CR among these three factors—tube, part, or image receptor—alters the shape of the part recorded in the image.

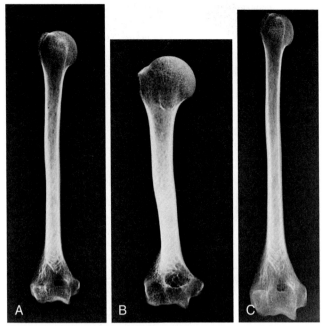

FIGURE 3-24 **A**, No distortion. **B**, Foreshortened. **C**, Elongated.

IMPORTANT RELATIONSHIP

Shape Distortion

Shape distortion can occur from inaccurate central ray (CR) alignment of the tube, the part being radiographed, or the image receptor. Elongation refers to images of objects that appear longer than the true objects. Foreshortening refers to images that appear shorter than the true objects.

Sometimes, shape distortion is advantageous in particular projections or positions. For example, CR angulation is sometimes required to elongate a part so that a particular anatomic structure can be visualized better. Also, rotating the part (and therefore creating shape distortion) is sometimes required to eliminate superimposition of objects that normally obstruct visualization of the area of interest. In general, shape distortion is not a necessary or desirable characteristic of radiographs.

The factors that determine the amount of image distortion are equally important for digital and film-screen imaging. Both SID and OID determine the amount of magnification of the anatomic structures on the image. In addition, improper alignment of the CR, anatomic part, image receptor, or a combination of these components distorts the shape of the image whether obtained with a digital or film-screen image receptor.

Scatter

Scatter radiation, as previously described, can add unwanted exposure to the radiographic image as a result of Compton interactions. Unwanted exposure or fog on the image does not provide information about the anatomic area of interest. Scatter degrades or decreases the visibility of the anatomic structures. The scatter or unwanted exposure recorded on the image has the effect of decreasing the contrast by masking the desired brightness of the image and changing the degree of difference (Figure 3-25).

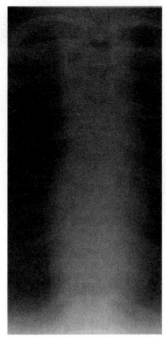

FIGURE 3-25 Scatter and fog.

Fog produced as a result of scatter reaching the image receptor can be visualized on both a digital and a film image. Even though the computer can change the contrast or gray levels displayed in a digital image, scatter radiation reaching the image receptor does not provide any information about the area of interest. Because digital image receptors can detect low levels of radiation intensity, they are more sensitive to scatter radiation than film.

Quantum Noise

Image noise contributes no useful diagnostic information and serves only to detract from the quality of an image. **Quantum noise** is a concern in digital imaging and is photon dependent. Quantum noise is visible as brightness or density fluctuations in the image. *Quantum mottle* is the term typically used when referring to noise on a film image. The fewer the photons reaching the image receptor to form the image, the greater the visibility of quantum noise on the digital image.

 IMPORTANT RELATIONSHIP
Number of Photons and Quantum Noise

Decreasing the number of photons reaching the image receptor may increase the amount of quantum noise within the radiographic image; increasing the number of photons reaching the image receptor may decrease the amount of quantum noise within the radiographic image.

Although quantum noise can be a problem for both digital and film-screen imaging, it is more likely to occur in digital imaging. As previously mentioned, the digital computer system can adjust for low or high x-ray exposures during image acquisition. When the x-ray exposure

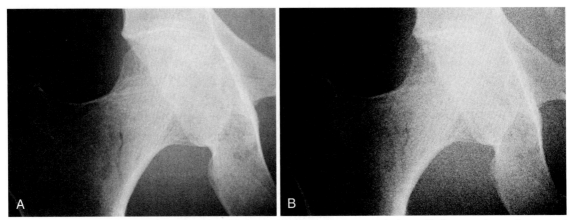

FIGURE 3-26 A, Image created using an appropriate x-ray exposure technique. **B,** Image shows increased quantum noise as a result of insufficient x-ray exposure to the image receptor.

to the image receptor is too low (i.e., when there is a decreased number of photons), computer processing alters the appearance of the digital image to make the brightness acceptable, but the image displays increased quantum noise (Figure 3-26). Certain postprocessing options may render quantum noise more or less noticeable.

The exposure technique should be selected on the basis of the requirements of the type of radiographic procedure being performed. A factor that differentiates digital from film-screen imaging is the ability of the computer to adjust the brightness of the image after exposure technique errors. Although the computer can adjust for both low- and high-exposure technique errors, the radiographer is still responsible for selecting exposure techniques that produce acceptable image quality while ensuring that the patient exposure remains *as low as reasonably achievable* (ALARA). In particular, exposures that are too low adversely affect the quantum noise of an image even though the computer can adjust the brightness. Exposures that are too high result in excessive radiation exposure to the patient. It is recommended that radiographers continue to select exposure techniques that produce diagnostic-quality radiographic images, regardless of whether the imaging system is digital or film-screen.

Image Artifacts

An **artifact** is any unwanted image on a radiograph. Artifacts are detrimental to radiographs because they can impede visibility of anatomy, pathologic conditions, or patient-identification information. They decrease the overall quality of the radiographic image.

Errors such as double-exposing an image receptor or the improper use of equipment can result in image artifacts and must be avoided. Foreign bodies are a class of artifacts imaged within a patient's body. Variation in exposure techniques may be necessary when imaging for a suspected foreign body.

Although the causes of some artifacts are the same regardless of the type of imaging system, others are specific to digital or film-screen imaging. Artifacts from patient clothing and items imaged that are not a part of the area of interest are the same for both film and digital systems. The radiographer must be diligent in removing clothing or items that could obstruct visibility of the anatomic area of interest (Figure 3-27). Scatter radiation or fog and image noise have also been classified as radiographic artifacts because they add unwanted information to the image.

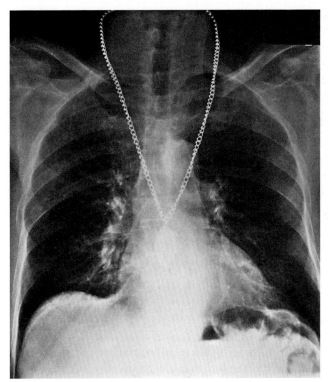

FIGURE 3-27 Image artifact.

   Digital image artifacts can be a result of errors during extraction of the latent image from the image receptor, inadequate CR imaging plate erasure, or performance of the electronic detectors. Artifacts specific to film-screen imaging are typically a result of film storage, handling, and chemical processing.

Digital versus Film-Screen Imaging

Although film-screen imaging served as a good medium for radiographic imaging for many decades, it has many limitations that can be overcome with digital imaging. One major deficiency is the limited **dynamic range** (the range of exposure intensities an image receptor can accurately detect). This limitation renders a film-screen radiograph very sensitive to underexposure or overexposure, which may necessitate image retakes. A limited dynamic range also restricts the visibility of structures that differ greatly in x-ray attenuation. An example is the difficulty of optimally visualizing both soft tissue and bony structures within a given film image.

 IMPORTANT RELATIONSHIP
Dynamic Range and Film-Screen Imaging

The range of exposure intensities that film can accurately detect is limited (limited dynamic range). This renders film more susceptible to overexposure and underexposure and restricts its ability to display tissues that vary greatly in x-ray attenuation.

Other drawbacks of film-screen imaging involve the cost of film itself, the necessity of developing the latent image into a manifest image via chemical processing and potential artifacts related to film handling and chemical processing. The time required to process the film before viewing the radiograph can delay the progress of an examination or diagnosis. Automatic film processors incur considerable equipment and maintenance costs and demand frequent quality-control procedures.

Another restriction associated with a film image is that once the film has been processed, the image is permanent, and further adjustments cannot be made. There is no option to alter the density or contrast of the manifest image. Therefore, the anatomic area that is to be optimally imaged must be selected at the time of exposure. For example, when an image is taken in the thoracic region, the exposure technique must be selected depending on whether the area of interest is the lungs or the ribs. A related issue is the limited contrast resolution, which is the ability to distinguish tissues of similar subject contrast, of film-screen receptors. Even if technique factors are chosen to optimize soft tissue contrast, the differential absorption among various soft tissues is slight and not well differentiated using film-screen imaging.

In addition, film images cannot be electronically stored or duplicated, displayed on computer monitors, or transmitted over computer networks. Traditional film archives consume significant space and are frequently prone to loss of films. In addition, personnel costs associated with maintaining the archive and the expense of storing radiographs and then retrieving them when needed for comparison is prohibitive. Film-screen imaging will be discussed more thoroughly in Chapter 5.

Digital imaging overcomes many limitations of film-screen radiography. Digital radiographic images can be quickly acquired and displayed and can be efficiently transmitted, processed, interpreted on a display monitor, stored, and retrieved via electronic means. Digital image acquisition, processing, and display are discussed more thoroughly in Chapter 4.

CHAPTER SUMMARY

- A radiographic image is a result of the differential absorption of the primary x-rays that interact with tissues of varying composition within the anatomic area of interest.
- Beam attenuation occurs when the primary x-ray beam loses energy as it interacts with anatomic tissues.
- X-rays have the ability to eject electrons (ionization) from atoms within anatomic tissue.
- Three primary processes occur during x-ray interaction with anatomic tissues: absorption, transmission, and scattering.
- Total absorption of the incoming x-ray photon is a result of the photoelectric effect.
- Scattering of the incoming x-ray photon is a result of the Compton effect.
- Scatter radiation reaching the image receptor provides no useful information and creates unwanted exposure or fog on the radiograph.
- The process of differential absorption remains the same for image formation regardless of the type of image receptor.
- A radiographic image is composed of varying brightness levels that structurally represent the anatomic area of interest.
- The visibility and accuracy of the recorded anatomic structural lines determine the overall quality of the radiographic image.
- Visibility of the recorded details is achieved by the proper balance of image brightness and contrast.
- Image contrast provides the ability to distinguish among the types of irradiated tissues.
- Gray scale is the number of different shades of gray that can be stored and displayed in a digital image.

- Spatial resolution refers to the accuracy of the recorded anatomic structural lines.
- Distortion describes the amount of magnification or misrepresentation in shape of the anatomic structures.
- Scatter radiation produces unwanted exposure on the image, known as fog.
- Quantum noise is a result of too few photons reaching the image receptor and is more of a concern in digital imaging.
- An artifact is any unwanted image on a radiograph.
- Digital image receptors have a wider dynamic range compared with film-screen image receptors.

REVIEW QUESTIONS

1. The process whereby a radiographic image is created by variations in absorption and transmission of the exiting x-ray beam is known as _____.
   A. attenuation
   B. the photoelectric effect
   C. the Compton effect
   D. differential absorption
2. Which of the following processes occur during the x-ray beam interaction with tissue?
   (1) Absorption
   (2) Photon transmission
   (3) Scattering
   A. 1 and 2 only
   B. 1 and 3 only
   C. 2 and 3 only
   D. 1, 2, and 3
3. The ability of an x-ray photon to remove an atom's electron is a characteristic known as

   _____.
   A. attenuation
   B. scattering
   C. ionization
   D. absorption
4. The x-ray interaction responsible for absorption is _____.
   A. differential
   B. photoelectric
   C. attenuation
   D. Compton
5. The x-ray interaction responsible for scattering is _____.
   A. differential
   B. photoelectric
   C. attenuation
   D. Compton
6. Remnant radiation is composed of which of the following?
   (1) Transmitted radiation
   (2) Absorbed radiation
   (3) Scattered radiation
   A. 1 and 2 only
   B. 1 and 3 only
   C. 2 and 3 only
   D. 1, 2, and 3

7. What interaction causes unwanted exposure to the image, known as fog?
   A. Compton
   B. Transmitted
   C. Photoelectric
   D. Absorption

8. Which of the following factors would affect beam attenuation?
   (1) Tissue atomic number
   (2) Beam quality
   (3) Fog
   A. 1 and 2 only
   B. 1 and 3 only
   C. 2 and 3 only
   D. 1, 2, and 3

9. The high brightness areas on a radiographic image are created by _____.
   A. transmitted radiation
   B. scattered radiation
   C. absorbed radiation
   D. primary radiation

10. An anatomic part that transmits the incoming x-ray photon would create an area of _____ on the radiographic image.
    A. fog
    B. high brightness
    C. low brightness
    D. noise

11. The process of creating a radiographic image by differential absorption varies for film-screen and digital imaging.
    A. True
    B. False

12. Which attribute(s) of a radiographic image affect(s) the *visibility* of sharpness?
    A. Distortion
    B. Contrast
    C. Brightness
    D. B and C

13. A radiographic image with many shades of gray but few differences among them is said to have _____.
    A. high contrast
    B. low contrast
    C. short-scale contrast
    D. excessive noise

14. Which of the following is defined as the range of exposure intensities that an image receptor can accurately detect?
    A. Long-scale contrast
    B. Spatial resolution
    C. Quantum noise
    D. Dynamic range

Digital Imaging

CHAPTER OUTLINE

Digital Image Characteristics
  Spatial Frequency and Spatial
    Resolution
  Modulation Transfer Func-
    tion (MTF)
Digital Image Receptors
  Computed Radiography
  Direct Radiography

Dynamic Range
Detective Quantum Efficiency
Signal-to-Noise Ratio
Contrast-to-Noise Ratio
Digital Image Processing
  Histogram Analysis
  Lookup Tables
Digital Imaging Artifacts

Image Display
  Display Monitors
  Laser Printers
Digital Communication
  Networks

OBJECTIVES

After completing this chapter, the reader will be able to perform the following:

1. Define all the key terms in this chapter.
2. State all the important relationships in this chapter.
3. Compare and contrast the attributes of a digital image.
4. Explain the digital characteristics of matrix and pixels.
5. Recognize the relationship among pixel size, field of view (FOV), and matrix size.
6. State the relationship between spatial frequency and spatial resolution.
7. Differentiate between computed radiography (CR) and direct radiography (DR) IRs.
8. Explain the relationship between sampling frequency and spatial resolution.
9. Describe how the size of a CR imaging plate can affect spatial resolution.
10. Recognize the differences between indirect and direct conversion digital IRs.
11. Explain the importance of dynamic range in exposure technique selection and image quality.
12. Define signal-to-noise ratio (SNR) and explain its importance to digital image quality.
13. Define contrast-noise ratio (CNR) and explain its importance to digital image quality.
14. Explain histogram analysis, automatic rescaling, and lookup tables and their role during image pre-processing to create a quality digital image.
15. Differentiate among the vendor-specific types of exposure indicators.
16. Compare and contrast the types of display monitors used for diagnostic interpretation and image viewing.
17. Identify the important features of monitors that may affect the quality of the displayed image.
18. Explain the difference between luminance and luminance ratio.
19. Recognize image display processing functions, including electronic masking, window level and width, subtraction, contrast enhancement, edge enhancement, smoothing, and equalization.
20. Define the acronyms PACS, DICOM, and HL7.

KEY TERMS

ambient lighting
automatic rescaling
bit
bit depth
brightness
byte
contrast resolution
contrast-to-noise ratio
detective quantum efficiency
    (DQE)
deviation index (DI)
digital imaging and com-
    munications in medicine
    (DICOM)

dynamic range
electronic masking
fill factor
flat-panel detectors (FPD)
grayscale
histogram analysis
imaging plate
latent image
lookup tables (LUT)
matrix
modulation transfer function
    (MTF)
photostimulable luminescence
photostimulable phosphor (PSP)

picture archival and communi-
    cation system (PACS)
pixel density
pixel pitch
pixels
sampling frequency
sampling pitch
scintillator
signal-to-noise ratio
spatial frequency
window level
window width

During radiographic imaging, the radiation exiting a patient is composed of a range of intensities that reflect the absorption and transmission characteristics of the anatomic tissues. The image receptor (IR) receives the exit radiation and creates the latent or invisible image. The latent image is differently acquired depending on the type of IR. This chapter describes the digital image characteristics, common types of digital IRs used in radiography, and how the image is formed, processed, and displayed.

DIGITAL IMAGE CHARACTERISTICS

In digital imaging, the **latent image** is stored as digital data and must be processed by a computer for viewing on a display monitor. Digital imaging can be accomplished using a specialized image receptor that can produce a computerized radiographic image. Two types of digital radiographic systems are in common use today: computed radiography (CR) and direct radiography (DR). Regardless of whether the imaging system is CR or DR, the computer can manipulate the radiographic image in various ways after the image has been digitally created.

Digital images are composed of numerical data that can be easily manipulated by a computer. When displayed on a computer monitor, there is tremendous flexibility in terms of altering the **brightness** and contrast of a digital image. The practical advantage of such capability is that regardless of the original exposure technique factors (within reason), any anatomic structure can be independently and well visualized. Computers can also perform various postprocessing image manipulations to further improve the visibility of the anatomic region.

A digital image is recorded as a **matrix** or combination of rows and columns (array) of small, usually square, "picture elements" called **pixels**. The size of a pixel is measured in microns (100 microns = 0.1 mm). Each pixel is recorded as a single numerical value, which is represented as a single brightness level on a display monitor. The location of the pixel within the image matrix corresponds to an area within the patient or volume of tissue (Figure 4-1).

Given the dimensions of an anatomic area, or field of view (FOV), a matrix size of 1024 × 1024 has 1,048,576 individual pixels; a matrix size of 2048 × 2048 has 4,194,304 pixels. Digital image quality is improved with a larger matrix size that includes a greater number of smaller pixels (Figure 4-2 and Box 4-1). Although image quality is improved for a larger matrix size and smaller pixels, computer processing time, network transmission time, and digital storage space increase as the matrix size increases.

1 Pixel

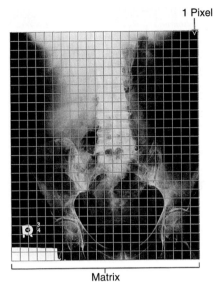

Matrix

FIGURE 4-1 Location of the pixel within the image matrix corresponds to an area within the patient or volume of tissue. *Note:* Pixel size is not to scale and is used for illustration only.

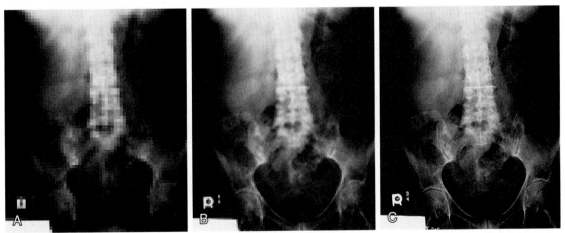

FIGURE 4-2 For a given field of view (FOV), the larger the matrix size, the greater the number of smaller individual pixels. Increasing the number of pixels improves the quality of the image. **A,** Matrix size is 64 × 64. **B,** Matrix size is 215 × 215. **C,** Matrix size is 2048 × 2048.

There is a relationship among pixel size, FOV, and matrix size, as demonstrated in the following formula:

$$\text{Pixel size} = \frac{\text{FOV}}{\text{Matrix size}}.$$

This relationship demonstrates that if the FOV is increased for a fixed matrix size, then the pixel size is also increased (direct relationship). However, if the matrix size is increased for a fixed FOV, then the pixel size is decreased (inverse relationship).

BOX 4-1 **Digital Imaging Terminology**

Matrix—image displayed as a combination of rows and columns (array); a larger matrix size improves spatial resolution

Pixel—smallest component of the matrix; a greater number of smaller pixels improves spatial resolution

Pixel bit depth—number of bits that determines the precision with which the exit radiation is recorded and controls the exact pixel brightness that can be displayed

---

 MATHEMATICAL APPLICATION

Pixel Size and FOV

FOV = 17 in (431.8 mm) and matrix size = 1024

$$\frac{431.8}{1024} = 0.42 \text{ mm pixel size}$$

If the FOV was decreased to 12 in (304.8 mm) for the same matrix size of 1024

$$\frac{304.8}{1024} = 0.30 \text{ mm pixel size}$$

Decreasing the FOV for a given matrix size will decrease the size of the pixels and increase spatial resolution.

 MATHEMATICAL APPLICATION

Pixel Size and Matrix Size

FOV = 17 in (431.8 mm) and matrix size = 1024:

$$\frac{431.8}{1024} = 0.42 \text{ mm pixel size}$$

If the matrix size was increased to 2,048 for the same FOV:

$$\frac{431.8}{2048} = 0.21 \text{ mm pixel size}$$

Increasing the matrix size for a given FOV will decrease the size of the pixels and increase spatial resolution.

 IMPORTANT RELATIONSHIP

Pixel Size, FOV, and Matrix Size

The pixel size is directly related to FOV and inversely related to matrix size. Increasing the FOV for the same matrix size will increase the size of the pixel and decrease spatial resolution, whereas increasing the matrix size for the same FOV will decrease the pixel size and increase spatial resolution.

The numerical value assigned to each pixel is determined by the relative attenuation of x-rays passing through the corresponding volume of tissue. Pixels representing highly attenuating tissues (increased absorption) such as bone are usually assigned a low value for higher brightness than pixels representing tissues of low x-ray attenuation (decreased absorption) (Figure 4-3). Each pixel also has a **bit depth,** or number of bits (Box 4-2), that determines the amount of precision in digitizing the analog signal and therefore the number of shades of gray that can be displayed in the image. Bit depth is determined by an analog-to-digital converter, which is an integral component of every digital imaging system. Because the binary system is used, bit depth is expressed as 2 to the power of n, or the number of bits (2^n). A larger bit depth allows a greater number of shades of gray to be displayed on a computer monitor. For example, a 12 bit depth (2^{12}) can display 4096 shades of gray, a 14 bit depth can display 16,384 shades of gray, and a 16 bit depth can display 65,536 shades of gray. A system that can digitize and display a greater number of shades of gray has better contrast resolution. An image with increased contrast resolution increases the visibility of anatomic details and the ability to distinguish among small anatomic areas of interest.

IMPORTANT RELATIONSHIP

Pixel Bit Depth and Contrast Resolution

The greater the pixel bit depth (i.e., 16 bit), the more precise the digitization of the analog signal, and the greater the number of shades of gray available for image display. Increasing the number of shades of gray available to display on a digital image improves its contrast resolution.

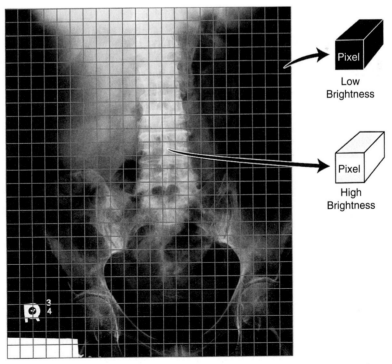

Pixel

Low Brightness

Pixel

High Brightness

FIGURE 4-3 Each pixel value represents a volume of tissue imaged.

> ### BOX 4-2   Binary Digits
>
> Computers operate and communicate through the binary number system, which uses combinations of zeros and ones to process and store information. A digital transistor can be operated in two states: off (0) or on (1). Each 0 and 1 is called a **bit** and refers to the computer's basic unit of information. When 8 bits are combined, they form a **byte**, and 2 bytes form a word.
>
> Binary digits are used to display the brightness level (grayscale) of a digital image. The greater the number of bits, the greater the number of shades of gray that can be displayed, and the quality of the image is improved.

Pixel size

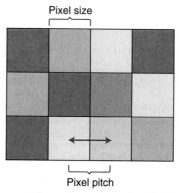

Pixel pitch

FIGURE 4-4 The distance measured from the center of a pixel to an adjacent pixel determines the pixel pitch or spacing.

A digital image is composed of discrete information in the form of pixels that display various shades of gray. As previously mentioned, the greater the number of pixels in an image matrix, the smaller their size. An image consisting of a greater number of pixels per unit area, or **pixel density**, provides improved spatial resolution. In addition to its size, the pixel spacing or distance measured from the center of a pixel to an adjacent pixel determines the **pixel pitch** (Figure 4-4). Smaller-sized pixels will have decreased pixel pitch and improved spatial resolution.

 IMPORTANT RELATIONSHIP

Pixel Density and Pitch and Spatial Resolution

Increasing the pixel density and decreasing the pixel pitch increases spatial resolution. Decreasing pixel density and increasing pixel pitch decreases spatial resolution.

Spatial Frequency and Spatial Resolution

Spatial resolution in digital imaging is primarily limited to the size of the pixel; however, when measuring an imaging system's ability to resolve small objects, it is important to understand the concept of spatial frequency and its relationship with spatial resolution. Anatomic details are composed of large and small objects and radiographic images display those details as variations from white-to-black brightness levels. Small objects have higher spatial frequency and large objects have lower spatial frequency. It is more difficult to accurately image small anatomic objects (high spatial frequency) compared to imaging large ones (low spatial frequency). **Spatial frequency** can be defined by the unit of line pairs per millimeter (lp/mm). A resolution test pattern is a device used to record and measure line pairs (Figure 4-5). An imaging system that can resolve a greater number of line pairs per millimeter (higher spatial frequency) has increased spatial resolution (Figure 4-6). In digital imaging systems, the

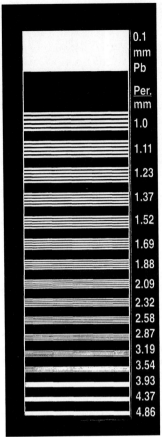

FIGURE 4-5 A resolution test pattern will record and measure line pairs per millimeter.

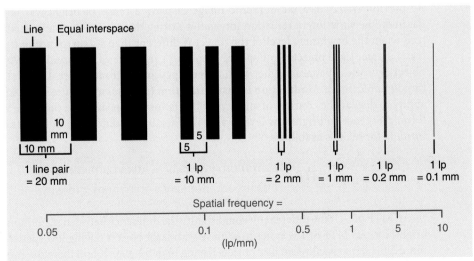

FIGURE 4-6 A line pair is a high-contrast line separated by an interspace of equal width. The spatial frequency is shown for each of the line pairs.

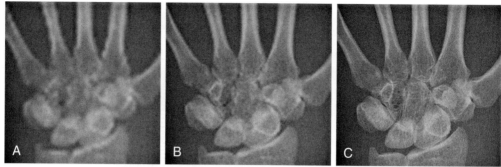

FIGURE 4-7 Images showing how pixel size affects spatial resolution. **A,** Image with 20 pixels per centimeter (cm) and therefore the pixel size is larger and the spatial resolution is poor. **B,** Image with 40 pixels per cm. **C,** Image with 100 pixels per cm and therefore the pixel size is smaller than that in images A and B and the spatial resolution is improved.

ability to resolve or demonstrate a specific spatial frequency is directly impacted by the size of the pixel. The images of the wrist (Figure 4-7) demonstrate the impact that pixel size has on the spatial resolution visualized in an image.

 IMPORTANT RELATIONSHIP

Spatial Frequency and Spatial Resolution

The unit of measure for spatial frequency is line pairs per millimeter (lp/mm). Increasing the number of line pairs per millimeter resolved in the imaging system (higher spatial frequency) results in improved spatial resolution.

Modulation Transfer Function (MTF)

As previously stated, a radiographic image displays a range of brightness levels (grayscale) based on the variation in radiation intensities exiting the tissue. Anatomic detail is best visualized when the brightness level of the object is different than its surrounding tissue (high contrast). Larger sized objects (low spatial frequency) are more easily visualized. As the size of the object decreases, it attains higher spatial frequency and becomes more difficult to visualize in a radiographic image. **Modulation transfer function (MTF)** is a measure of the imaging system's ability to display the contrast of anatomic objects varying in size, and the value will be between 0 (no difference in brightness levels) and 1.0 (maximum difference in brightness levels). The formula for MTF is as follows:

$$\text{MTF} = \frac{(\text{maximum intensity} - \text{minimum intensity})}{(\text{maximum intensity} + \text{minimum intensity})}$$

An MTF of 1 (100% difference) would signify the difference between maximum and minimum brightness. An MTF of 1 is easier to achieve with large objects having low spatial frequency. It is more difficult to visualize smaller objects having high frequency, and therefore most digital imaging systems' MTFs would measure much lower than 1.0.

> ### ◢ IMPORTANT RELATIONSHIP
> #### *Modulation Transfer Function (MTF) and Anatomic Detail*
>
> MTF is a measure of the imaging system's ability to accurately display small anatomic objects having high spatial frequency. An imaging system that has a high MTF can display anatomic detail with improved visibility.

Different types of digital image receptors use various methods of transforming the continuous exit radiation intensities into the array of discrete pixels for image display. Some digital image receptors use a sampling technique, whereas others have fixed detector elements that are used to capture the exit radiation intensities. Regardless of the type used, a major determinant of the spatial resolution of digital images is the pixel size and spacing.

The device used for digital image display also affects the ability to view anatomic details. High-resolution (2048 × 2560) monitors are required to maximize the amount of spatial resolution viewed in digital images.

DIGITAL IMAGE RECEPTORS

Two types of digital IRs are typically used in radiography: computed radiography (CR) and direct radiography (DR). These IRs differ in their construction and how they acquire latent images. Once the latent image is acquired and the raw data are digitized, image processing and display are essentially the same, regardless of the type of IR.

Computed Radiography

CR IRs can be portable or fixed in a table or upright x-ray unit. The CR IR includes a **cassette** that houses the **imaging plate** (IP) (Figure 4-8). The radiation exiting the patient interacts with the IP, where the photon intensities are absorbed by the phosphor. Although some of the absorbed energy is released as visible light (luminescence), a sufficient amount of energy is stored in the phosphor to produce a latent image. **Luminescence** is the emission of light when stimulated by radiation.

The IP primarily consists of support, phosphor, and protective layers (Figure 4-9). The phosphor layer is composed of barium fluorohalide crystals doped with europium, referred to as the **photostimulable phosphor (PSP).** This type of phosphor emits visible light when stimulated by a high-intensity laser beam, a phenomenon termed **photostimulable luminescence**.

CR imaging requires a two-step process for image acquisition: image capture in the IP and image readout. The latent image is formed in the PSP when the exit x-ray intensities are absorbed

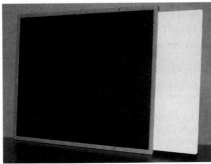

FIGURE 4-8 Typical CR cassette showing the imaging plate housed within.

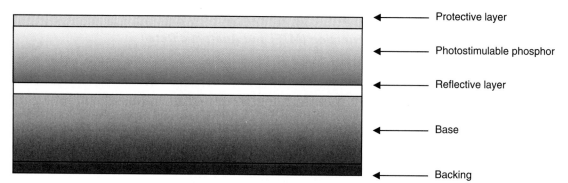

FIGURE 4-9 Cross-section of a CR imaging plate.

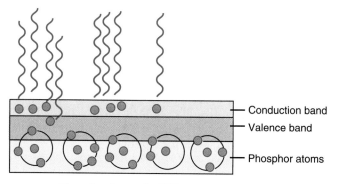

**Phosphor layer of a PSP
plate during exposure**

FIGURE 4-10 During exposure of the PSP phosphor layer, the higher-energy electrons will become trapped in the conduction band. A percentage of the higher-energy electrons will return to their normal state and release the excess energy as visible light.

by the phosphor and the europium atoms become ionized by the photoelectric effect. The absorbed energy excites the electrons, elevating them to a higher energy state where they become stored or trapped in the conduction band (Figure 4-10). The conduction band is an energy level just beyond the valence band (outermost energy band of an atom). The number and distribution of these trapped electrons are proportional to the tissue's differential x-ray absorption and form the latent image. Some of these excited electrons immediately return to their normal state and the excess energy is released as visible light. A percentage of electrons remain in this higher-energy state until released during laser beam scanning of the readout stage. The acquired image data (released energy) are extracted from the digital receptor, converted to digital data, and computer processed for image display. Exposed IPs should be processed within a relatively short amount of time (within 1 h) because the latent image dissipates over time.

> ### IMPORTANT RELATIONSHIP
> #### Computed Radiography Digital Image Receptors
>
> The CR latent image is acquired in the PSP layer of the IP. Most energy from the exit radiation intensities is stored in the PSP for extraction in the reader unit.

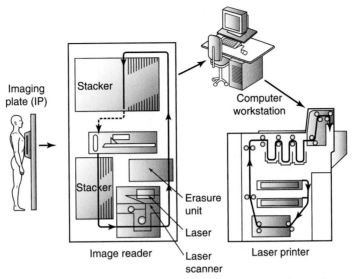

FIGURE 4-11 The exposed CR imaging plate is placed in a reader unit to release the stored image, convert the analog image to digital, and send the data to a computer monitor, laser printer for a hard copy, or both. The reader unit also erases the exposed imaging plate in preparation for the next exposure.

The exposed IP is placed in or sent to a reader unit that converts the analog data into digital data for computer processing (Figure 4-11). Reader units are available in single- or multi-plate configurations. The major components of a typical reader unit are a drive mechanism to move the IP through the scanning process; an optical system, which includes the laser, beam-shaping optics, collecting optics, and optical filters; a photodetector, such as a photomultiplier tube (PMT); and an analog-to-digital converter (ADC). Manufacturers differ in the CR reader mechanics. Some devices move the IP and some move the optical components. There are three important stages in digitizing the CR latent image: scanning, sampling, and quantization.

The purpose of scanning is to convert the latent image into an electrical signal (voltage) that can be subsequently digitized and displayed as a manifest digital image. Once in the reader unit, the IP is removed from the cassette and scanned with a helium–neon laser beam or a solid-state laser diode to release the stored energy as visible light (Figure 4-12). Absorption of the laser beam energy releases the trapped electrons, and they return to a lower energy state. During this process, the excess energy is emitted as visible light (photostimulable luminescence). The scanning of the plate results in a continuous pattern of light intensities being sent to the PMT or photodetector, whose output is directed to the ADC for sampling and quantization.

A PMT collects, amplifies, and converts the visible light to an electrical signal proportional to the range of energies stored in the IP. The signal output from the PMT is digitized by an ADC in order to produce a digital image. To digitize the analog signal from the PMT, it must first be sampled. An important performance characteristic of an ADC is the **sampling frequency**, which determines how often the analog signal is reproduced in its discrete digitized form. Increasing the sampling frequency of the analog signal increases the pixel density of the digital data and improves the spatial resolution of the digital image (Figure 4-13). The closer the samples are to each other (increased sampling frequency), the smaller the **sampling pitch**, or distance between the sampling points (Figure 4-14). Increasing the sampling frequency decreases the sampling pitch and results in smaller-sized pixels. The distance between the midpoint of one pixel to the midpoint of an adjacent

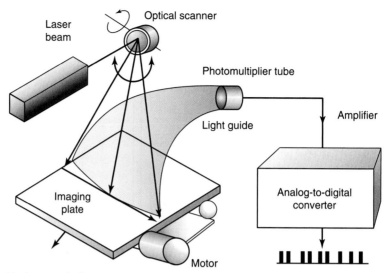

FIGURE 4-12 A neon–helium laser beam scans the exposed CR imaging plate to release the stored energy as visible light. The photomultiplier tube collects, amplifies, and converts the light to an electrical signal. The analog-to-digital converter converts the analog data to digital data.

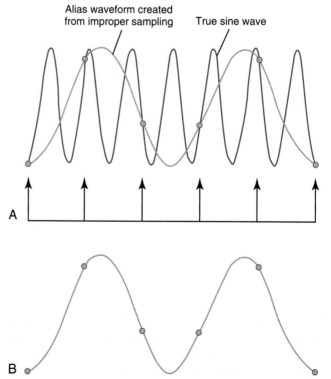

FIGURE 4-13 CR sampling and its effect on the digital data. **A** represents the sampling points of the analog waveform. **B** shows the improper digital waveform that results from low sampling frequency.

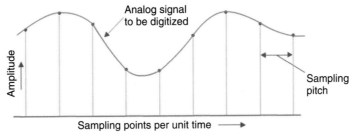

FIGURE 4-14 Sampling and pixel pitch. The sampling frequency determines the distance between the midpoint of one pixel and the midpoint of an adjacent pixel.

pixel describes the **pixel pitch**. Spatial resolution is improved with an increased number of smaller pixels resulting in a more faithful digital representation of the acquired analog image.

 IMPORTANT RELATIONSHIP

Sampling Frequency and Spatial Resolution

Increasing the sampling frequency results in a smaller sampling and pixel pitch, which improves the spatial resolution of the digital image. Decreasing the sampling frequency results in a larger sampling and pixel pitch and decreased spatial resolution.

Manufacturers of CR equipment vary in the method of sampling IPs of different sizes. Some manufacturers fix the sampling frequency to maintain a fixed spatial resolution, whereas others vary the sampling frequency to maintain a fixed matrix size. If the spatial resolution is fixed, the image matrix size is simply proportional to the IP size. A larger IP has a larger matrix to maintain spatial resolution (Figure 4-15). If the matrix size is fixed, changing the size of the IP would affect the spatial resolution of the digital image. For example, under a fixed matrix size system, changing from a 14 × 17 in (35 × 43 cm) IP size to a 10 × 12 in (25 × 30 cm) one would result in improved spatial resolution for the same field of view (FOV) (Figure 4-16). Spatial resolution is improved because in order to maintain the same matrix size and number of pixels, the pixels must be smaller in size. It is recommended to use the smallest IP size reasonable for the anatomic area of interest.

 IMPORTANT RELATIONSHIP

Imaging Plate Size and Matrix Size

For a fixed matrix size CR system, using a smaller IP for a given field of view (FOV) results in improved spatial resolution of the digital image. Increasing the size of the IP for a given FOV results in decreased spatial resolution.

Another important ADC performance characteristic is degree of quantization or pixel bit depth, which controls the number of gray shades or contrast resolution of the image. During the process of quantization, each pixel, representing a brightness value, is assigned a numerical value. Quantization reflects the precision with which each sampled point is recorded. As previously discussed, the pixel size and pitch determine the spatial resolution and the pixel bit depth determines the system's ability to display a range of shades of gray to represent anatomic tissues. Pixel bit depth is fixed by the choice of ADC, and CR systems manufactured with a greater pixel

FIXED SAMPLING FREQUENCY

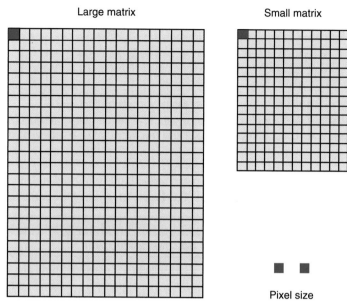

FIGURE 4-15 Fixed sampling frequency. A fixed sampling frequency will maintain a fixed spatial resolution. A larger IP size will have a larger matrix to maintain the same pixel size. *Note*: Pixel size is not to scale and is used for illustration only.

FIXED MATRIX SIZE

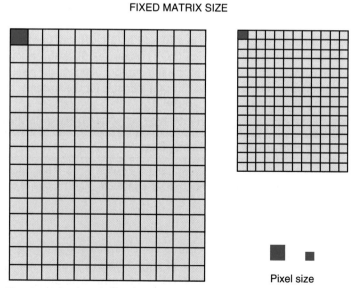

FIGURE 4-16 Fixed matrix size. A fixed matrix size will vary the sampling frequency for a different IP size. A larger IP size will result in a larger pixel size and decreased spatial resolution. *Note*: Pixel size is not to scale and is used for illustration only.

bit depth (i.e., 16-bit [where 2^{16} bits can display 65,536 shades of gray]) improve the contrast resolution of the digital image.

Before the IP is returned to service, the plate is exposed to an intense white light to release any residual energy that could affect future exposures. PSPs can be reused and are estimated to have a life of 10,000 readings before requiring replacement. Advancements in PSP material, laser beam technology, and dual-sided IP scanning will continue to improve the process of CR image acquisition.

Direct Radiography

DR IRs have a self-scanning readout mechanism that employs an array of x-ray detectors that receive the exit radiation and convert the varying x-ray intensities into proportional electronic signals for digitization. In contrast to CR, which requires a two-step image acquisition process and results in a longer delay between image capture and image readout, DR imaging combines the two processes. As a result, DR images are available almost instantly after exposure. However, DR receptors are more fragile and much more expensive than CR IRs. Several types of electronic detectors are available for DR.

Flat-Panel Detectors

Flat-panel detectors are solid-state IRs employing a large-area active matrix array of electronic components ranging in size from 43 × 35 cm to 43 × 43 cm (17 × 14 in to 17 × 17 in). Flat-panel detectors are constructed with layers in order to receive x-ray photons and convert them to electrical charges for storage and readout (Figure 4-17). Signal storage, signal readout, and digitizing electronics are integrated into the flat-panel device. The first layer is composed of an x-ray converter, the second layer houses the thin-film transistor (TFT) array, and the third layer is a glass substrate. The TFT array is divided into square detector elements (DEL), each having a capacitor to store electrical charges and a switching transistor for readout. Electrical charges are separately read out from each detector element. The electronic signal is then sent to the ADC for digitization.

The DEL has an x-ray-sensitive area representing each pixel in the image matrix. The pixel is therefore smaller than the DEL and can only capture a percentage of the x-rays reaching the

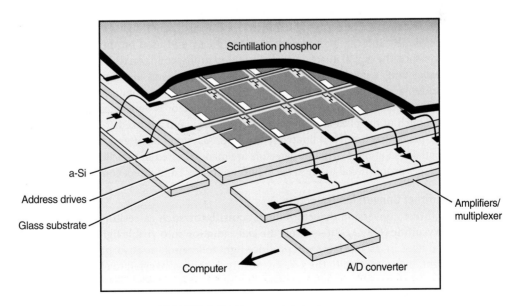

FIGURE 4-17 Flat-panel-detector array.

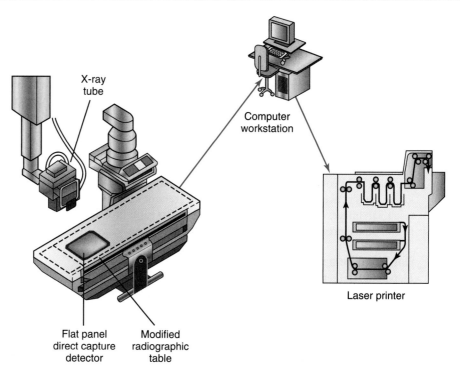

FIGURE 4-18 Flat-panel digital detector fixed in a modified x-ray table.

detector. This percentage of x-ray capture (~80%) is known as the **fill factor**. Although flat-panel detectors with smaller DELs have smaller pixel sizes and therefore improved spatial resolution, the fill factor is decreased and becomes a limitation. Efforts to further decrease the DEL for improved spatial resolution would require more radiation exposure to reach the IR to create the digital image.

The detector system is usually dedicated to a single room and can be permanently mounted within the table or an upright Bucky system. Flat-panel digital detectors are also available as mobile IRs and can be removed from the Bucky and used on the tabletop or a stretcher. After exposure, the digital image is available within milliseconds on a viewing monitor, and no separate reader unit is involved (Figure 4-18). Flat-panel systems are highly dose efficient and provide quicker access to images compared with CR. The spatial resolution of flat-panel receptors is generally superior to that of CR. Because a pixel detector is built into the DR flat-panel IR, the size and pitch of the pixel are determined by the DEL and are fixed. Therefore, spatial resolution for flat-panel-detector IRs is limited to the DEL. A system that uses a smaller DEL size has improved spatial resolution. Flat-panel detectors are manufactured in two different ways to create electrical charges proportional to the x-ray exposure: indirect and direct conversion methods.

Indirect Conversion Detectors

Indirect conversion detectors use a **scintillator** such as cesium iodide (CsI) or gadolinium oxysulfide (Gd_2O_2S) to convert the exit radiation into visible light. This phosphor-type material used in a scintillator will produce light following the absorption of the x-rays. The visible light, in proportion to the x-ray exposure, is then converted to electrical charges by photodetectors (layer of amorphous silicon in the TFT array). The electrical charges are temporarily stored by capacitors in the TFT array before being digitized and processed in the computer (Figure 4-19).

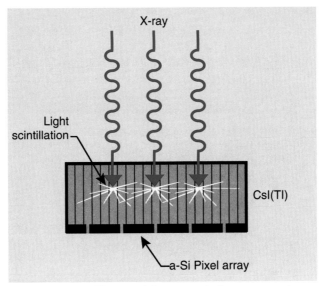

FIGURE 4-19 Flat-panel detector—indirect conversion.

The design of the scintillator used to convert the x-ray intensities into visible light can be structured or unstructured. Structured scintillator phosphors (in the form of needles or columns), usually crystalline CsI, reduce the spread of visible light, thus yielding images with higher spatial resolution than that of images obtained from unstructured scintillators. *Indirect conversion detectors* are so named because they involve a two-stage process of converting x-ray intensities first to visible light and then to electrical charges during image acquisition. The electrical signals are then directed to amplifiers and the ADC to produce a raw digital image.

Direct Conversion Detectors

Direct conversion detectors use an amorphous selenium-coated (a-Se) detector to directly convert the exit radiation to electrical charges (Figure 4-20). To compensate for the moderately low atomic number of selenium ($Z = 34$), the thickness of the amorphous selenium is relatively high (approximately 1 mm). An electrical field is applied across the selenium layer to limit the lateral diffusion of electrons as they migrate toward the thin-film transistor array. By this means, excellent spatial resolution is maintained. Similar to indirect conversion detectors, the electronic charge is stored in a TFT array before it is amplified, digitized, and processed in the computer.

Regardless of the type of digital imaging system, the varying electrical signals are sent to the ADC for conversion into digital data. The digitized pixel intensities are patterned in the computer to form the image matrix. The image matrix is a digital composite of the varying x-ray intensities exiting the patient. Each pixel has a brightness level representing the attenuation characteristic of the volume of tissue imaged. Once the varying x-ray intensities are converted to numeric data, the digital image can be electronically processed, manipulated, transported, or stored.

Dynamic Range

The **dynamic range** of a digital imaging system refers to the ability of a detector to accurately capture the range of photon intensities that exit the patient. Compared with film-screen detectors,

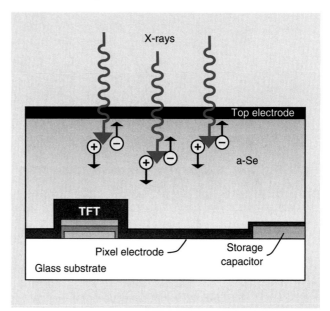

FIGURE 4-20 Flat-panel detector—direct conversion.

digital IRs have a much wider dynamic range (Figure 4-21). In practical terms, this wide dynamic range means that a small degree of underexposure or overexposure would still result in acceptable image quality. This characteristic of digital receptors is advantageous in situations where automatic exposure control (AEC) is not normally available, such as in portable radiography. During ADC, a numerical value (digital data) is assigned to the pixel that represents the attenuation characteristics of that volume of tissue. Processing the digital data yields a radiographic image that can be viewed on a display monitor and altered in various ways. Even if optimal exposure techniques are not used, the image rescaling that occurs during this processing step can produce images with the appropriate brightness levels.

The ability of the IR to capture a wide range of exit photon intensities does not mean a quality image is always created. Although lower-than-necessary x-ray exposures can be detected and processed, image quality suffers because there is insufficient exposure to the IR and quantum noise results. The computer can process the data resulting from an IR exposed to higher-than-necessary radiation and produce a quality image but at the expense of patient overexposure. It is the responsibility of the radiographer to determine the amount of exposure necessary to produce a quality digital image within the *as low as reasonably achievable* (ALARA) principle.

IMPORTANT RELATIONSHIP

Digital Detectors and Dynamic Range

Digital IRs have a wide dynamic range; that is, they can accurately capture a wide range of x-ray intensities exiting the patient. The computer then processes the raw pixel data to compensate for exposure errors and create a radiographic image. However, lower- or higher-than-necessary exposure techniques do not guarantee a quality digital image with reasonable radiation exposure to the patient.

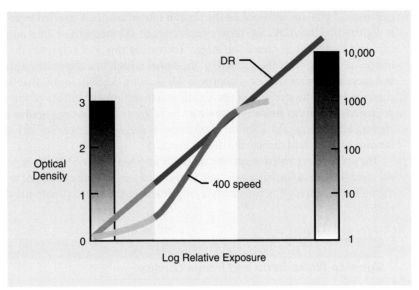

FIGURE 4-21 Digital image receptors have a wider dynamic range compared with radiographic film.

! Radiation Protection Alert

Digital Detectors and Dynamic Range

Because digital image receptors have a wide dynamic range, a quality image can be produced when using more radiation exposure than necessary. Radiographers must take extra precautions to not unnecessarily overexpose patients.

Detective Quantum Efficiency

Detective quantum efficiency (DQE) is a measurement of the efficiency of an image receptor in converting the x-ray exposure it receives to a quality radiographic image. If an image receptor system is able to convert x-ray exposure into a quality image with 100% efficiency (meaning no information loss), the DQE would measure 100% or 1.0. However, no imaging system has 100% conversion efficiency. Nevertheless, the higher the DQE of a system, the lower the radiation exposure required to produce a quality image, thereby decreasing patient exposure. The system's DQE value is impacted by both the type of material used in the image receptor to capture the exit radiation and the energy of the x-ray. For example, the DQE is higher for DR when compared to CR.

IMPORTANT RELATIONSHIP

Detective Quantum Efficiency (DQE) and X-ray Exposure

An image receptor with a higher DQE requires less x-ray exposure to produce a quality radiographic image when compared to an image receptor with a lower DQE value.

Signal-to-Noise Ratio

Signal-to-noise ratio (SNR) is a method of describing the strength of the radiation exposure compared with the amount of noise apparent in a digital image. Image noise is a concern with any electronic digital image. Because the photon intensities are converted to an electronic signal that is digitized by the ADC, the term *signal* refers to the strength or amount of radiation exposure captured by the IR to create the image. Increasing the SNR improves the quality of the digital image; this means that the strength of the signal is high in comparison with the amount of noise, and therefore, image quality is improved. Decreasing the SNR means that there is increased noise compared with the strength of the signal, and therefore, the quality of the radiographic image is degraded. **Quantum noise** results when there are too few x-ray photons captured by the IR to create a latent image. In addition to quantum noise, sources of noise include the electronics that capture, process, and display the digital image.

The ability to visualize anatomic tissues is affected by the SNR. Noise interferes with the signal strength just as background static would interfere with the clarity of music heard. When the digital image displays increased noise, regardless of the source, anatomic details have decreased visibility.

 IMPORTANT RELATIONSHIP

Signal-to-Noise Ratio and Image Quality

Increasing the SNR increases the visibility of anatomic details, whereas decreasing the SNR decreases the visibility.

Contrast-to-Noise Ratio

Contrast-to-noise ratio (CNR) is a method of describing the contrast resolution compared with the amount of noise apparent in a digital image. Just as increased noise affects the SNR and visibility of the anatomic details, it also impacts the contrast displayed within the digital image. Brightness differences in the digital image are a result of varying exit-radiation intensities from the attenuation of the x-ray beam in anatomic tissue (differential absorption). As previously stated, digital imaging systems have higher contrast resolution than film-screen images. A system with higher contrast resolution means that anatomic tissues that attenuate the x-ray beam similarly (low subject contrast) can be better visualized. However, if the image has increased noise, the low subject contrast tissues will not be as well visualized. Digital images with a higher CNR will increase the visibility of anatomic tissues (see Figure 4-22).

 IMPORTANT RELATIONSHIP

Contrast-to-Noise Ratio and Image Quality

Increasing the CNR increases the visibility of anatomic details, whereas decreasing the CNR decreases the visibility.

DIGITAL IMAGE PROCESSING

After the raw image data are extracted from the digital receptor and converted to digital data, the image must be computer processed before its display and diagnostic interpretation. The term *digital image processing* refers to various computer manipulations applied to digital images for the purpose of optimizing their appearance. Although several possible digital image processing operations are outside the scope of this textbook, several highly important and commonly used processing steps are described.

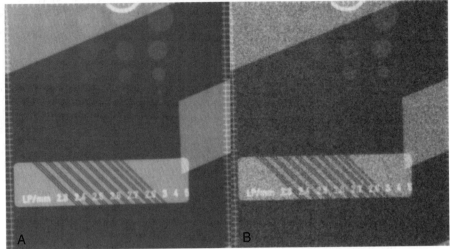

FIGURE 4-22 Contrast-to-noise ratio. **A,** Image of a contrast detail phantom showing an increased contrast-to-noise ratio. Phantom objects are more visible. **B,** Image of contrast detail phantom showing a decreased contrast-to-noise ratio. Phantom objects are less visible.

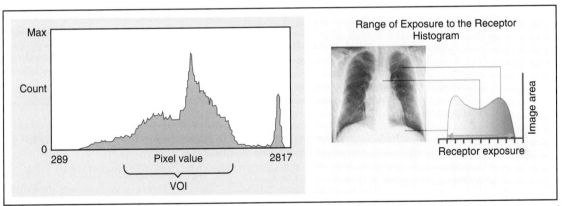

FIGURE 4-23 The histogram represents the number of digital pixel values versus the relative prevalence of those values in the latent image. The *x*-axis represents the amount of exposure and the *y*-axis the incidence of pixels for each exposure level. Each image has its own histogram.

Histogram Analysis

Histogram analysis is an image-processing technique commonly used to identify the edges of an image and assess the raw data prior to image display. In this method, the computer first creates a histogram (or graphic representation of a data set) of the image (Figure 4-23). A data set includes all the pixel values that represent the image before edge detection and rescaling. This graph represents the number of digital pixel values versus the relative prevalence of the pixel values in the image. The *x*-axis represents the amount of exposure, and the *y*-axis represents the incidence of pixels for each exposure level. The computer analyzes the histogram using processing algorithms and compares it with a pre-established histogram specific to the anatomic part being imaged. This process is called **histogram analysis**. The computer software has stored histogram models, each having a shape characteristic of the selected anatomic region and projection. These stored

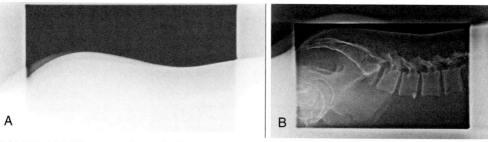

FIGURE 4-24 Histogram-Analysis Error. **A,** Poor quality CR image resulting from a histogram error due to incorrect collimation. **B,** Image showing correctly collimated borders resulting in a quality CR image.

histogram models have **values of interest (VOI)**, which determine the range of the histogram data set that should be included in the displayed image.

In CR imaging, the entire imaging plate is scanned to extract the image from the photostimulable phosphor. The computer identifies the exposure field and the edges of the image, and all exposure data outside this field are excluded from the histogram. Ideally, all four edges of a collimated field should be recognized. If at least three edges are not identified, all data, including raw exposure or scatter outside the field, may be included in the histogram, resulting in a histogram-analysis error. In newer CR imaging systems, the collimated borders may not have the same impact on the histogram as in older CR systems. Histogram-analysis errors are less likely to occur with DR IRs compared with CR IRs because the image data are extracted only from the exposed detectors. See Figure 4-24 for an example of a histogram-analysis error.

▧ IMPORTANT RELATIONSHIP

Histogram Analysis

With digital systems, the computer creates a histogram of the data set. The histogram is a graph of the exposure received to the pixel elements and the prevalence of the exposures within the image. This created histogram is compared with a stored histogram model for that anatomic part; VOIs are identified and the image is displayed.

Histogram analysis is also employed to maintain consistent image brightness despite overexposure or underexposure of the IR. This procedure is known as **automatic rescaling**. The computer rescales the image on the basis of the comparison of the histograms, which is actually a process of mapping the grayscale to the VOI to present a specific display of brightness (Figure 4-25). Although automatic rescaling is a convenient feature, radiographers should be aware that rescaling errors occur for a variety of reasons and can result in poor-quality digital images.

Exposure Indicator

An important feature of digital image processing is its ability to create an image with the appropriate amount of brightness, regardless of the exposure to the IR. As a result of the histogram analysis, valuable information is provided to the radiographer regarding the exposure to the digital IR. The **exposure indicator** provides a numeric value indicating the level of radiation exposure to the digital IR. See Table 4-1 for a list of CR vendor-specific exposure indicators.

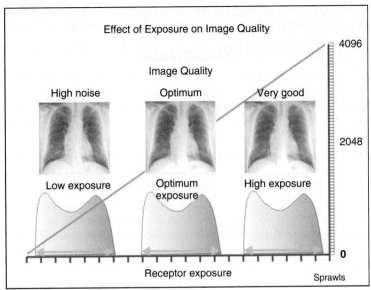

FIGURE 4-25 Automatic rescaling is employed during histogram analysis to maintain a consistent image brightness despite overexposure or underexposure of the IR.

TABLE 4-1	Computed Radiography Vendor-Specific Exposure Indicators			
Vendor	**Exposure Indicator**	**Value = 1 mR exposure**	**2x Exposure**	**½ Exposure**
Fuji and Konica	Sensitivity (S)	200	100	400
Carestream (Kodak)	Exposure index (EI)	2000	2300	1700
Agfa	Log median value (lgM)	2.5	2.8	2.2

In CR, the exposure indicator value represents the exposure level to the imaging plate, and the values are vendor specific. Fuji and Konica use sensitivity (S) numbers, and the value is inversely related to the exposure to the IR. An S number of 200 is equal to 1 mR of exposure to the IR. If the S number increases from 200 to 400, this would indicate a decrease in exposure to the IR by half. Conversely, a decrease in the S number from 200 to 100 would indicate an increase in exposure to the IR by a factor of 2, or doubling of the exposure. Carestream (Kodak) uses exposure index (EI) numbers; their value is directly related to the exposure to the plate and the changes are logarithmic expressions. For example, a change in EI from 2000 to 2300, a difference of 300, is equal to a factor of 2 and represents twice as much exposure to the plate. Agfa uses log median (lgM) numbers; their value is directly related to exposure to the plate and the changes are logarithmic expressions. For example, a change in lgM from 2.5 to 2.8, a change of 0.3, is equal to a factor of 2 and represents twice as much exposure to the IR. Optimal ranges of the exposure indicator values are vendor specific and vary among the types of procedures, such as abdomen and chest imaging versus extremity imaging. DR imaging systems also display an exposure indicator that varies according to the manufacturer's specifications.

This variability among the manufacturer specific exposure indicator values and relationship to the IR exposure has been challenging to radiographers. As a result, the industry has recommended a universal standard exposure indicator. Although there are some variations between the standard exposure indicators, there is common terminology. The **Deviation**

Index (DI) is a value that reflects the difference between the desired or target exposure to the IR and the actual exposure to the IR. A DI of 0 would indicate there is no difference between the desired EI and the actual EI. A DI that is above 0 indicates there is increased exposure to the IR, and a DI below 0 indicates there is decreased exposure to the IR. It is important to note that all EIs, even the recommended standard DI, have limitations. Variables such as collimation, kVp, and centering may influence the EI, and therefore the level of noise and image quality should be evaluated along with the EI or DI value. The radiographer needs to be knowledgeable about the EI value on the equipment she/he uses in digital imaging and how exposure techniques can be altered to correct for exposure errors. In addition, the Department standards should be followed for how over- and under-exposures are to be handled before repeating the image.

The radiographer should monitor the exposure indicator values as a guide for proper exposure techniques. If the exposure indicator value is within the acceptable range, adjustments can be made for contrast and brightness with postprocessing functions, and this will not degrade the image. However, if the exposure is outside of the acceptable range, attempting to adjust the image data with postprocessing functions would not correct for improper IR exposure and may result in noisy or suboptimal images that should not be submitted for interpretation.

The radiographer has a role in the selection of the appropriate anatomic part and projection before computer processing. This step prepares the computer for the type of data being supplied for histogram analysis. If the radiographer selects a part other than the imaged one, a histogram-analysis error may occur. In addition, any errors that occur, such as during data extraction from the IR or rescaling during computer processing, could affect the exposure indicator and provide a false value. It is important for radiographers not only to consider the exposure indicator value carefully but also to recognize its limitations.

 IMPORTANT RELATIONSHIP

Exposure Indicators

The radiographer should strive to select techniques that result in exposure indicator values falling within the indicated optimum range for the corresponding digital imaging system. However, the radiographer also needs to recognize the limitations of exposure indicators for providing accurate information.

Lookup Tables

Following histogram analysis, **lookup tables** provide a method of altering the image to change the display of the digital image in various ways. Because digital IRs have a linear exposure response and a very wide dynamic range, raw data images exhibit low contrast and must be altered to improve the visibility of anatomic structures. Lookup tables provide the means to alter the brightness and grayscale of the digital image using computer algorithms. Further, they are sometimes used to reverse or invert image grayscale. Figure 4-26 visually compares pixel values of the original image with those of a processed image. If the image is not altered, the graph would be a straight line. If the original image is altered, the original pixel values would be different in the processed image and the graph would no longer be a straight line but might resemble a characteristic curve for radiographic film (Figure 4-27).

For example, each pixel value could be altered to display the digital image with a change in contrast. New pixel values would be calculated that result in the image being displayed with

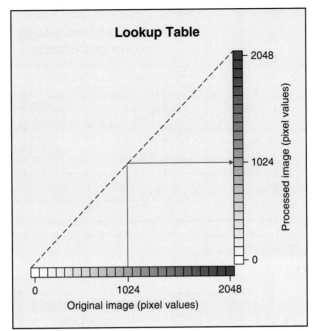

FIGURE 4-26 Straight line graph demonstrating no change in the pixel values from the original to the processed image.

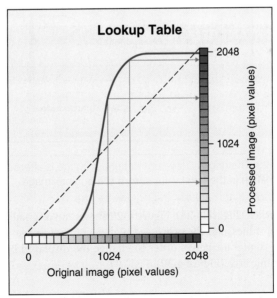

FIGURE 4-27 Graph demonstrating a change in pixel values from the original image to the processed image. The shape of the graph is similar to the characteristic curve for radiographic film.

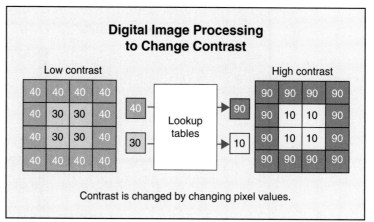

FIGURE 4-28 Lookup table altering the pixel values of a low-contrast image to display an image with higher contrast.

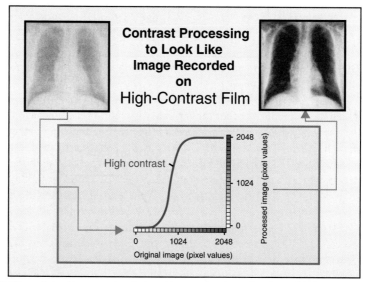

FIGURE 4-29 The original low-contrast chest image is altered to have higher contrast. The graph shows a change in the pixel values from the original image.

higher contrast (Figure 4-28). Figure 4-29 shows the original image, the graph following changes in the pixel values, and the processed higher-contrast image. Lookup tables provide a method of processing digital images in order to change the displayed brightness and contrast required for each anatomic area (Figure 4-30).

IMPORTANT RELATIONSHIP

Lookup Tables

Lookup tables provide the means to alter the original pixel values to improve the brightness and contrast of the image.

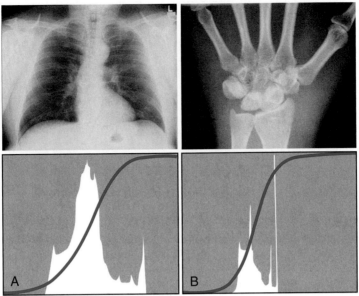

FIGURE 4-30 A, Chest image with its histogram and LUT graph, which differs from **B,** image of the wrist with its histogram and LUT graph.

DIGITAL IMAGING ARTIFACTS

Digital imaging artifacts occur for various reasons and generally have a bright or dark appearance. The complexity of the electronics involved in creating the digital image often make it difficult to isolate the cause of the problem. Unlike the +/− density artifacts found on film images, the level of brightness of digital artifacts does not necessarily provide an indication of the source. Digital artifacts may be classified as detectors (CR plate, TFT array), occurring during image data extraction prior to the ADC or during the ADC process and subsequent signal processing performed by the computer up to the point of image display. Examples of CR-detector-related artifacts would be IP stains, particulates, scratches, cracks, and fogging. Artifacts occurring during data extraction on CR systems are related to issues with the laser optics, transport mechanisms, light guide, and laser sampling and stationary grid frequencies. See Figure 4-31 for examples of CR artifacts.

DR detector artifacts may be related to calibration of an individual detector element (DEL), row, or column of the detector matrix. Artifacts occurring during data extraction are related to electronic readout mechanisms associated with the rows and columns of the DELs comprising the detector matrix.

If the source of the artifact is not related to the detector or extraction of image data up to the ADC, the remaining sources are likely to be the electronic components starting within the ADC and subsequent circuits that are involved with transmitting the digital signal to the computer for processing or processed image data sent to the display monitor. A discussion of artifacts related to the electronic readout mechanisms or occurring within the ADC and subsequent components of the imaging system is beyond the scope of this book.

IMAGE DISPLAY

Following computer processing, the digital image is ready to be displayed for viewing. *Soft-copy viewing* refers to the display of the digital image at a computer workstation as opposed

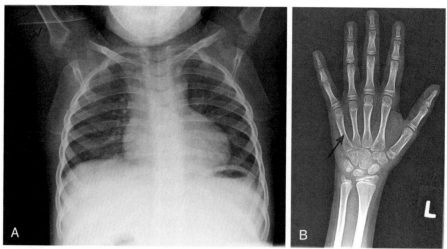

FIGURE 4-31 CR Image Artifacts. **A,** bright lines in the shoulder region as a result of scratches on the imaging plate; **B,** bright specs between the 4th and 5th metacarpals as a result of dirt on the image plate.

to viewing images on film or another physical medium (hard copy). The quality of the digital image is also affected by important features of the display monitor, such as its luminance, resolution, and viewing conditions such as ambient lighting and monitor placement. Specialized postprocessing software is used at the display workstation to aid the radiologist in image interpretation. In addition to soft-copy viewing, the digital image can be printed on specialized film by a laser printer.

Display Monitors

As previously discussed, the quality of the digital image is affected by its acquisition parameters and subsequent computer processing. In addition, the quality of the digital image is affected by the performance of the display monitor. The quality of display monitors may not be equal among all those used for viewing digital images. Monitors used by radiologists for diagnostic interpretation, referred to as *primary*, must be of higher quality than the monitors used only for routine image review. However, the radiographer's monitor should be of sufficiently high quality in order to accurately discern all the image quality characteristics before sending the image to the radiologist for diagnostic interpretation. Display monitors used for diagnostic interpretation are typically monochrome high-resolution monitors and can be set to portrait or landscape formats and configured with one, two, or four monitors (Figure 4-32). A display monitor having diagonal dimensions of 54 cm (21 in) is adequate for viewing images sized 35 × 43 cm (14 × 17 in).

Types of Monitors

Cathode ray tubes (CRTs) and liquid crystal displays (LCDs) are types of monitors typically used for viewing digital images. LCDs are replacing CRTs, and newer technology, such as plasma-type monitors, continues to develop.

A CRT monitor creates an image by accelerating and focusing electrons to strike the faceplate composed of a fluorescent screen (Figure 4-33). Because the image is scanned on the screen in lines, the number of lines affects the quality of the displayed image. It is recommended that CRT monitors scan at least 525 lines per 1/30 of a second. The major components of the CRT monitor are the electron gun encasing a cathode, focusing and deflecting coils, and the anode. This type of display monitor typically has a curved faceplate, and its dimensions are thicker.

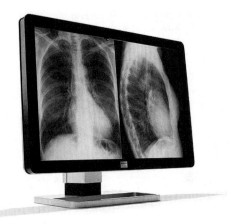

FIGURE 4-32 A set of portrait display monitors used for soft-copy viewing.

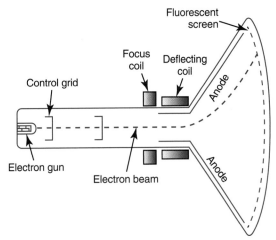

FIGURE 4-33 The CRT monitor creates an image by accelerating and focusing electrons to strike a faceplate composed of a fluorescent screen.

The LCD monitor passes light through liquid crystals to display the image on the glass faceplate. Additional components include a source for the electrical signal and light waveforms and polarizing filters (Figure 4-34). The electrical signals can vary the light waveforms that pass through the crystals for viewing on the faceplate. The LCD monitor has a flat faceplate, and its dimensions are thinner.

Plasma monitors may also be a modern option for display monitors. Plasma monitors are very similar in construction to LCD monitors, but instead of a liquid crystal layer, there is a thin layer of pixels.

Several important features of monitors can affect the quality of the displayed image. Spatial resolution (as determined by screen size and matrix size), luminance, and contrast resolution are just some important characteristics of display monitors.

Viewing Conditions

Placement of the display monitors and the level of light in the room, referred to as **ambient lighting**, can affect soft-copy viewing of digital images. Positioning the monitor away from any direct light sources reduces the amount of reflection on the faceplate of the monitor. In addition, maintaining a low level of ambient lighting can help enhance the viewer's perception of image brightness and

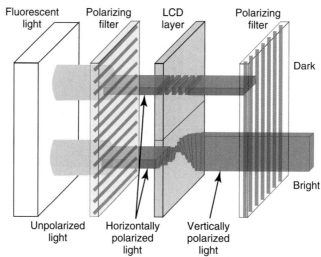

FIGURE 4-34 The LCD monitor passes light through liquid crystals to display the image on the glass faceplate.

contrast displayed on the monitor. Display monitors with thicker faceplates, such as CRTs, have a tendency to reflect more ambient lighting than monitors with thinner faceplates, such as LCDs.

Performance Criteria

Several important features of display monitors affect their performance. Digital images are captured and processed to display a specific matrix size. As previously discussed, an image created with a large matrix having many smaller-sized pixels improves the spatial resolution of the digital image (pixel image). If the monitor used for viewing the digital image cannot display a matrix of that size (because it has too few display pixels), image quality is decreased. Therefore, the monitor matrix size should be at least as large as the image matrix size. It is recommended that a high-resolution 5-megapixel (2048 × 2560 pixels) display monitor be used for diagnostic interpretation.

Because anatomic tissue is visualized using various brightness levels, the amount of light emitted from the monitor (luminance) affects the quality of the displayed image. **Luminance** is a measurement of the light intensity emitted from the surface of the monitor and is expressed in units of candela per square meter (cd/m^2). Primary display monitors should exhibit an average luminance between 300 and 500 cd/m^2. A ratio of the maximum to minimum luminance is evaluated as a part of display monitor quality control and is recommended to be at least 250/100.

The contrast resolution of a digital image is determined by the pixel bit depth. A digital imaging system capable of displaying 16,384 shades of gray (14 bit) requires a monitor capable of displaying a large grayscale range. Monitors that have a higher luminance ratio are capable of displaying a greater grayscale range. The DICOM Grayscale Standard Display Function (GSDF) as recommended by the American Association of Physicists in Medicine (AAPM) Task Group 18 should not vary by more than 10%.

Additional concerns of display monitors include geometrical distortions, such as concavity and convexity; veiling glare, which adversely affects image contrast; and display noise, which is typically a result of statistical fluctuations or luminance differences in the image. Routine quality control of the display monitor is just as important as monitoring the digital imaging acquisition and processing devices. Box 4-3 describes quality-control methods for evaluating digital imaging systems.

BOX 4-3   Quality Control Check: Digital Imaging Systems

Manufacturers of digital imaging equipment have developed quality control procedures specific to their equipment; however, there are basic universal procedures for CR, DR, and display monitors.

Several QC Phantom devices are available to assess the performance of the photostimulable phosphor (PSP) and flat-panel detector (FPD) imaging systems.

- Image receptors (IR) need to be visually inspected for any dirt or scratches that could result in image artifacts. In addition, they should be regularly cleaned according to the manufacturer's specifications.
- The sensitivity of each PSP and FPD should be routinely checked to ensure the consistency of the exposure indicator value calibration.
- Shading or uniformity evaluates brightness consistency throughout the image.
- Linearity of the system can be evaluated by proportionally increasing and decreasing the radiation exposure to the IR and validating that the exposure indicator responds accordingly.
- Contrast resolution can be measured by imaging a contrast detail phantom to assess the visibility of low-contrast objects.
- Spatial resolution can be monitored by imaging a line-pair resolution test tool.
- For CR systems, the laser beam performance can be evaluated by imaging an opaque straight-edged object and visually checking for any jitter along the edges of the object.
- The measurement tool available at the workstation should be checked for accuracy.
- The thoroughness of the IP erasure function can be evaluated by performing a secondary erasure on the IP and checking for any residual exposure (ghosting). The FPD can be evaluated to confirm that no charges remain from the previous exposure.

Display Monitor

QC test devices for evaluating the performance of the display monitor include the American Association of Physicists in Medicine (AAPM) TG18-QC test pattern and the Society of Motion Picture and Television Engineers test pattern (SMPTE). Several aspects of a display monitor can be evaluated with these test patterns, including geometric distortion, luminance, resolution, contrast resolution, noise, and veiling glare.

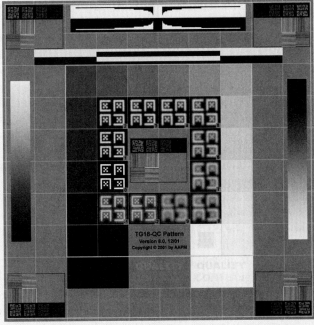

American Association of Physicists in Medicine (AAPM) TG18-QC test pattern

Continued

BOX 4-3   Quality Control Check: Digital Imaging Systems—cont'd

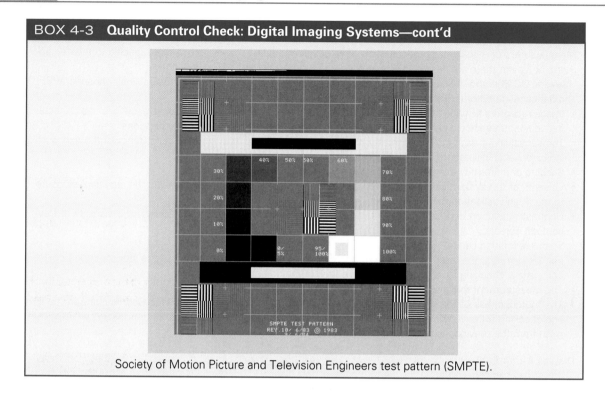

Society of Motion Picture and Television Engineers test pattern (SMPTE).

Postprocessing

Postprocessing functions are computer software operations available to the radiographer and radiologist that allow manual manipulation of the displayed image. These functions allow the operator to manually adjust many presentation features of the image to enhance the diagnostic value.

Electronic Masking. Once the image is processed, regions viewed on the image can be altered further by **electronic masking**, also known as *shuttering*. For example, when the area of interest is properly collimated, the image may display increased brightness surrounding the radiation-exposed field. This region of brightness provides no useful information and can be removed from the displayed image. In addition, electronic masking can remove regions within the radiation-exposed field that provide no useful information. Electronic masking has no effect on the overall image quality or on patient exposure.

Brightness. Because the image is composed of numerical data, the brightness level displayed on the computer monitor can be easily altered to visualize the range of the recorded anatomic structures. This adjustment is accomplished using the windowing function. The **window level** (or center) sets the midpoint of the range of brightness visible in the image. Changing the window level on the display monitor allows the image brightness to be increased or decreased throughout the entire range. When the range of brightness displayed is less than the maximum, the processed image presents only a subset of the total information contained within the computer (Figure 4-35).

Assume that pixel values from 0 to 2048 are used to represent the full range of digital image brightness levels. A high pixel value (e.g., 1078) could represent a volume of tissue that attenuates fewer x-ray photons and is displayed as a decreased brightness level. Therefore, a low pixel value (e.g., 350) represents a volume of tissue that attenuates more x-ray photons and is displayed as increased brightness.

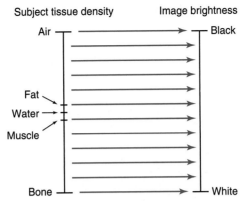

FIGURE 4-35 Changing the window level increases or decreases the image brightness throughout the range of densities recorded in the image.

Moving the window level up to a high pixel value increases the visibility of the darker anatomic regions (e.g., lung fields) by increasing the overall brightness on the display monitor. Conversely, to better visualize an anatomic region represented by a low pixel value, one would decrease the window level to decrease the brightness on the display monitor.

IMPORTANT RELATIONSHIP

Window Level and Image Brightness

A direct relationship exists between window level and image brightness on the display monitor. Increasing the window level increases the image brightness; decreasing the window level decreases the image brightness.

Contrast. The number of different shades of gray that can be stored and displayed by a computer system is termed **grayscale**. **Contrast resolution** is another term associated with digital imaging and is used to describe the ability of the imaging system to distinguish between objects that exhibit similar densities because they attenuate the x-ray beam similarly. An important distinguishing characteristic of a digital image is its improved contrast resolution compared with a film-screen image. As previously mentioned, the contrast resolution of a pixel is determined by the bit depth or number of bits (i.e., 12, 14, or 16), which affects the number of shades of gray available for image display. Increasing the number of shades of gray increases the contrast resolution within the image. An image with increased contrast resolution, when optimally windowed, increases the visibility of very subtle anatomic features.

Once the digital image is processed, radiographic contrast can be adjusted to vary the visualization of the area of interest; this is necessary because the contrast resolution of the human eye is limited. **Window width** is a control that adjusts the radiographic contrast. Because the digital image can display shades of gray ranging from black to white, the display monitor can vary the range or number of shades of gray visible on the image to show the desired anatomy. Adjusting the range of visible shades of gray varies the image contrast. When the entire number of shades of gray are displayed (wide window width), the image has lower contrast; when a smaller number of shades of gray are displayed (narrow window width), the image has higher contrast (Figure 4-36).

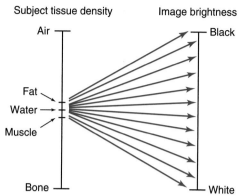

FIGURE 4-36 Changing the window width increases or decreases the range of visible brightness levels. A narrow window width decreases the range of brightness levels and increases contrast. Wider window width increases the range of brightness levels and reduces contrast.

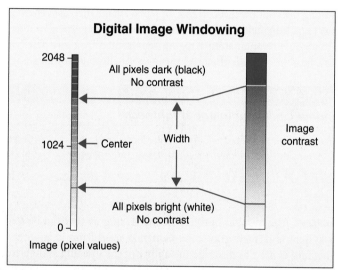

FIGURE 4-37 The level or center of the window and the window width change the visual display of the digital image.

In digital imaging, an inverse relationship exists between window width and image contrast. A wide window width displays an image with lower contrast than the same area of interest displayed with a narrow window width.

The center or midpoint of the window level and the width of the window determine the brightness and contrast of the displayed image (Figure 4-37). Figure 4-38 demonstrates how the image is altered when the window level is changed for a given window width.

IMPORTANT RELATIONSHIP

Window Width and Image Contrast

A narrow (decreased) window width displays higher radiographic contrast, whereas a wider (increased) window width displays lower radiographic contrast.

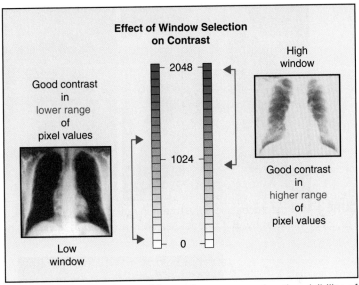

FIGURE 4-38 Changing the window level for a chest x-ray varies the visibility of the anatomic detail or contrast for both low- and high-density areas.

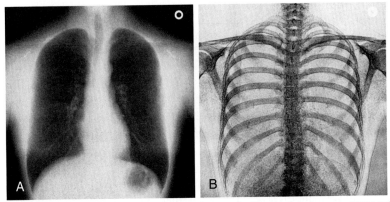

FIGURE 4-39 Subtraction postprocessing techniques. **A,** Skeletal areas are removed. **B,** Lungs and soft tissue are removed.

The ability to optimize image display in real time using the window level and width controls is a major advantage of soft-copy (versus hard copy) viewing of digital images. It is important to note that windowing does not alter the original stored pixel values of an image but rather alters only how they are displayed.

Depending on the software available during soft-copy viewing, a digital image can be additionally manipulated in a variety of ways. The following are six common postprocessing techniques:

1. *Subtraction* (Figure 4-39) is a technique that can remove superimposed structures so that the anatomic area of interest becomes more visible. Because the image is in a digital format, the computer can subtract selected brightness values to create an image without superimposed structures.
2. *Contrast enhancement* (Figure 4-40) is a postprocessing technique that alters the pixel values to increase image contrast.

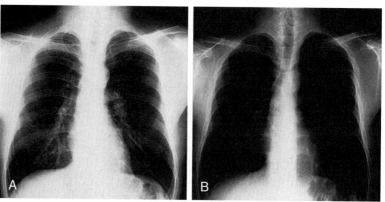

FIGURE 4-40 Postprocessing adjustment in radiographic contrast. **A,** Longer-scale contrast typical of chest radiography. **B,** Contrast has been adjusted to present a higher scale.

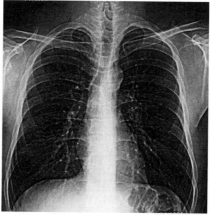

FIGURE 4-41 A radiographic image demonstrates an edge-enhancement postprocessing technique.

3. *Edge enhancement* (also known as high-pass filtering) (Figure 4-41) is a postprocessing technique that improves the visibility of small, high-contrast structures. However, image noise may be slightly increased.
4. *Inversion* (also known as black/white reversal) (Figure 4-42) is a postprocessing technique that reverses the grayscale from the original radiograph.
5. *Smoothing* (also known as low-pass filtering) (Figure 4-43) is a postprocessing technique that suppresses image noise (quantum noise). However, spatial resolution is degraded.
6. **Equalization** (Figure 4-44) is a postprocessing function whereby underexposed areas (light areas) are made darker and overexposed areas (dark areas) are made lighter. The effect is an image that appears to have lower contrast so that dense and lucent structures can be better seen within the same image.

Other postprocessing functions include region of interest (ROI), which provides calculation of selected pixel values within the area of interest to provide quantitative information about the tissue. Additional software can provide stitching of the images for viewing anatomic areas that require more than one image such as for a scoliosis series.

A word of caution is warranted regarding postprocessing: overuse of these functions can drastically and negatively alter the data set, which is the digital image. Overwriting the original image

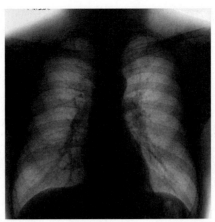

FIGURE 4-42 Radiographic image demonstrates a black/white reversal postprocessing technique.

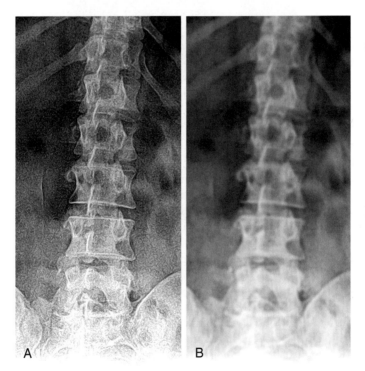

FIGURE 4-43 Smoothing (also known as low-pass filtering). **A,** Image without applying smoothing processing. **B,** Image following smoothing processing.

with a postprocessed replica may reduce the diagnostic and archival quality of the data. One should also keep in mind that in many facilities, the radiographers' workstations use monitors of significantly lower quality and viewing conditions that are very different compared with the radiologists' workstations. How an image looks on the radiographer's workstation in a brightly lit work area may be very different from the way it looks on the radiologist's high-resolution monitor in a darkened reading room. Therefore, care should be taken in the postprocessing of an image before forwarding it for interpretation.

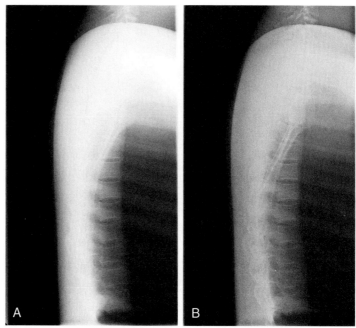

FIGURE 4-44 Equalization. **A,** Image without equalization. **B,** Image with equalization.

Laser Printers

Although not commonly needed for interpretation, hard-copy records of digital images may still occasionally be desired. Digital images can be windowed while being viewed on a display monitor and then printed onto film by a laser camera. Multiple images can be printed on a single sheet, and multiple copies of images processed differently can be printed. Laser printers that use either wet or dry printing methods are available. Wet laser printers use liquid chemicals (developer and fixer) to process the image. In dry processing, the chemicals are part of the film. The image is created by use of heat instead of liquid chemicals.

DIGITAL COMMUNICATION NETWORKS

Modern radiology practice requires efficient and simple acquisition, storage, retrieval, transmission, and display of digital image data from multiple imaging modalities. Digital communication needs in radiology also include the processing and delivery of patient data and subsequent interpretation of radiological procedures. The ability to simultaneously integrate image, voice, and medical information involves a more complex system. A **picture archival and communication system (PACS)** is a computer system designed for digital imaging that can receive, store, distribute, and display digital images; radiology information systems (RIS) and hospital information systems (HIS) are computer systems that provide medical information.

Integration of these systems can be accomplished by networks. A network system links all of these computer systems so that images, patient data, and interpretations can be viewed simultaneously by people at different workstations (Figure 4-45). An important goal of a radiology

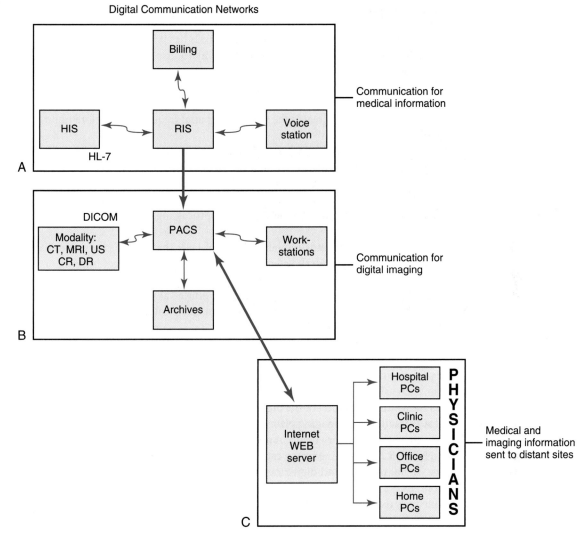

FIGURE 4-45 A, Communication among the computer systems for medical information. **B,** Communication among the computer systems for imaging. **C,** Referring physicians can receive radiology reports, patient data, and radiographic images through the Internet.

network system is to provide the referring physician with the radiology report, patient data, and radiographic images at a convenient location and in a timely manner.

Digital Imaging and Communications in Medicine (DICOM) is a communication standard for information sharing between PACS and imaging modalities. The **Health Level Seven standard (HL7)** is a communication standard for medical information. Connectivity and communication among these systems are necessary for radiology to realize the full potential of digital communication. Network systems are currently being marketed to meet the demands in radiology. A well-integrated system would improve patient care through cost-effective, reliable, secure, and timely delivery of diagnostic information.

CHAPTER SUMMARY

- A digital image with a larger matrix and smaller-sized pixels has improved quality.
- A pixel's bit depth determines the available shades of gray to display the digital image or its contrast resolution.
- Spatial resolution is improved by increasing the pixel density and decreasing the pixel pitch.
- Line pairs per millimeter (lp/mm) is the unit of measurement for spatial frequency. Increasing the number of resolved lp/mm increases the visualized spatial frequency, therefore improving the spatial resolution.
- The modulation transfer function (MTF) is a measure of an imaging system's ability to display contrast of anatomic objects varying in size, and the value ranges between 0 (no difference in brightness levels) and 1.0 (maximum difference in brightness levels).
- CR and DR IRs differ in their construction and how they acquire latent images. Once the latent image is acquired and the raw data are digitized, image processing and display are essentially the same for CR and DR.
- In CR, the imaging plate has a photostimulable phosphor layer that absorbs the exit radiation and excites electrons, which become elevated to a higher energy state and get trapped.
- The exposed imaging plate is placed in a reader unit where the trapped electrons are released during the laser beam scanning, and the excess energy is emitted as visible light. A photodetector collects, amplifies, and converts the visible light to an electrical signal proportional to the range of energies stored in the imaging plate.
- The signal output from the photodector is digitized by an ADC converter to produce a digital image.
- The sampling frequency determines how often the analog signal is reproduced in its discrete digitized form. Increasing the sampling frequency increases the pixel density of the digital data and improves the spatial resolution of the digital image.
- Following data extraction, CR imaging plates must be erased by exposure to an intense white light to release any residual energy before reuse.
- In contrast to CR, DR IRs combine image capture and readout.
- Signal storage, signal readout, and digitizing electronics are integrated into a solid-state flat-panel detector.
- Flat-panel detectors use both indirect and direct conversion methods to create proportional electrical charges that are sent to the ADC for conversion to digital data.
- Indirect conversion detectors use a scintillator to convert the exit radiation to visible light, and then the visible light is converted to electrical charges for storage in the TFTs.
- Direct conversion detectors directly convert the exit radiation into electrical charges for storage in the TFTs.
- Once the varying x-ray energies are converted to numerical data, the digital image can be electronically processed, manipulated, transported, or stored.
- Digital IRs have a wide dynamic range, which means that they can accurately capture the wide range of photon energies that exit a patient. However, lower- or higher-than-necessary exposure techniques do not guarantee a quality digital image with reasonable radiation exposure to the patient.
- Detective quantum efficiency (DQE) is a measurement of the efficiency of an image receptor in converting the x-ray exposure it receives to a quality radiographic image. The higher the DQE of a system, the lower the radiation exposure required to produce a quality image, and therefore, patient exposure is decreased.
- SNR is a method of describing the strength of the radiation exposure compared with the amount of noise apparent in a digital image. When the digital image displays increased noise, regardless of the source, anatomic details will have decreased visibility.

- CNR is a method of describing the contrast resolution compared with the amount of noise apparent in a digital image. Digital images having a higher CNR will increase the visibility of anatomic tissues.
- With digital systems, computers create histograms or graphs of the exposure received to the IR and the prevalence of those exposures within the image.
- Histogram analysis is an image-processing technique used to identify the data of the image and to compensate for image overexposure and underexposure.
- The computer analyzes the histogram using processing algorithms and compares it with a preestablished histogram specific to the anatomic part being imaged.
- Automatic rescaling is a process employed to maintain a consistent image brightness despite overexposure or underexposure.
- During histogram analysis, the exposure indicator provides a numerical value that indicates the level of radiation exposure to the digital IR.
- Following histogram analysis, lookup tables provide the means to alter the original pixel values to improve the brightness and contrast of the image.
- Display monitors provide soft-copy viewing of digital radiographs. Primary monitors are high-quality monitors used for diagnostic interpretation.
- Two commonly used display monitors are CRT and LCD. CRT monitors create an image by accelerating and focusing electrons to strike a faceplate comprising a fluorescent screen. LCD monitors pass light through liquid crystals to display the image on a glass plate.
- Important features regarding display monitors are viewing conditions, matrix size, luminance, luminance ratio, and contrast resolution.
- Postprocessing functions, such as electronic masking, cropping, window level and width, subtraction, contrast enhancement, edge enhancement, smoothing, and equalization allow manipulation of the displayed image.
- Laser printers that use either wet or dry methods to print hard-copy images are available.
- PACS is the communication system for digital imaging modalities and can receive, store, distribute, and display digital images.
- DICOM is a communication standard for information sharing between PACS and imaging modalities, and HL7 is a communication standard for medical information.

REVIEW QUESTIONS

1. Which of the following would improve digital image quality?
   A. Small matrix and large pixel size
   B. Decreased pixel density and increased pixel pitch
   C. Large matrix and large pixel size
   D. Large matrix and increased pixel density
2. The type of image receptor that uses a photostimulable phosphor to acquire the latent image is _____.
   A. an intensifying screen
   B. a flat-panel detector
   C. computed radiography
   D. radiographic film
3. Which of the following is used to extract the latent image from an imaging plate?
   A. Laser beam
   B. Photomultiplier tube
   C. Analog-to-digital converter
   D. Thin-film transistor

4. Which of the following will improve the quality of the digital image?
   A. Decreased sampling frequency and increased sampling pitch
   B. Decreased sampling frequency and decreased sampling pitch
   C. Increased sampling frequency and increased sampling pitch
   D. Increased sampling frequency and decreased sampling pitch
5. Which of the following would improve the quality of the digital image for a given field of view (FOV)?
   A. A fixed matrix size and larger imaging plate
   B. A decreased sampling frequency and larger imaging plate
   C. A small matrix size and larger pixel size
   D. A fixed matrix size and small imaging plate
6. What is the process of assigning a numerical value to represent a brightness value?
   A. Dynamic range
   B. Signal-to-noise ratio
   C. Quantization
   D. Spectral sensitivity
7. Which of the following pixel bit depths would display a greater range of shades of gray to represent anatomic tissues?
   A. 8 bit
   B. 10 bit
   C. 14 bit
   D. 16 bit
8. Digital imaging systems have a wide dynamic range.
   A. True
   B. False
9. A lower signal-to-noise ratio improves the quality of a digital image.
   A. True
   B. False
10. Which of the following is a measurement of the efficiency of an image receptor in converting the x-ray exposure it receives to a quality radiographic image?
    A. CNR
    B. MTF
    C. DQE
    D. SNR
11. Which of the following is defined as a graphic representation of the pixel values?
    A. Automatic rescaling
    B. Values of interest
    C. Histogram
    D. Exposure indicator
12. What process is employed to maintain consistent digital image brightness for overexposure or underexposure?
    A. Automatic rescaling
    B. Histogram
    C. Exposure indicator
    D. Lookup tables

13. Which of the following is *not* a numerical value indicating the level of radiation exposure to a digital image receptor?
    A. Sensitivity number
    B. Exposure indicator
    C. Window level
    D. Exposure index

14. What digital process alters image brightness and grayscale to improve the visibility of anatomic structures?
    A. Automatic rescaling
    B. Histogram analysis
    C. Exposure indicator
    D. Lookup tables

15. What type of monitor passes light through liquid crystals to display a digital image?
    A. TFT
    B. LCD
    C. CRT
    D. PACS

16. Maintaining a low level of ambient lighting can improve soft-copy viewing of digital images.
    A. True
    B. False

17. Display monitors used for soft-copy viewing of digital images should have _____.
    A. increased ambient lighting
    B. decreased matrix size
    C. low spatial resolution
    D. high luminance

18. Which of the following is *not* a function during post-processing of a displayed digital image?
    A. Automatic rescaling
    B. Electronic masking
    C. Windowing
    D. Edge enhancement

19. A wider window width _____.
    A. increases brightness
    B. decreases brightness
    C. increases contrast
    D. decreases contrast

20. What is the communication standard for information sharing between PACS and imaging modalities?
    A. DQE
    B. DICOM
    C. SMPTE
    D. HL7

5

Film-Screen Imaging

CHAPTER OUTLINE

Film-Screen Imaging
  Radiographic Film
  Intensifying Screens
Radiographic Film Processing
  Automatic Film Processing
  Quality Control
  Silver Recovery
Sensitometry

Equipment
  Penetrometer
  Sensitometer
  Densitometer
Optical Density
  Diagnostic Range
Sensitometric Curve
  Log of Relative Exposure
  Regions

Film Characteristics
  Speed
  Contrast
  Exposure Latitude
Clinical Considerations
  Optimal Density
  Maximum Film Contrast
  Image Display

OBJECTIVES

After completing this chapter, the reader will be able to perform the following:

1. Define all the key terms in this chapter.
2. State all the important relationships in this chapter.
3. Compare film-screen and digital IRs in terms of their dynamic range and explain the importance of dynamic range in exposure technique selection and image quality.
4. Explain how latent images are formed on film.
5. State the purpose of intensifying screens in film-screen imaging.
6. Explain how intensifying screens can be characterized on the basis of the type of phosphor, spectral emission, spectral sensitivity, and screen speed.
7. Recognize the effect intensifying screens have on image quality and patient radiation exposure.

8. Explain how latent images are converted to manifest images during automatic film processing.
9. State the developing and fixing agents used in chemical processing.
10. List the sequential stages and systems needed to process a quality radiographic film image.
11. State methods to maintain the archival quality of film radiographs.
12. Discuss the role of chemical replenishment, temperature control, and silver recovery during film processing.
13. State the requirements for darkroom safelights, temperature, and humidity control.
14. Define sensitometry and discuss film speed, contrast, and latitude.

KEY TERMS

active layer	illuminators	screen speed
automatic film processor	immersion heater	sensitometer
average gradient	intensifying screen	sensitometric curve
base plus fog (B + F)	intensity of radiation	sensitometric strip
cassette	exposure	sensitometry
D_{max}	latent image centers	shoulder region
D_{min}	latent image formation	silver halide
densitometer	luminescence	silver recovery
developing agents	maximum contrast	slope
double-emulsion film	optical density (OD)	spectral emission
dynamic range	optimal density	spectral matching
emulsion layer	penetrometer	spectral sensitivity
exposure latitude	phosphor layer	speed
feed tray	rare earth elements	speed exposure point
film contrast	recirculation system	speed point
film speed	reducing agents	standby control
fixing agent	relative speed	step-wedge densities
fluorescence	replenishment	straight-line region
gradient point	screen film	toe region

FILM-SCREEN IMAGING

Before the development of digital IRs, radiographic images were acquired, processed, and displayed on film. Film is placed in a cassette housing two intensifying screens for the purpose of reducing patient exposure. To create and display a radiographic image, an **active layer** or **emulsion** is adhered to a sheet of polyester plastic. The emulsion contains crystals suspended in gelatin that serve as the latent imaging centers. To reduce patient exposure, radiographic film is placed between two intensifying screens. The intensifying screens convert the exit radiation intensities into visible light, and the light exposes the crystals in the emulsion.

The film must be chemically processed in an automatic processor before it is visualized on the sheet of polyester plastic. Once it is chemically processed, the film image displays densities ranging from dark to light that correspond to the variations in the intensities of radiation exiting the anatomic tissues. The dark densities are created when the exposed crystals are converted to black metallic silver. The light or clear areas on the film result from the removal of unexposed crystals during chemical processing. The resulting image represents a range of densities created as a result of the x-ray attenuation characteristics of the anatomic structures. Anatomic tissues through which radiation is transmitted are visualized as dark densities and those in which radiation is absorbed are visualized as light or clear areas on the film.

Although film-screen served as a good medium for radiographic images for many decades, it has many limitations that can be overcome with digital imaging. One major deficiency is the limited **dynamic range** (i.e., the range of exposure intensities that an image receptor can accurately detect) of film. This limitation renders a film very sensitive to underexposure or overexposure, which may necessitate image retakes. A limited dynamic range also restricts the visibility of structures that differ greatly in x-ray attenuation. An example is the difficulty of optimally visualizing both soft tissue and bony structures within a given film image. Box 5-1 presents limitations of film.

IMPORTANT RELATIONSHIP

Dynamic Range and Film-Screen Imaging

> The range of exposure intensities that film can accurately detect is limited (limited dynamic range). This renders film more susceptible to overexposure and underexposure and restricts its ability to display tissues that vary greatly in x-ray attenuation.

Although film-screen IRs are being replaced with digital IRs, knowledge of the former remains useful.

Radiographic Film

Radiographic film acquires the latent image and must be chemically processed before it is visible. Consequently, film serves as the medium for image acquisition, processing, and display. Several types of radiographic film are still used in medical imaging departments. Depending on the specific application, film manufacturers produce film in a variety of sizes ranging from 20 × 25 cm (8 × 10 in) to 35 × 43 cm (14 × 17 in). The composition of film can be described in layers (Box 5-2). The most important layer for creating the image is the **emulsion layer**. This is a radiation- and light-sensitive layer of the film. The emulsion of film consists of silver halide crystals suspended

---

BOX 5-1   Limitations of Film

- Limited dynamic range that renders a film sensitive to underexposure or overexposure
- Restricts the visibility of optimally visualizing both soft tissue and bony structures within a given image
- Film cost
- Necessity for chemical processing
- Potential artifacts due to film handling and chemical processing
- Film processing time, cost, maintenance, and delay in viewing the image
- No adjustment in image postprocessing
- Limited contrast resolution
- Cannot be electronically stored or duplicated, displayed on computer monitors, or transmitted over computer networks
- Traditional film archives consume significant space and are frequently prone to loss of films
- Storage and retrieval costs

BOX 5-2   Composition of Radiographic Film

- *Supercoat*—durable protection layer
- *Emulsion*—radiation- and light-sensitive layer
- *Adhesive*—adheres layers together
- *Film base*—polyester layer that gives the film physical stability

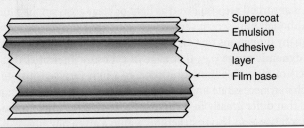

in gelatin. **Silver halide** is a material that is sensitive to radiation and light. The emulsion layer is fragile and must have a layer composed of a polyester base so that the film can be handled and processed while remaining physically strong after processing. Most film used in radiographic procedures has a dye or tint added to the base layer to decrease eye strain when viewed on a view (illuminator) box.

Screen film is the most widely used radiographic film. As its name implies, it is intended to be used with one or two intensifying screens. Screen film is more sensitive to light and less sensitive to x-rays. Screen film can have either a single- or double-emulsion coating. **Double-emulsion film** has an emulsion coating on both sides of the base. Film-screen imaging typically uses double-emulsion film with two intensifying screens.

Latent Image Formation

The specific way in which latent images are formed is unknown, but the Gurney–Mott theory of **latent image formation** is most widely believed to explain best the manner in which this process occurs. To explain latent image formation, it is necessary to describe what happens at the molecular level in the emulsion layer of the film—specifically, what happens to silver halide crystals when exposed to x-rays and light.

Physical imperfections, known as *sensitivity specks*, in the silver halide crystals are the sites of the latent image formation (Figure 5-1). Exposure to x-rays and light ionizes the silver halide crystals, and the freed electrons become trapped at the sensitivity specks. The negatively charged sensitivity

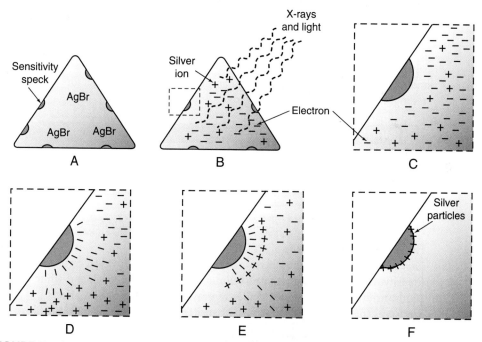

FIGURE 5-1 Latent image formation theory. **A,** Before exposure, silver halide (AgBr and AgI) is suspended in gelatin in the emulsion layer. Sensitivity specks exist as physical imperfections in the film lattice. **B,** Exposure to x-rays and light ionizes the silver halide. **C,** Negatively charged electrons and positively charged silver ions float freely in the emulsion gelatin. **D,** Sensitivity specks trap electrons. **E,** Each trapped electron attracts a silver ion. **F,** Metallic silver clumps around the sensitivity specks.

specks attract the freed silver ions. Every silver ion that combines with an electron is neutralized by that electron, thereby becoming metallic silver. Several sensitivity specks with many silver ions attracted to them become **latent image centers**. These latent image centers appear as areas of radiographic density on the manifest image after processing. It is believed that for a latent image center to appear, it must contain at least three sensitivity specks with at least three silver atoms each. With more exposure to the film, more metallic silver is visualized as radiographic density.

 IMPORTANT RELATIONSHIP

Sensitivity Specks and Latent Image Centers

Sensitivity specks serve as the focal points for the development of latent image centers. After exposure, these specks trap the free electrons and then attract and neutralize the positive silver ions. After enough silver is neutralized, the specks become a latent image center and are converted into metallic silver after chemical processing.

Current manufacturers of radiographic film offer a wide variety of films. These differ not only in size and general type but also in film speed, film contrast, exposure latitude, and spectral sensitivity.

Film Speed
Film speed is the degree to which the emulsion is sensitive to x-rays or light. The greater the speed of a film, the more sensitive it is. Because sensitivity increases, less exposure is necessary to produce a specific density. Two primary factors, both relating to the silver halide crystals found in the emulsion layers, affect the speed of radiographic film. The first factor is the number of silver halide crystals present and the second factor is the size of these crystals. Radiographic film manufacturers control film speed by manipulating both of these factors during the production of radiographic films with specific speeds.

 IMPORTANT RELATIONSHIP

Silver Halide and Film Sensitivity

As the number and/or size of silver halide crystals increase, film sensitivity or speed increases. A faster film speed requires less radiation exposure to produce a specific density.

Film Contrast and Latitude
Film contrast refers to the ability of radiographic film to provide a certain level of image contrast (density differences). High-contrast film accentuates more black and white areas, whereas low-contrast film primarily shows shades of gray. The latitude of film affects the range of radiation exposures that can provide diagnostic densities. A radiographic film capable of responding to a wide range of exposures to produce diagnostic densities is considered to be a *wide-latitude film*.

Spectral Sensitivity
Spectral sensitivity refers to the color of light to which a particular film is most sensitive. In radiography, there are generally two categories of spectral sensitivity films: blue sensitive and green sensitive (orthochromatic). When radiographic film is used with intensifying screens, it is important to match the spectral sensitivity of the film with the spectral emission of the screens.

Spectral emission refers to the color of light produced by a particular intensifying screen. In radiography, two categories of spectral emission generally exist: blue light-emitting screens and green light-emitting screens. It is critical to use blue-sensitive film with blue light-emitting screens and green-sensitive film with green light-emitting screens. **Spectral matching** refers to correctly matching the color sensitivity of the film to the color emission of the intensifying screen. An incorrect match of film and screens based on spectral emission and sensitivity results in radiographs that display inappropriate levels of radiographic density.

Intensifying Screens

An **intensifying screen** is a device found in radiographic cassettes that contains phosphors to convert x-ray energy into light, which then exposes the radiographic film (Figure 5-2). The purpose of this device is to intensify the action of the x-rays and permit much lower x-ray exposures compared with film alone.

As with radiographic film, the construction of screens can be described in layers (Box 5-3). The **phosphor layer**, or active layer, is the most important screen component because it contains

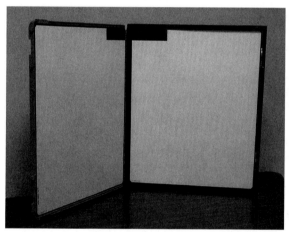

FIGURE 5-2 Typical set of intensifying screens inside a cassette.

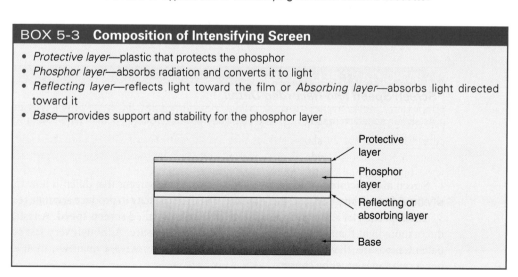

BOX 5-3   Composition of Intensifying Screen

- *Protective layer*—plastic that protects the phosphor
- *Phosphor layer*—absorbs radiation and converts it to light
- *Reflecting layer*—reflects light toward the film or *Absorbing layer*—absorbs light directed toward it
- *Base*—provides support and stability for the phosphor layer

Protective layer
Phosphor layer
Reflecting or absorbing layer
Base

the phosphor material that absorbs the transmitted x-rays and converts them to visible light. The most common phosphor materials consist of chemical compounds of elements from the rare earth group. **Rare earth elements** are elements that range in atomic number from 57 to 71 on the periodic table; they are referred to as *rare earth elements* because they are relatively difficult and expensive to extract from the Earth.

Intensifying screen systems used in cassettes generally include two screens. The screen that is mounted on the side of the cassette facing the x-ray tube is called the *front screen*, and the screen that is mounted on the opposite side is called the *back screen*. With two screens, the film (double-emulsion) is exposed to approximately twice as much light as that in a single-screen system because the film is exposed to light from both sides. Some screen systems use only a single screen and are used with single-emulsion film. When a single screen is used, it is mounted as a back screen on the side of the cassette that is opposite from the tube side. When loading a single-emulsion film into the appropriate cassette with a single screen, the emulsion side of the film must be placed against the intensifying screen.

Film is much more sensitive to visible light than to x-rays. By converting each absorbed high-energy x-ray photon into thousands of visible light photons, intensifying screens amplify film optical density. Without screens, the total amount of energy to which the film is exposed comprises only x-rays. With screens, the total amount of energy to which the film is exposed is divided between x-rays and light. When intensifying screens are used, approximately 90%–99% of the total energy to which the film is exposed is light. X-rays account for the remaining 1%–10% of the energy.

Intensifying screens operate by a process known as *luminescence*. **Luminescence** is the emission of light from the screen when stimulated by radiation. The desired type of luminescence in imaging is *fluorescence*. **Fluorescence** refers to the ability of phosphors to emit visible light only while exposed to x-rays (with little or no afterglow). An undesired type of luminescence is phosphorescence. *Phosphorescence* is the emission of light after x-ray exposure has terminated. Phosphorescence or afterglow causes unwanted exposure to the film.

Screen Speed

The purpose of intensifying screens is to decrease the radiation dose to the patient. Because screen phosphors can intensify the action of x-rays by converting them to visible light, the use of such screens allows the radiographer to use considerably lower mAs values. The disadvantage of using screens is the reduction in recorded detail. The reason for the reduction is that visible light photons created within the screen tend to disperse before reaching the film emulsion; this blurs the image.

 IMPORTANT RELATIONSHIP

Screen Speed and Recorded Detail

> As screen speed increases, recorded detail decreases; as screen speed decreases, recorded detail increases.

Screen manufacturers produce a variety of intensifying screens that differ in how well they intensify the action of the x-rays and therefore differ in their capacity to produce accurate recorded detail.

The capability of a screen to produce visible light is called **screen speed**. A faster screen produces more light than a slower screen for the same exposure. Although very fast screens reduce patient exposure, they also degrade recorded detail and increase quantum mottle (noise), and hence, a balance must be chosen.

IMPORTANT RELATIONSHIP

Screen Speed, Light Emission, and Patient Dose

> The faster an intensifying screen, the more light is emitted for the same intensity of x-ray exposure. As the screen speed increases, less radiation is necessary, and the radiation dose to the patient is decreased; as screen speed decreases, more radiation is necessary, and the radiation dose to the patient is increased.

Several factors affect how fast or slow an intensifying screen is, including absorption efficiency, conversion efficiency, thickness of the phosphor layer, and size of the phosphor crystal (Table 5-1). The presence of a reflecting layer, an absorbing layer, or dye in the phosphor layer also affects screen speed.

Absorption efficiency refers to the ability of the screen to absorb the incident x-ray photons. A rare earth phosphor screen absorbs approximately 60% of the incident photons. *Conversion efficiency* describes how well the screen phosphor takes these x-ray photons and converts them to visible light. Increased absorption and conversion efficiency mean that rare earth phosphors have increased speed compared with a previously used screen phosphor, calcium tungstate. This increased speed allows the radiographer to substantially reduce the x-ray exposure required to produce images with the appropriate amount of density.

In addition, the thickness of the phosphor layer and the size of the crystal affect the screen speed. A thicker phosphor layer contains more phosphor material than a thinner one. Phosphor converts x-rays into light; hence, if more phosphor material is present in a screen, more light is produced, increasing the screen speed. The size of the phosphor material crystals also affects screen speed. Larger phosphor crystals produce more light than smaller phosphor crystals. Again, more light being produced means that the screen is faster.

The final factors that affect screen speed are the presence or absence of a reflecting layer, a light-absorbing layer, or light-absorbing dyes in the phosphor layer. When present, a reflecting layer increases screen speed (at the expense of decreased recorded detail) by redirecting retrograde light back toward the film emulsion. Conversely, a light-absorbing layer or light-absorbing dyes present in the phosphor layer are used to decrease screen speed (and increase recorded detail) by absorbing light that would otherwise reach and expose the film.

The ability of the screen to produce visible light can also be described in terms of its **relative speed** (RS). RS results from comparing film-screen systems on the basis of the amount of light produced for a given exposure. Film-screen relative speeds range from 50 to 800 RS. Most radiology departments that use film-screen technology have at least two different speeds of intensifying screen systems. A fast system is usually available with an RS of approximately 400. A 400 RS system is a good compromise between the beneficial effect of decreasing the patient dose and the detrimental effect of decreasing the recorded detail. A slower system is usually available, and it

TABLE 5-1 Summary of Effects of Screen Factors on Screen Speed, Recorded Detail, and Patient Dose

Screen Factor	Screen Speed	Recorded Detail	Patient Dose
Thicker phosphor layer	↑	↓	↓
Larger phosphor crystal size	↑	↓	↓
Reflective layer	↑	↓	↓
Absorbing layer	↓	↑	↑
Dye in phosphor layer	↓	↑	↑

is sometimes labeled on the outside of the cassette as *detail* or *extremity*. Typically, the RS of this system is 100. Detail or extremity screen systems are relatively slow and require greater exposure and result in higher patient doses. However, the anatomic parts imaged with detail or extremity screen systems are generally small; therefore, they do not require large exposures. Detail or extremity screen systems produce excellent recorded detail. The radiographer must be careful in selecting the appropriate screen system for the ordered examination. Cassettes with extremity and detail screens should be used only for tabletop examinations. They should never be used in the Bucky tray because of the excessive amount of exposure required. (Box 5-4)

Because the film-screen system speed affects radiographic density, the mAs should be adjusted if the film-screen speed is changed. Increasing the film-screen system speed requires a decrease in the mAs to maintain radiographic density. A decrease in the film-screen system speed requires an increase in the mAs to maintain density.

 IMPORTANT RELATIONSHIP

Film-Screen System Speed and mAs

Increasing the film-screen speed requires a decrease in the mAs to maintain density. Decreasing the film-screen speed requires an increase in the mAs to maintain density.

The RS classification of film-screen systems provides a method whereby exposure techniques can be adjusted for changes in film-screen speed. The relative film-screen speed conversion formula is a mathematical formula for adjusting the mAs for changes in the film-screen system speed:

$$\frac{mAs_1}{mAs_2} = \frac{RS_2}{RS_1}$$

The correct relative film-screen speed factors must be used to calculate the new mAs required to compensate for the change in density. The new mAs then produces an exposure comparable with that of the original exposure technique.

 MATHEMATICAL APPLICATION

Adjusting mAs for Changes in Film-Screen System Speed

A quality radiograph is obtained using 10 mAs at 65 kVp and a 100-speed film-screen system. What new mAs is used to maintain radiographic density when changing to a 400-speed film-screen system?

$$\frac{10 \text{ mAs}}{X} = \frac{400 \text{ speed}}{100 \text{ speed}}$$

$$10 \text{ mAs} \times 100 \,; 1000 = 400X \,; \frac{1000}{400} = 2.5 \text{ mAs} = X$$

The remaining component in the film-screen IR is the **cassette**. Serving as a container for both the intensifying screens and the film, the cassette must be light-proof, lightweight for portability,

---

BOX 5-4   Quality-Control Check: Intensifying Screens

- Intensifying screens should produce an image with uniform density, provide uniform resolution, and not create image artifacts. Several simple quality-control procedures can be performed to monitor the performance of intensifying screens.
- A step wedge or homogeneous phantom can be imaged to evaluate the uniformity of optical densities within one screen and compare optical densities for screens of the same speed. Optical densities should be within ±0.05 throughout each image and within ±0.20 among screens of the same speed.
- A resolution test tool can be imaged to measure the spatial resolution of each screen. Intensifying screens with the same speed should visualize the same number of line pairs per millimeter.
- An ultraviolet lamp can be used to evaluate the condition of the surface of the screen. The surface should be free of dirt, stains, and defects.

---

and rigid enough not to bend under a patient's weight, all while allowing the maximum amount of radiation to pass through and reach the screens. Low x-ray-absorbing materials, such as thermoset plastic, magnesium, or even graphite carbon fiber, can be found inside the fronts of cassettes. Inside the backs of cassettes may be found thin sheets of lead foil designed to absorb backscatter before it exposes the film.

RADIOGRAPHIC FILM PROCESSING

Following the exposure of the film to radiant energy from x-rays and the light from intensifying screens, the film must be chemically processed to view the radiographic image. Automatic film processing is the method used to produce a visible permanent image.

Automatic Film Processing

The purpose of radiographic film processing is to convert the latent image into a manifest image. According to the Gurney-Mott theory, exposure of the silver bromide crystals in the film emulsion by light or x-ray photons creates the latent image and initiates the conversion process. Chemical processing of the exposed film completes the conversion process and transforms the image into a permanent visible image.

Processing Stages

An **automatic film processor** (Figure 5-3) is a device that includes chemical tanks, a roller transport system, and a dryer system for the processing of radiographic film. The processing of a radiograph occurs in four stages: developing, fixing, washing, and drying. Each stage has its specific function and implementation method (Table 5-2).

Developing

The primary function of developing is to convert the latent image into a manifest (or visible) image. The purpose of the **developing agents**, or **reducing agents**, is to reduce exposed silver halide to metallic silver and to add electrons to the exposed silver halide. Two chemicals are used to accomplish this purpose: phenidone and hydroquinone. *Phenidone* is said to be a fast reducer, producing gray (lower) densities. *Hydroquinone* is said to be a slow reducer, producing black (higher) densities. The developer solution needs an alkaline pH environment for the chemicals to properly function.

IMPORTANT RELATIONSHIP

Developing or Reducing Agents

The developing agents are responsible for reducing the exposed silver halide crystals to metallic silver, visualized as radiographic densities. Phenidone is responsible for creating the lower densities, and hydroquinone is responsible for creating the higher densities. Their combined effect results in a range of visible densities on the radiograph.

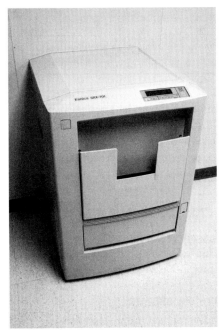

FIGURE 5-3 Type of automatic film processor used in radiography.

TABLE 5-2   Automatic Film Processing Stages
Developing
Converts latent image to a manifest or visible image
Developing or Reducing Agents
• Phenidone—faster and produces gray densities
• Hydroquinone—slower and produces black densities
Fixing
Removes unexposed silver halide from film; stops the development process; hardens the emulsion
Fixing Agent
• Ammonium thiosulfate
Washing
Removes fixing solution from surface of film
Drying
Removes 85%–90% of moisture from film

During the development process, a developer solution donates additional electrons to the sensitivity specks, or electron traps, in the emulsion layers of the film. These additional electrons attract more silver to these areas, amplifying the amount of atomic silver at each latent image center. Exposed silver halide is reduced to metallic silver when bromide and iodide ions are removed from the emulsion. The atomic silver that was exposed to radiant energy (light and x-rays) is converted to metallic silver and presented as radiographic densities. Unexposed silver halide does not immediately react to the developer because it has not been ionized and does not accept electrons from the developer. Given extended exposure to developing solution or exposure to excessively heated developing solution, however, even unexposed areas of film can react to developing solution.

Fixing

The primary functions of the fixing stage are to remove unexposed silver halide from the film and to make the remaining image permanent. In addition, there are two secondary functions of fixing. One is to stop the development process; the other is to harden the emulsion further. Fixing solution must function to remove all undeveloped silver halide while not affecting the metallic silver image.

The purpose of the **fixing agent** is to clear undeveloped silver halide from the film. A thiosulfate (sometimes referred to as *hypo*), such as ammonium thiosulfate, is the chemical used as this agent. The fixer solution needs an acidic pH environment for the chemicals to properly function.

 IMPORTANT RELATIONSHIP

Clearing the Unexposed Crystals

The fixing agent, ammonium thiosulfate, is responsible for removing the unexposed crystals from the emulsion.

Washing

The purpose of the washing process is to remove fixing solution from the surface of the film. This is a further step in making the manifest image permanent. If not properly washed, the resulting radiograph will show a brown staining of the image, resulting in image loss and a decrease in its diagnostic value. This staining is caused by thiosulfate (fixing agent) that remains in the emulsion layers. A certain amount of thiosulfate always remains within the film, but the goal of washing is to remove enough so that the radiograph can be used for an extended period.

 IMPORTANT RELATIONSHIP

Archival Quality of Radiographs

Maintaining the archival (long-term) quality of radiographs requires most of the fixing agent to be removed (washed) from the film. Staining or fading of the permanent image results when too much thiosulfate remains on the film.

The process by which washing works is referred to as *diffusion*. Diffusion exposes the film to water, which has a lower concentration of thiosulfate than the film; thus, the fixing agent diffuses into the water.

Eventually, thiosulfate concentrations in the wash water can become greater than the concentrations in the films being processed; therefore, the wash water must be frequently replaced.

Water flows freely from the input water supply through the wash tank and down the drain while the roller transport system is operating. This type of system provides a constant supply of fresh wash water to aid in the diffusion process. The moving water also causes agitation and increases diffusion.

Drying

The final process in automatic processing is drying. The purpose of drying films is to remove 85%–90% of the moisture from the film so that it can be easily handled and stored while maintaining the quality of the diagnostic image. As a result, finished radiographs should retain 10%–15% of their moisture when processing is complete. If films are excessively dried, the emulsion layers can crack, decreasing the diagnostic quality of the radiograph.

 IMPORTANT RELATIONSHIP

Archival Quality of Radiographs

> Permanent radiographs must retain a moisture content of 10%–15% to maintain archival quality. Excessive drying can cause the emulsion layers to crack.

Increased relative humidity decreases the efficiency of dryers in processors, so an increased drying temperature is necessary. Processors are equipped with thermostatic controls to allow selection of a wide range of dryer temperatures.

To chemically process a radiographic image, specialized equipment and systems must perform concurrently to move the film through the processing stages according to the manufacturer's specifications.

Processor Systems

Automatic processors use a vertical transport system of rollers that advance the film through the various stages of film processing (Figure 5-4). A film is introduced into the processor on the feed tray. The **feed tray** is a flat metal surface with an edge on either side that permits the film to easily enter the processor while remaining correctly aligned. Automatic processors use different types of rollers to move the film through the processor. Transport and crossover rollers ensure that the film is moved into and through the tanks at a constant speed.

An electric motor provides power for the roller assemblies to transport the film through the processor. The on–off switch that provides electrical power to the processor activates this motor. Most processors are also equipped with a **standby control**, which is an electrical circuit that shuts off power to the roller assemblies when the processor is not being used. Pushing the standby control switch when one is ready to process a film can reactivate the roller assemblies and water intake.

Replenishment refers to the replacement of fresh chemicals (specifically, developer solution and fixer solution) after chemical losses during processing. The replenishment of the chemicals used in the automatic processor is necessary because these chemicals eventually become exhausted or inactive, and their ability to perform their functions decreases. Developing solution becomes exhausted from both use and exposure to air, which reduces its chemical strength.

Fixer solution becomes exhausted for several reasons: it becomes weakened from use as a result of accumulations of silver halide removed from the film during the fixing process and because developer solution remains in the film, which decreases the strength and activity of the fixer solution.

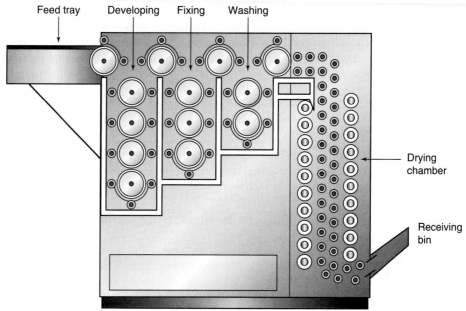

FIGURE 5-4 Cross-section of an automatic processor showing the vertical transport system of rollers.

![icon] **IMPORTANT RELATIONSHIP**

Replenishment and Solution Performance

The replenishment system provides fresh chemicals for the developing and fixing solutions to maintain their chemical activity and volume when they become depleted during processing.

The amount of solution that is replenished is preset and based on the size of the film or occurs at timed intervals. Replenishment systems are usually adjusted so that more fixer solution is replenished per film compared with developer solution.

Automatic processors have a recirculation system for the developer and fixer tanks. Each tank has a separate system that consists of a pump and connecting tubing. The **recirculation system** acts to circulate the solutions in each of these tanks by pumping solution out of one portion of the tank and returning it to a different location within the same tank from which it was removed. The recirculation system keeps the chemicals mixed, which helps to maintain solution activity and provides agitation of the chemicals around the film to facilitate fast processing.

Recirculation also helps to maintain the proper temperature of the developer solution. The developer recirculation system includes an in-line filter that removes impurities as recirculation takes place.

Temperature control of the developer solution is important because the activity of this solution depends directly on its temperature. An increase or decrease in developer temperature can adversely affect the quality of the radiographic image.

In most 90 s automatic processors, the developer temperature must be maintained at 93°F–95°F (33.8°C–35°C). An **immersion heater** is a heating coil that is immersed in the bottoms of the developer and fixer tanks. Most automatic processors are thermostatically controlled to heat the developer solution to its proper temperature and maintain that temperature as long as the processor is turned on.

> ### IMPORTANT RELATIONSHIP
> #### *Developer Temperature and Radiographic Quality*
>
> Variations in developer temperature can adversely affect the quality of the radiographic image. Increasing the developer temperature increases the density, and decreasing it decreases the density. Further, radiographic contrast may be adversely affected by changes in the developer temperature.

Radiographs must be properly dried to be viewed and stored. The film is dried by hot air that is blown onto both surfaces of the film as it moves through the dryer. This air is forced through the dryer by a blower and is directed onto the film by air tubes. The temperature of the air that is used for drying films is thermostatically monitored for accurate control of moisture removal from the film.

Inadequate processing is evidenced by certain appearances of the finished radiograph. Particular problems can be pinpointed by analyzing the radiographs. These problems and the radiographic appearances that indicate them are summarized in Table 5-3.

TABLE 5-3   Indicators of Inadequate Processing

Radiographic Appearance	Processing Problem
Decrease in density	Developer exhausted
	Developer under-replenishment
	Processor running too fast
	Low developer temperature
	Developer improperly mixed
Increase in density	Developer over-replenishment
	High developer temperature
	Light leak in processor
	Developer improperly mixed
Pinkish stain (dichroic fog)	Contamination of developer by fixer
	Developer or fixer under-replenishment
Brown stain (thiosulfate stain)	Inadequate washing
Emulsion removed by developer	Insufficient hardener in developer
Milky appearance	Fixer exhausted
	Inadequate washing
Streaks	Dirty processor rollers
	Inadequate washing
	Inadequate drying
Water spots	Inadequate drying
Minus-density scratches	Scratches from guide plates caused by roller or plate misalignment

Quality Control

Unexposed film should be stored in its original packaging so that important information about it, such as its expiration date and lot number, can be retained. Film boxes should be vertically and not horizontally stored to prevent pressure artifacts from forming on the film. Film should be stored away from heat sources and ionizing radiation. Both heat and radiation can cause the silver halide in the film emulsion to break down, resulting in fogged film. The shelf life of film, as expressed by its expiration date, must be observed. Film should not be used beyond its expiration date.

The manner in which film is handled in the darkroom can have a profound effect on radiographs. Common hazards to radiographic quality that can be found in the darkroom are white-light exposure, safelight exposure, ionizing radiation exposure, and other potential hazards.

Darkrooms must be free from all outside white-light exposure. A white-light source may be located inside the darkroom, but it should be connected to an interlock system whereby the film bin may not be opened as long as the darkroom white-light source is on. In addition, temperature and humidity can adversely affect the film. Film should be stored and handled at temperatures ranging from 55°F to 75°F (14°C to 24°C) with a relative humidity of 30%–60%. Without moisture in the air (low humidity), any build-up of static charges can expose the film.

Countertops must be clean and static-free to avoid the formation of radiographic artifacts on the films. Several brands of commercial cleaning fluids contain an antistatic component ideal for cleaning darkroom countertops and processor feed trays.

Other potential hazards to film in the darkroom include heat and chemical exposure. Film stored within the darkroom should not be near any heat source. Processing chemicals must be kept away from film and film-handling areas to prevent exposure and contamination of these areas.

Ionizing radiation exposure to film in the darkroom is a potential hazard because many darkrooms share common walls with radiographic rooms. The walls that are common between the darkroom and a radiographic room must be lined with lead as required by law for standard protection from radiographic exposures. The bin where film is stored and available for immediate use should also be lined with lead to prevent fog that may result from radiation exposure.

Safelights used in the darkroom must be equipped with a safelight filter appropriate for the type of film being handled. Commonly used filters include Kodak Wratten 6B for blue-sensitive film and Kodak GBX for orthochromatic film, which is sensitive to both blue-violet and green visible light. Safelight filters must be free of cracks, because white light that leaks from the safelight could expose the film. The power rating of the light bulbs used in safelights should be no greater than that recommended by film manufacturers (generally 7.5–15 W), which is indicated on the outside of the box of radiographic film.

Good radiographic quality cannot be achieved when film is improperly stored, mishandled before or after exposure, or incorrectly processed. Common film artifacts resulting from improper storage, darkroom handling, or improper processing are shown in Figure 5-5. Furthermore, a quality-control program must be implemented and systematically followed to ensure proper processing of radiographic film. Box 5-5 describes quality-control methods for evaluating the darkroom and film processor.

Silver Recovery

Because fixer solution is used to remove unexposed silver halide from the film, used fixer solution contains a high concentration of accumulated silver. Some type of silver recovery must be used under such conditions. **Silver recovery** refers to the removal of silver from used fixer solution. For some facilities that regularly process large volumes of radiographs, the financial rewards of silver recovery may be an added incentive.

Silver-recovery units are available for on-site silver recovery and generally require servicing by an outside contractor familiar with the equipment and its method of removing silver. These silver-recovery units are directly connected to the drain system of the fixer tank to remove silver as used fixer solution passes through the unit. After the silver has been recovered, the used fixer is drained.

Silver-recovery units work by one of two methods. The first is called *metallic replacement*. There are two types of metallic replacement silver-recovery units: one uses steel wool and the other uses a silver-extraction filter. A steel wool metallic replacement unit uses steel wool to filter the used fixer solution. Silver replaces the iron in the steel wool and can then be easily removed after significant accumulation in a canister or replacement cartridge occurs. A silver-extraction unit uses a foam filter that is impregnated with steel wool. Again, the silver from used fixer solution replaces the iron in the steel wool. A silver-extraction filter is more efficient at removing silver from used fixer and lasts longer than a simple steel wool metallic replacement unit.

The second method of silver recovery is the *electrolytic method*, and it is the most efficient one; however, the units needed for this process are more expensive than metallic replacement units. Electrolytic units have an electrically charged drum or disc that attracts silver. The silver plates onto the drum or disc and can be removed when a substantial amount of silver has been collected.

Silver is considered a heavy metal, and its disposal is regulated by local and state agencies. In many locales, strict limits are placed on the concentrations of silver in used fixer that can be

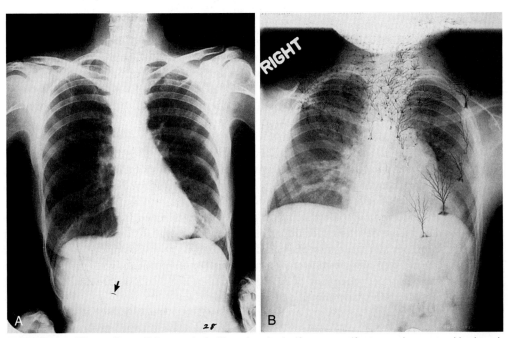

FIGURE 5-5 Film artifacts (5 images). **A,** Plus-density half-moon artifacts can be caused by bending or kinking the film *(arrow)* **B,** Plus-density static discharge artifact can be caused by sliding a film over a flat surface.

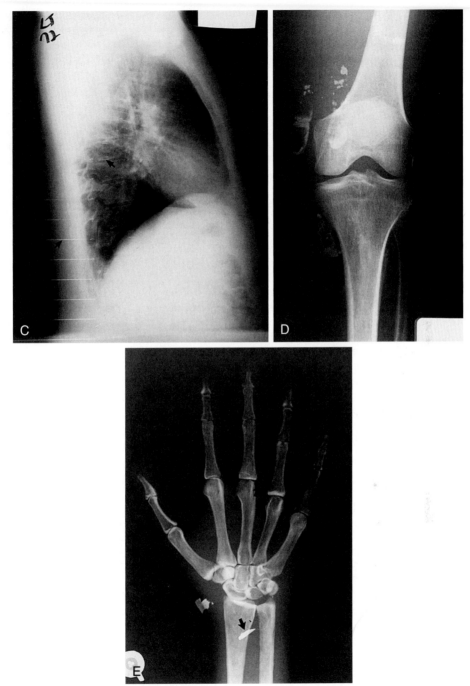

FIGURE 5-5 CONT'D C, Minus-density scratch artifacts can be caused by transport rollers *(arrows)* **D,** Minus-density caused by moisture on finger. **E,** Dirty screens or cassettes can cause nonspecific minus-density artifacts.

BOX 5-5   Quality Control: Darkroom and Film Processor

A quality-control program must be implemented and systematically followed to ensure proper processing of radiographic film. A good quality-control program should include steps for monitoring all the equipment and activities required for the production of quality radiographic images, including (but not limited to) the following:

- Sensitometric monitoring of the film processor for providing valuable information about the daily functioning of the processor.
- Following the establishment of baseline measurements, daily exposure and processing of a sensitometric strip, measurement of the appropriate optical density points with a densitometer, and plotting them on a control chart with predetermined upper and lower acceptable limits. The graph provides a visual indicator of any acute or evolving processor malfunction.
- Typically, a processor control chart should monitor B + F, medium optical density or speed, and upper and lower density differences to evaluate contrast.
- Speed and contrast indicators should not have an optical density value that varies more than ±0.15 from baseline measurements.
- B + F should not have an optical density value greater than +0.05 from the baseline measurement.
- Developer temperature should be measured daily with a digital thermometer and should not vary by more than ±0.5°F (0.3°C).
- The darkroom environment should be well ventilated, clean, organized, and safe.
- A safelight fog test should be performed semi-annually and result in an optical density of less than +0.05 due to added fog.
- Replenishment rates should be checked weekly and fall within ±5% of manufacturer's specification.
- Recommended quarterly quality-control checks include the following:
  - Developer solution pH should be maintained between 10 and 11.5.
  - Fixer pH should be maintained between 4 and 4.5.
  - Developer specific gravity should not vary by more than ±0.004 from the manufacturer's specifications.

---

disposed of via the sewer system. Silver recovery is an important process in radiology because silver is a natural resource that can be toxic to the environment and has monetary value.

 IMPORTANT RELATIONSHIP

Silver Recovery

Silver is a natural resource, is a heavy metal that can be toxic to the environment, and it must be removed from the used fixer.

SENSITOMETRY

In film-screen imaging, **sensitometry** is the study of the relationship between the intensity of radiation exposure to a film and the amount of blackness produced after processing (density). The **intensity of radiation exposure** is the measure of the quantity of radiation reaching an area of the film. Sensitometry provides a method for evaluating the characteristics of film and film-screen combinations used in radiography. Radiographic film and intensifying screen manufacturers are capable of designing film and screens to respond differently to a given intensity of radiation exposure. In particular, film and screens designed for radiography of the chest or extremities respond differently to equal amounts of radiation exposure. The radiographer should understand how the selected film and film-screen system will respond to a given intensity of exposure.

Sensitometry is also a method of evaluating the performance of automatic film processors. Because automatic film processors affect a radiograph's density and contrast, the variability of their performance can be monitored by sensitometric methods.

EQUIPMENT

Several pieces of equipment are needed to evaluate the relationship between the intensity of radiation exposure and the density produced after processing. The radiographic film should be exposed to a range of radiation intensities to evaluate its response to low, middle, and high exposures. This can be accomplished easily by passing radiation through an object that varies in thickness using a radiographic x-ray unit. The resultant effect is an image of varying uniform densities that correspond to specific intensities of radiation exposure.

Penetrometer

A **penetrometer** is a device constructed of uniform absorbers of increasing thicknesses, such as aluminium or tissue-equivalent plastic (Figure 5-6). When radiographed, the penetrometer produces a series of uniform densities that resemble a step wedge (Figure 5-7). When **step-wedge densities** are produced with a penetrometer and a radiographic x-ray unit, the variability of the output of the equipment could affect the range of densities produced.

Sensitometer

A device known as a **sensitometer** is designed to produce consistent step-wedge densities by eliminating the variability of the x-ray unit (Figure 5-8). It uses a controlled light source to expose an optical step-wedge template. The step-wedge template transmits light in varying intensities to expose the radiographic film. After the film has been processed, a density step-wedge image, or **sensitometric strip**, is produced. Penetrometers and sensitometers are available in 11-, 15-, or 21-step densities.

Densitometer

A **densitometer** is a device used to numerically determine the amount of blackness on a film after processing (i.e., it measures radiographic density). This device is constructed to emit a constant intensity of light (incident) onto an area of film and then measure the amount of light transmitted through the film (Figure 5-9). The densitometer determines the amount of light transmitted and calculates a measurement known as **optical density (OD)**.

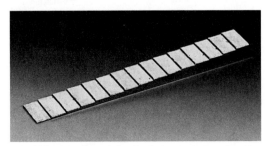

FIGURE 5-6 Penetrometer. When radiographed, a penetrometer produces an image showing a series of uniform densities.

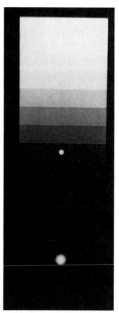

FIGURE 5-7 Radiograph of a penetrometer showing step-wedge densities.

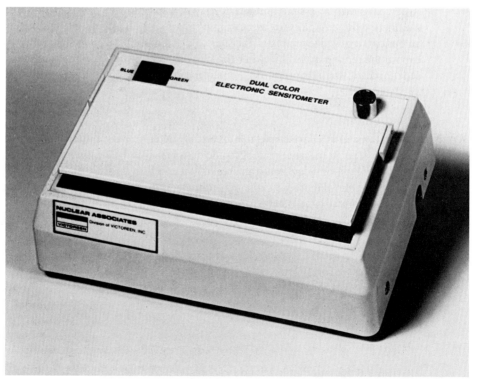

FIGURE 5-8 A sensitometer is designed to produce consistent step-wedge densities.

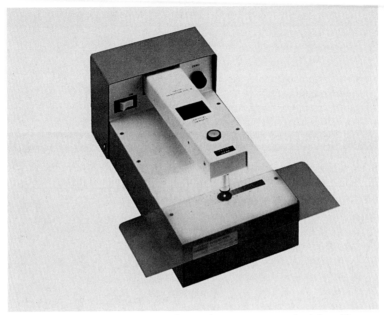

FIGURE 5-9 A densitometer is used to measure optical densities.

OPTICAL DENSITY

Optical density is represented as a numerical calculation that compares the amount of light transmitted through an area of radiographic film to the amount of light originally striking (incident on) the film. Box 5-6 shows the mathematical formula used for light transmittance. Because the range of radiographic densities is large, the calculation of radiographic densities is compressed onto a logarithmic scale (Table 5-4) for easier management.

A film that allows 100% of the original incident light to be transmitted has a logarithmic value of 0. A film that allows only 1% of the original incident light through has a logarithmic value of 2.0. This logarithmic value of light transmittance is termed *optical density*. The formula used to calculate optical density is shown in Box 5-7.

Notice the relationship between light transmittance and optical density (Table 5-4). When 100% of the light is transmitted, the optical density equals 0.0. When 50% of the light is transmitted, the optical density is equal to 0.3, and when 25% of the light is transmitted, the optical density equals 0.6. When a logarithmic scale base of 10 is used, every change of 0.3 in optical density corresponds to a change in the percentage of light transmitted by a factor of 2 ($\log_{10}$ of 2 = 0.3).

Optical densities can range from 0.0 to 4.0 OD. Because most radiographic film has a tint added to its base and processing adds a slight amount of fog, the lowest amount of optical density is usually between 0.10 and 0.20 OD. This minimum amount of density on the radiographic film is termed **base plus fog (B + F)**.

Diagnostic Range

The useful range of optical densities is between 0.25 and 2.5 OD. However, the diagnostic range of optical densities for general radiography usually falls between 0.5 and 2.0 OD. This desired range of optical densities is found between the extreme low and high densities produced on the film.

TABLE 5-4 **Percentage of Light Transmittance and Calculated Optical Densities**

Percentage of Light Transmitted ($I_t/I_o \times 100$)	Fraction of Light Transmitted (I_t/I_o)	Optical Density ($\log I_o/I_t$)
100	1	0
50	$1/2$	0.3
32	$8/25$	0.5
25	$1/4$	0.6
12.5	$1/8$	0.9
10	$1/10$	1
5	$1/20$	1.3
3.2	$4/125$	1.5
2.5	$1/40$	1.6
1.25	$1/80$	1.9
1	$1/100$	2
0.5	$1/200$	2.3
0.32	$2/625$	2.5
0.125	$1/80$	2.9
0.1	$1/1000$	3
0.05	$1/2000$	3.3
0.032	$2/3125$	3.5
0.01	$1/10,000$	4

SENSITOMETRIC CURVE

When the optical density measurements from a sensitometric strip are graphed on semilogarithmic paper, the result is a curve characteristic of the radiographic film type. Box 5-8 lists other terms used for the **sensitometric curve**.

This sensitometric curve visually demonstrates the relationship between the intensity of radiation exposure (x-axis) and the resultant optical densities (y-axis) (Figure 5-10). The position of the curve on the x-axis and its shape can vary greatly and depends on the type of radiographic film used.

BOX 5-8 **Other Terms for Sensitometric Curve**

Characteristic curve
D log E curve
H & D curve
Hurter & Driffield curve

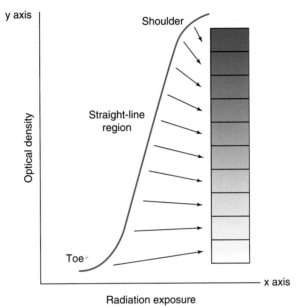

FIGURE 5-10 Plotting optical densities corresponding to the change in intensity of exposure results in a curve characteristic of the type of the film.

Log of Relative Exposure

When sensitometric methods are used to evaluate the characteristics of radiographic film, it is more useful to measure the intensity of radiation exposure in increments of a constant change, such as doubling or halving. For every doubling or halving change in the percentage of light transmitted, a change of 0.3 occurs in optical density. Along the x-axis, for every change of 0.3 in log relative exposure, the intensity of radiation exposure changes by a factor of 2 (Figure 5-11). When Figure 5-11 is used as an example, the relative mAs (the product of milliamperage and exposure time) value is 32 for a log of exposure of 1.5, and the relative mAs value is 64 for a log of exposure of 1.8. This relationship can be demonstrated throughout the log relative exposure scale on the sensitometric curve. Two exposures, one double the other, will always be separated by 0.3 on the logarithmic exposure scale.

Regions

A sensitometric curve demonstrates three distinct regions (Figure 5-12). When the characteristics of different types of radiographic film are evaluated, differences will be demonstrated within any of these regions.

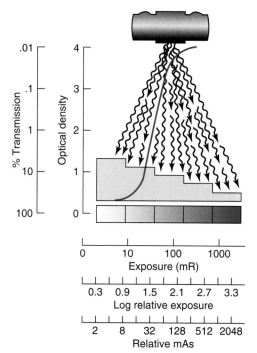

FIGURE 5-11 A sensitometric curve is created by plotting the optical density values obtained from the range of exposures that are used to create the step-wedge densities. The logarithmic relative exposure value representing the change in exposure by a factor of 2 is a more useful value than the milliroentgen (mR) exposure or relative mAs.

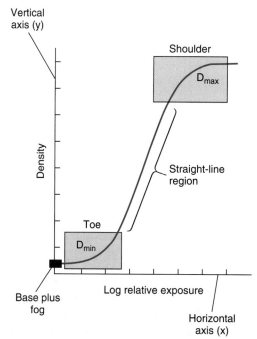

FIGURE 5-12 The sensitometric curve demonstrates three distinct regions: toe, straight-line, and shoulder.

Toe Region

The **toe region** of the sensitometric curve represents the area of low density. The point on the sensitometric curve where a minimum amount of radiation exposure produced a minimum optical density is known as D_{min}. Generally, D_{min} will be equal to B + F even though they represent two different measurements. Changes in exposure intensity in this region have little effect on the optical density.

Straight-Line Region

At a certain point along the x-axis, changes in exposure begin to have a much greater effect on the optical density. This **straight-line region** is where the diagnostic or most useful range of densities is produced.

Shoulder Region

There is a point on the sensitometric curve where changes in exposure intensity no longer affect the optical density. In this **shoulder region**, the point on the curve where maximum density has been produced is known as D_{max}. Once the maximum density achievable within the film has been reached (D_{max}), continued increases in exposure intensity begin to reverse the optical density. This process is called *solarization*, and it is used in the design of duplicating film.

FILM CHARACTERISTICS

Comparing sensitometric curves in these regions provides information about three important characteristics of radiographic film. Each film characteristic plays an important role in radiographic imaging.

Speed

An important characteristic of radiographic film is its sensitivity to radiation exposure, which is referred to as its **speed**. The speed of a film indicates the amount of optical density produced for a given amount of radiation exposure. It is a characteristic of the film's sensitivity to the intensity of radiation exposure.

Speed Point

Typically, the speed of radiographic film is determined by locating the point on a sensitometric curve that corresponds to the optical density of 1.0 plus B + F. This point is called the **speed point** (Figure 5-13). This optical density point is used because it is within the straight-line portion of the sensitometric curve. The speed point serves as a standard method of indicating film speed.

Speed Exposure Point

When comparing film types, the radiographer must determine what log of exposure produces the speed point. This can be determined by drawing a line from the sensitometric curve speed point to the area on the x-axis (log of exposure) that produced the optical density at 1.0 plus B + F (Figure 5-14). This important point, called the **speed exposure point**, indicates the intensity of exposure needed to produce a density of 1.0 plus B + F (speed point). A film that has a speed exposure point of 0.9 is faster than a film having a speed exposure point of 1.2.

Figure 5-15 presents two sensitometric curves and their respective speed and speed exposure points. A faster-speed film is positioned to the left (closer to the y-axis) of slower-speed film.

It is important to remember that the speed of the film is determined by the amount of exposure (log of exposure) needed to produce an optical density of 1.0 plus B + F, regardless of the shape of the sensitometric curve (Figure 5-16).

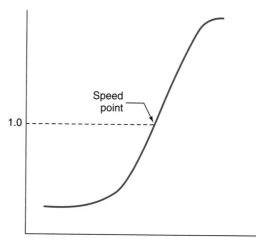

FIGURE 5-13 The sensitometric curve speed point indicates the intensity of exposure needed to produce a density of 1.0 plus B + F.

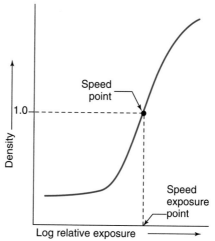

FIGURE 5-14 The speed exposure point indicates the intensity of exposure needed to produce a density of 1.0 plus B + F (speed point).

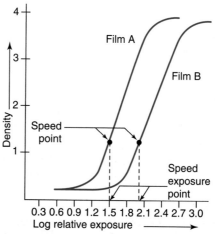

FIGURE 5-15 Obtaining the same speed point requires that *Film A* should have a log of exposure of 1.5 and *Film B* should have a log of exposure of 2.0. Faster-speed films are located to the left of slower-speed films.

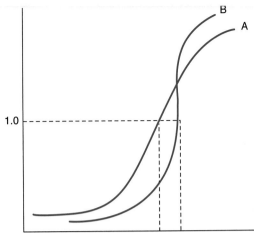

FIGURE 5-16 As the shape of the sensitometric curve varies, the speed can also vary if it is measured at points other than the standard of 1.0 plus B + F.

BOX 5-9 Determining the Slope of a Line

$$\text{Slope} = \frac{Y\,(\text{rise})}{X\,(\text{run})}, \quad \frac{y_2 - y_1}{x_2 - x_1}$$

The slope of a line mathematically indicates its tilt or slant. Comparisons of the slope (mathematical calculation) can be made among different lines. For radiography, the higher the number, the steeper the slope, and the lower the number, the lesser the slope.

Contrast

Radiographic contrast is a result of both the subject contrast and the **film contrast**. Film contrast is controlled by the design and manufacture of film components and the effects of processing. The ability of a radiographic film to provide a level of contrast can be evaluated by the steepness, or **slope**, of the sensitometric curve. The slope of this line mathematically indicates the ratio of the change in y (optical density) for a unit change in x (log relative exposure) (Box 5-9).

Visually comparing the steepness (slope) of the straight-line region of the curve provides a method of evaluating the level of contrast produced by a film (Figure 5-17). Radiographic film capable of producing higher contrast will have a more vertical straight-line region (steeper slope). General-purpose radiographic film is categorized as either high contrast or medium contrast.

Gradient Point

Determining the slope along any portion of the sensitometric curve provides information about the contrast produced at that point, which is called the **gradient point**. Gradient points can be determined for any region of the sensitometric curve, such as the toe, middle, and shoulder. The gradient point can be determined by calculating the slope of the line (change in optical density divided by the change in log exposure) at any portion of the curve.

Average Gradient

When comparing films, the radiographer typically determines contrast by calculating the sensitometric curve's **average gradient** of the slope of the straight-line region (Figure 5-18). A standard used in sensitometry is to determine the film contrast between the optical densities of 0.25 and 2.0

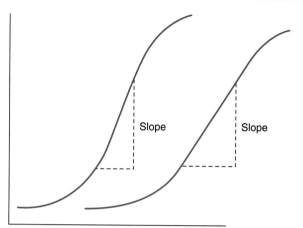

FIGURE 5-17 The slope of the straight-line region determines the inherent film contrast. Steeper slopes indicate higher contrast.

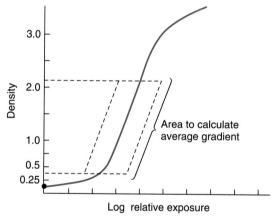

FIGURE 5-18 A film's average gradient is calculated between a low density (0.25 plus B + F) and a high density (2.0 plus B + F).

plus B + F. Finding the difference between these two points and dividing by the difference between their respective logarithms of exposure provides a numerical calculation for film contrast. Most radiographic films have an average gradient between 2.5 and 3.5; film contrast is higher for a film with an average gradient of 3.0 than one with an average gradient of 2.7.

Exposure Latitude

Exposure latitude refers to the range of exposures that produce optical densities within the straight-line region of the sensitometric curve (Figure 5-19). Radiographic films that are capable of responding to a wide range of exposures to produce optical densities within the straight-line region are considered wide-latitude films. When comparing a film with narrow latitude to one with wide latitude, it is apparent that a film with narrow latitude is a higher-contrast film and a film with wide latitude is a lower-contrast film (Figure 5-20). A steep slope has a small range of exposures available to produce densities within the straight-line region, whereas a less steep slope has a greater range of such exposures.

When selecting what type of radiographic film to use, the radiographer should evaluate its characteristics in terms of speed, contrast, and latitude. Radiographic film used in chest

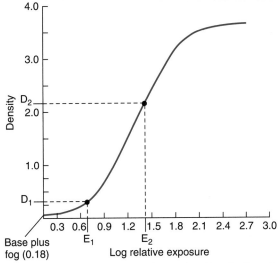

FIGURE 5-19 A film's exposure latitude can be determined by finding the range of exposures that will produce densities within the straight-line region of the curve. The use of a low and high density similar to those used to calculate average gradient would provide optical densities within the straight-line region of the sensitometric curve.

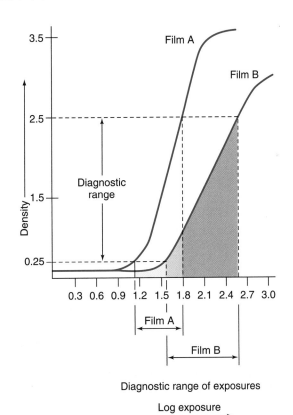

Diagnostic range of exposures

FIGURE 5-20 A higher-contrast film, *Film A*, has a narrower range of exposures available to pro-duce optical densities within the straight-line region compared with a lower-contrast film, *Film B*.

radiography typically requires lower contrast and wider-exposure latitude, whereas film designed for use in extremity radiography requires higher contrast, resulting in a narrow exposure latitude. The speed of radiographic film is considered in combination with the intensifying screen speed to provide a film-screen system speed.

CLINICAL CONSIDERATIONS

To provide radiographic images of optimal quality, the radiographer must appropriately control the visibility factors of density and contrast. A relationship exists between density and contrast to maximize the amount of visible recorded detail.

Optimal Density

For a given anatomic area to be radiographed, the selected exposure techniques should produce radiographic densities that lie within the straight-line region of the sensitometric curve. Optical densities within this range maximize the amount of information visible within the radiographic image, resulting in **optimal density**.

The challenge for radiographers is to determine the amount of radiation exposure necessary to produce optical densities within the straight-line region of a film's sensitometric curve. Different types of radiographic film may require different amounts of exposure to produce such densities. As previously demonstrated, it may take more or less radiation exposure to produce an optical density of 1.0 plus B + F for Film A as compared with Film B. Therefore, the relationship between radiation exposure and optical density depends on the shape and position of a film's sensitometric curve.

For a given type of radiographic film, when optical densities lie within the straight-line region of the sensitometric curve, a change in the exposure technique has a direct effect on optical density (Figure 5-21). When optical densities lie outside the straight-line region, a greater or lesser change in exposure technique may be needed to move the optical densities back within the diagnostic range (0.5–2.0 OD); therefore, when evaluating a radiograph with a density error, the radiographer must determine the amount of change needed in the exposure technique.

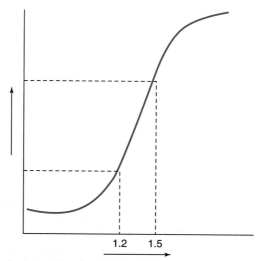

1.2   1.5

FIGURE 5-21 When optical densities lie within the straight-line region of the curve, a change in log exposure of 0.3 (change by a factor of 2) directly affects optical densities.

In diagnostic radiology, one type of film is typically used for most procedures. Access to a film's sensitometric curve for the purpose of calculating exposure changes is not practical. Therefore it is the radiographer's responsibility to use the standard guidelines (discussed in Chapter 6) regarding exposure changes to correct for density errors.

Maximum Film Contrast

Film contrast is the difference in optical density between two points anywhere along the sensitometric curve (Figure 5-22). If these differences in optical density were to be plotted as points between the x- and y-axes, the result would be a film's contrast curve (Figure 5-23). When the contrast curve is evaluated, it is apparent that **maximum contrast** (the greatest difference in optical densities) is achievable within the straight-line region of the sensitometric curve. When optical densities of the anatomic area of interest lie outside the straight-line region, film contrast is decreased. When optical densities lie within the straight-line region of the sensitometric curve, the film has reached its maximum capability in visualizing recorded detail.

In summary, sufficient radiographic density is needed to visualize recorded detail. A film's maximum radiographic contrast can be visualized only when optical densities lie within the straight-line region of the sensitometric curve. When optical densities lie outside this region, film contrast is decreased. When both optimum density and maximum contrast have been achieved, the visibility of recorded details is of optimal radiographic quality. See Box 5-10 for Practical Tips.

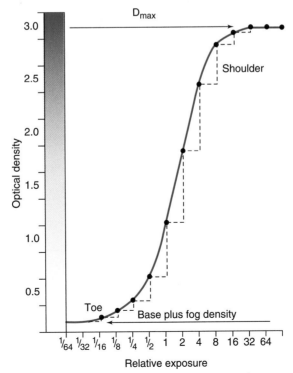

FIGURE 5-22 Density differences calculated along the sensitometric curve can be used to evaluate film contrast.

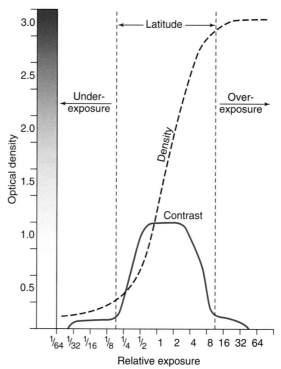

FIGURE 5-23 Plotting the density differences of a sensitometric curve results in a contrast curve. Maximum film contrast is achieved within the straight-line region.

BOX 5-10 Practical Tips

Sensitometric Curve Position Along the X-Axis
Sensitometric curves of faster-speed film are positioned to the left of slower-speed film, and sensitometric curves of slower-speed film are positioned to the right of faster-speed film.

Changes in Exposure Technique to Correct for Density Errors
To correct for the density error, optical densities that lie outside the straight-line region of the sensitometric curve (toe or shoulder region) require a greater or lesser change in exposure than those that lie within the straight-line region.

Achieving Maximum Film Contrast
To achieve the maximum contrast that the film is capable of producing, the radiographer must ensure that the optical densities lie within the straight-line region of the sensitometric curve.

Image Display

In order to view a processed film image, it must be displayed on an illuminator. **Illuminators**, or viewboxes, are devices that provide light illumination so that the anatomy, displayed as various shades of optical densities, can be visualized.

Illuminators

The dimensions of an illuminator are typically 14 × 17 in (35 × 43 cm) and can be individually arranged or combined in rows as a bank of illuminators (Figure 5-24). The most important

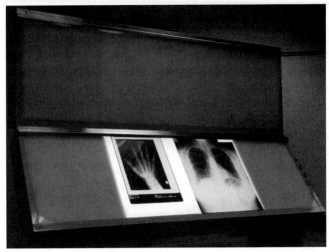

FIGURE 5-24 Bank of illuminators.

performance criterion of film illuminators is the uniformity of light intensity within and among viewboxes. Variations in light emission can affect the visibility of anatomic detail, and therefore, maintaining clean and damage-free viewboxes along with proper bulb wattage is essential for quality control.

CHAPTER SUMMARY

- In film-screen imaging, film serves as the medium for image acquisition, processing, and display.
- A film image is displayed on a polyester sheet of plastic composed of densities resulting from exposed crystals converted to black metallic silver after chemical processing.
- Silver halide crystals suspended in a film's emulsion layer absorb the radiant energy (x-rays and visible light) and form a latent image.
- Film is placed in a cassette between two intensifying screens, permitting lower x-ray exposures compared with film alone.
- The intensifying screen phosphors emit visible light (fluoresce) in proportion to the exit radiation to expose the film.
- Intensifying screens can be manufactured to have varying speeds. Increasing intensifying screen speed reduces not only the required radiation exposure but also the recorded detail in the image.
- Automatic film processing incorporates several chemical stages and systems to convert a latent image into a manifest image.
- Hydroquinone and phenidone are chemical reducing agents used during the developing stage to convert the exposed silver halide crystals to black metallic silver.
- Ammonium thiosulfate is the chemical fixing agent to clear undeveloped crystals from the film's emulsion.
- Maintaining the archival quality of radiographs requires that most of the fixing agent be washed from the film.
- During the drying stage, 85%–90% of the moisture needs to be removed from the film for long-term storage.

- Important systems for processing films include replenishment, chemical recirculation, temperature control, and a transport system to move the film through the tanks at a constant speed.
- Film should be stored and handled in a darkroom at temperatures ranging from 55°F to 75°F (14°C to 24°C) and with a relative humidity of 30%–60%. Without moisture in the air (low humidity), any build-up of static charges can expose the film.
- Safelights used in the darkroom must be equipped with a safelight filter appropriate for the type of film being handled.
- Silver recovery can be accomplished by the electrolytic method or metallic replacement and is an important process because silver is a natural resource, is a heavy metal that can be toxic to the environment, and must be removed from the used fixer.
- Sensitometry is the study of the relationship between radiation exposure and the amount of density produced after a film is chemically processed.
- Optical density is a measurement of the amount of light transmitted through an area on the film.
- Radiographic film can be manufactured to differ in terms of speed, contrast, latitude, and spectral sensitivity.
- Speed is the sensitivity of film to radiation and has a direct relationship with optical density. The location of the sensitometric curve along the x-axis indicates its speed.
- The slope of the straight-line portion of a sensitometric curve (average gradient) will indicate the film's level of contrast; the steeper the slope, the higher the contrast.
- Exposure latitude refers to the range of exposures that produce optical densities in the straight-line portion of the sensitometric curve and is inversely related to contrast. Higher-contrast films have narrower exposure latitudes.
- When both optimum density and maximum contrast have been achieved, the visibility of recorded detail is of optimal radiographic quality.
- Radiographic films are displayed on illuminators that emit uniform light intensity.

REVIEW QUESTIONS

1. Which of the following is the latent image center for radiographic film?
   A. Phosphor layer
   B. Polyester base
   C. Detector element
   D. Sensitivity speck
2. Which of the following describes a film's sensitivity to x-rays or light?
   A. Gamma
   B. Speed
   C. Contrast
   D. Latitude
3. Intensifying screens are used to _____.
   A. decrease patient exposure
   B. increase recorded detail
   C. increase film latitude
   D. decrease contrast
4. The ability to emit light only when stimulated by x-rays is known as _____.
   A. phosphorescence
   B. sensitometry
   C. conversion efficiency
   D. fluorescence

5. What reducing agent acts slowly to produce the higher densities on a film radiograph?
   A. Ammonium thiosulfate
   B. Hydroquinone
   C. Phenidone
   D. Cesium iodide

6. What chemical agent is responsible for clearing the unexposed silver halide crystals during film processing?
   A. Ammonium thiosulfate
   B. Hydroquinone
   C. Phenidone
   D. Cesium iodide

7. Which automatic processing system primarily maintains the chemical activity level?
   A. Replenishment
   B. Standby control
   C. Recirculation
   D. Quality control

8. Why is silver recovery necessary during film processing?
   A. It is a natural resource.
   B. It is toxic to the environment.
   C. It has monetary value.
   D. All of the above

9. What term is defined as a measure of the amount of light transmitted through the film?
   A. Sensitometry
   B. Film contrast
   C. Film speed
   D. Optical density

10. What is the diagnostic range of optical densities?
    A. 0.15 to 4.0
    B. 0.5 to 1.25
    C. 0.5 to 2.0
    D. 0.10 to 2.0

11. A change of _____ in optical density results from a change in the percentage of light transmittance by a factor of 2.
    A. 0.03
    B. 0.3
    C. 3.0
    D. 30

12. Changes in radiation exposure have the greatest effect on optical densities in which sensitometric region?
    A. Toe
    B. Shoulder
    C. Straight-line
    D. Toe and Shoulder

13. When the exposure technique used produces densities outside the straight-line portion of a sensitometric curve, how was contrast affected?
    A. Increased
    B. No effect
    C. Decreased
    D. Improved

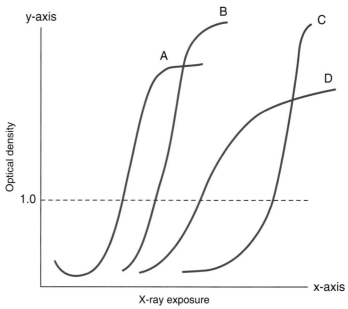

FIGURE 5-25 Film types and sensitometric graphs (A–D). The shape and position of the graph along the x-axis displays the differing characteristics of film speed, contrast, and latitude.

14. Compare the sensitometric curves in Figure 5-25. Which film is faster?
    A. Film A
    B. Film B
    C. Film C
    D. Film D
15. Compare the sensitometric curves in Figure 5-25. Which film has lower contrast?
    A. Film A
    B. Film B
    C. Film C
    D. Film D
16. Film B has an exposure speed point of 1.5, and Film A has an exposure speed point of 1.2. Is there a difference in speed?
    A. Film A is twice as fast as Film B.
    B. Film A and B have equal speed.
    C. Film A is half as fast as Film B.
    D. Film B is twice as fast as Film A.

Exposure Technique Factors

CHAPTER OUTLINE

Primary Factors
  Milliamperage and Exposure
    Time
  Kilovoltage Peak
Secondary Factors
  Focal Spot Size

Source-to-Image-Receptor
  Distance
Object-to-Image-Receptor
  Distance
Calculating Magnification
Central Ray Alignment
Grids

Beam Restriction
Generator Output
Tube Filtration
Compensating Filters
Patient Factors
  Body Habitus
  Part Thickness

OBJECTIVES

After completing this chapter, the reader will be able to perform the following:

1. Define all the key terms in this chapter.
2. State all the important relationships in this chapter.
3. Explain the relationship between milliamperage and exposure time with radiation production and image receptor (IR) exposure.
4. Calculate changes in milliamperage and exposure time to change or maintain exposure to the IR.
5. Compare the effect of changes in milliamperage (mA) and exposure time on digital and film-screen images.
6. Recognize how to correct exposure factors for a density error.
7. Explain how kilovoltage peak (kVp) affects radiation production and IR exposure.
8. Calculate changes in kVp to change or maintain exposure to the IR.
9. Compare the effects of changes in kVp on digital and film-screen images.
10. Recognize the factors that affect spatial resolution and distortion.
11. Calculate changes in mAs for changes in source-to-image-receptor distance.
12. Calculate the magnification factor, and determine image and object size.
13. Describe the use of grids and beam restriction and their effect on IR exposure and image quality.
14. Calculate changes in mAs when adding or removing a grid.
15. Recognize patient factors that may affect IR exposure.
16. Identify exposure factors that can affect patient radiation exposure.
17. State exposure technique modifications for the following considerations: body habitus and patient thickness.

KEY TERMS

15% rule
body habitus
exposure indicator
inverse-square law
magnification factor (MF)

mAs/distance compensation
formula
object-to-image-receptor
distance (OID)

source-to-image-receptor
distance (SID)
source-to-object distance
(SOD)

In Chapter 2, variables that affect both the quantity and the quality of the x-ray beam were presented. Milliamperage and exposure time affect the quantity of radiation produced, and kilovoltage affects both the quantity and the quality. Chapter 3 emphasized that a good-quality radiographic image accurately represents the anatomic area of interest. The characteristics evaluated for image quality are brightness, contrast, spatial resolution, distortion, and noise. This chapter focuses on exposure techniques and the use of accessory devices and their effects on the radiation reaching the image receptor (IR) and the image produced. Radiographers have the responsibility of selecting the combination of exposure factors to produce a good-quality image. Knowledge of how these factors affect the exposure to the IR individually and in combination assists the radiographer in producing a radiographic image with the amount of information desired for a diagnosis.

Because various types of IRs respond differently to the radiation exiting the patient, these differences are noted throughout this chapter. Digital IRs separate acquisition from processing and image display; their response to changes in radiation exposure does not affect the amount of brightness displayed on the image. The level of brightness and contrast can be altered during computer processing and image display. However, the amount of exposure to the digital IR needs to be carefully selected, as with film-screen IRs, to produce a quality image with the lowest amount of exposure to the patient. Radiographic film acquires the latent image and needs to be chemically processed before the image can be displayed. Changes in the quantity and quality of radiation exposure to a film-screen IR affect the amount of density and contrast visible on the processed radiograph. This chapter discusses all the primary and secondary factors and their effects on the radiation reaching the IR.

PRIMARY FACTORS

The primary exposure technique factors selected by the radiographer on the control panel are milliamperage (mA), exposure time, and kilovoltage peak (kVp). Depending on the type of control panel, milliamperage and exposure time may be selected separately or combined as one factor, milliamperage·second (mAs). Regardless, it is important to understand how changing each factor separately or in combination affects the radiation reaching the IR and the radiographic image.

Milliamperage and Exposure Time

The quantity of radiation reaching the patient affects the amount of remnant radiation reaching the IR. The product of milliamperage and exposure time is directly proportional to the quantity of x-rays produced. Once an anatomic part is adequately penetrated, the exposure to the IR will increase in proportion to increases in the quantity of x-rays (Figure 6-1). Conversely, when the quantity of x-rays is decreased, the exposure to the IR decreases. Therefore, exposure to the IR can be increased or decreased by adjusting the amount of radiation (mAs).

 IMPORTANT RELATIONSHIP

mAs and Quantity of Radiation

As mAs increases, the quantity of radiation reaching the IR increases. As mAs decreases, the amount of radiation reaching the IR decreases.

Because the mAs is the product of milliamperage and exposure time, increasing either milliamperage or time will have the same effect on the radiation exposure.

 MATHEMATICAL APPLICATION

Adjusting Milliamperage or Exposure Time

$$200 \text{ mA} \times 0.1 \text{ s} = 20 \text{ mAs}$$

To increase the mAs to 40, one could use the following formulas:

$$400 \text{ mA} \times 0.1 \text{ s} = 40 \text{ mAs}$$

$$200 \text{ mA} \times 0.2 \text{ s} = 40 \text{ mAs}$$

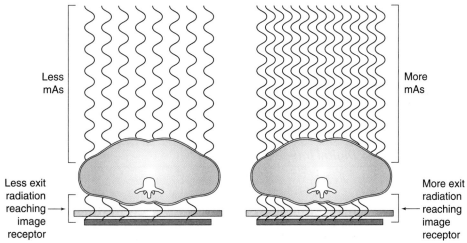

FIGURE 6-1 The mAs and radiation exposure. As the quantity of x-rays is increased (mAs), the exposure to the image receptor proportionally increases.

As demonstrated in the Mathematical Application, mAs can be doubled by doubling either the milliamperage or the exposure time. A change in either milliamperage or exposure time proportionally changes the mAs. To maintain the same mAs, the radiographer must increase the milliamperage and proportionally decrease the exposure time.

IMPORTANT RELATIONSHIP

Milliamperage and Exposure Time

Milliamperage and exposure time have an inversely proportional relationship when maintaining the same mAs.

 MATHEMATICAL APPLICATION

Adjusting Milliamperage and Exposure Time to Maintain mAs

$$200 \text{ mA} \times 100 \text{ ms} \ (0.1 \text{ s}) = 20 \text{ mAs}$$

To maintain mAs, use the following formulas:

$$400 \text{ mA} \times 50 \text{ ms} \ (0.05 \text{ s}) = 20 \text{ mAs}$$

$$100 \text{ mA} \times 200 \text{ ms} \ (0.2 \text{ s}) = 20 \text{ mAs}$$

It is important for the radiographer to determine the appropriate mAs level needed to produce a diagnostic image. This is not an easy task because there are so many variables that can affect the required mAs. For example, single-phase generators produce less radiation with the same mAs compared with high-frequency generators. A patient's age, the general condition of the patient, and the thickness of the anatomic part also affect the mAs required for a procedure. In addition, IRs respond differently for a given mAs level. Digital IRs can detect a wide range of radiation intensities (wide dynamic range) exiting the patient and are not as dependent on the mAs as film-screen IRs. However, exposure errors can adversely affect the quality of a digital image. If the mAs is too low (low exposure to the digital IR), image brightness is adjusted during computer processing to achieve the desired level. Even after adjusting the level of brightness, there may be increased quantum noise visible within an image (Figure 6-2). If the selected mAs is too high (high exposure to the digital IR), the brightness can also be adjusted; however, the patient will receive more radiation than necessary.

 IMPORTANT RELATIONSHIP

mAs and Digital Image Brightness

The level of mAs does not directly affect image brightness when using digital IRs. During computer processing, image brightness is maintained when the mAs is too low or too high. A lower-than-needed mAs produces an image with increased quantum noise, and a higher-than-needed mAs exposes a patient to unnecessary radiation.

The brightness of a digital image can be altered during image processing; hence, information about the exposure to the IR is important. Manufacturers of each type of digital system specify the expected range of x-ray exposure sufficient to produce a quality image. A numerical value (**exposure indicator**) is displayed on the processed image to indicate the level of x-ray exposure received (incident exposure) on the digital IR. It is important for the radiographer to consider the indicated value because exposure errors, as previously stated, affect the quality of the digital image and the radiation dose to the patient. Exposure errors are not obvious by simply looking at the digital image, because the digital data are normalized to provide images with diagnostic density and brightness. Most manufacturers of digital IRs suggest a range for the exposure indicator on the basis of the radiographic procedure. If the exposure indicator value falls outside this range, image quality, patient exposure, or both could be compromised.

IMPORTANT RELATIONSHIP

Exposure Indicator Value

A numerical value or exposure indicator is displayed on the processed digital image to indicate the level of x-ray exposure received (incident exposure) on the IR. If the exposure indicator value falls outside the manufacturer's suggested range, image quality, patient exposure, or both could be compromised.

For film-screen IRs, the mAs directly controls the density produced in the image. When mAs is increased, density is increased; when the mAs is decreased, density is decreased (Figure 6-3).

When a film image is too light (insufficient density), an increase in mAs may be needed to correct the density; when a film image has excessive density, the mAs may need to be decreased. When using a film-screen IR, radiographers need to assess the level of density produced on the processed image and determine whether the density is sufficient to visualize the anatomic area of interest. The radiographer must decide how much of a change in mAs is needed to correct the density error.

Generally, for repeat radiographs necessitated by density errors, the mAs is adjusted by a factor of 2; therefore, a minimum change involves doubling or halving the mAs. This change typically changes the film densities to best visualize the anatomic area of interest. Usually, radiographs with sufficient but not optimal density are not repeated. In addition, if a radiograph must be repeated because of another error, such as positioning, the radiographer may use the opportunity to adjust the density to produce a radiograph of optimal quality. Making a visible change in radiographic density requires the minimum amount of change in mAs to be approximately 30% (depending on equipment, this may vary between 25% and 35%). Radiographic images generally are not repeated to make only a slight visible change. A radiographic image repeated because of insufficient or excessive density requires a change in mAs by a factor of at least 2.

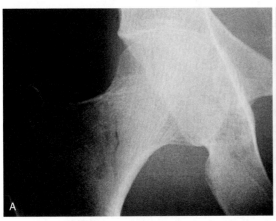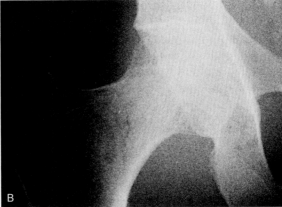

FIGURE 6-2 A, Radiograph obtained with high mAs showing decreased quantum noise. **B,** Radiograph obtained with low mAs showing increased quantum noise.

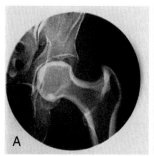 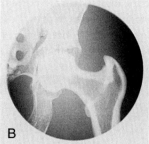 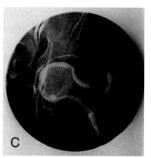

FIGURE 6-3 Changes in mAs have a direct effect on density. **A,** Original image. **B,** Decrease in density when the mAs is decreased by half. **C,** Increase in density when the mAs is doubled.

 IMPORTANT RELATIONSHIP

mAs and Film-Screen Density

The amount of mAs has a direct effect on the amount of radiographic density produced when using a film-screen IR. The minimum change needed to correct a density error is determined by multiplying or dividing the mAs by 2.

To best visualize the anatomic area of interest, the selected mAs must produce a sufficient amount of radiation that reaches the IR, regardless of type. An excessive or insufficient amount of mAs adversely affects image quality and patient radiation exposure.

Kilovoltage Peak

The kVp affects the exposure to the IR because it alters the amount and penetrating ability of the x-ray beam. The area of interest must be adequately penetrated before the mAs can be adjusted to produce a quality radiographic image. When adequate penetration is achieved, increasing the kVp further results in more radiation reaching the IR. In addition to affecting the amount of radiation exposure to the IR, the kVp affects image contrast.

IMPORTANT RELATIONSHIP

kVp and the Radiographic Image

Increasing or decreasing the kVp changes the amount of radiation exposure to the IR and the contrast produced within the image.

Kilovoltage Peak and Exposure to the Image Receptor

Because kVp affects the amount of radiation reaching the IR, its effect on the digital image is similar to the effect of mAs. Assuming that the anatomic part has been adequately penetrated, too much radiation reaching the IR (within reason) will still produce a digital image with the appropriate level of brightness as a result of computer adjustment during image processing; however, the patient will be overexposed. Similarly, too little radiation reaching the IR (within reason) will produce a digital image with the appropriate level of brightness, but the increased quantum noise will decrease the image quality. Excessive or insufficient radiation exposure to the digital IR, as a result of the mAs or kVp, should be reflected in the exposure indicator value.

IMPORTANT RELATIONSHIP

Exposure Errors in Digital Imaging

kVp and mAs exposure errors should be reflected in the exposure indicator value; however, image brightness can be maintained during computer processing.

 Radiation Protection Alert

Excessive Radiation Exposure and Digital Imaging

Although the computer can adjust image brightness for technique exposure errors, routinely using more radiation than required for the procedure in digital radiography unnecessarily increases patient exposure. Even though the digital system can adjust overexposure, it is an unethical practice to knowingly overexpose a patient.

The kVp has a greater effect on the image when using film-screen IRs. Increasing the kVp increases the IR exposure and density produced on a film image, and decreasing the kVp decreases the IR exposure and density produced on a film image (Figure 6-4).

For film-screen IRs, kVp has a direct relationship with density; however, the effect of the kVp on density is not equal throughout the range of kVp (low, middle, and high). A greater change in the kVp is needed when operating at a high kVp (>90) compared with operating at a low kVp (<70) (Figure 6-5).

 IMPORTANT RELATIONSHIP

Exposure Errors and Film-Screen Imaging

kVp directly affects the density produced on a film-screen image; however, its effect is not equal throughout the range of kVp (low, middle, and high).

Kilovoltage is not a factor that is typically manipulated to vary the amount of IR exposure because the kVp also affects contrast. However, it is sometimes necessary to manipulate the kVp

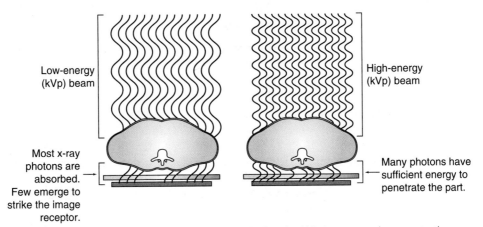

FIGURE 6-4 The kVp and radiation exposure. Increasing the kVp increases the penetrating power of the radiation and increases the exposure to the image receptor.

to maintain the required exposure to the IR. For example, using portable or mobile x-ray equipment may limit the choice of mAs settings, and the radiographer must adjust the kVp to maintain sufficient exposure to the IR.

Maintaining or adjusting exposure to the IR can be accomplished with kVp using the **15% rule**. The 15% rule states that increasing or decreasing the kVp by 15% has the same effect as doubling or halving the mAs; for example, increasing the kVp from 82 to 94 (15%) produces a similar exposure to the IR as increasing the mAs from 10 to 20.

 IMPORTANT RELATIONSHIP

kVp and the 15% Rule

A 15% increase in kVp has the same effect on exposure to the IR as doubling the mAs. A 15% decrease in kVp has the same effect on exposure to the IR as halving the mAs.

Increasing the kVp by 15% increases the exposure to the IR, unless the mAs is decreased. In addition, decreasing the kVp by 15% decreases the exposure to the IR, unless the mAs is increased.

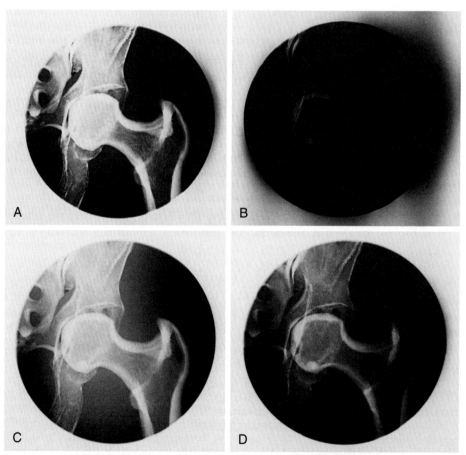

FIGURE 6-5 The kVp range and radiographic density. **A–D,** Radiographs produced at 50 kVp **(A)** and at 90 kVp with the mAs adjusted to maintain radiographic density **(C)**; a 10 kVp increase at 50 kVp **(B)** produces a greater change in density than a 10 kVp increase at 90 kVp **(D)**.

As mentioned earlier, the effects of changes in the kVp are not uniform throughout the range of kVp. When a low or high kVp is used, the amount of change required to maintain the exposure to the IR may be greater or less than 15%.

 MATHEMATICAL APPLICATION

Using the 15% Rule

To increase exposure to the IR, multiply the kVp by 1.15 (original kVp + 15%):

$$75 \text{ kVp} \times 1.15 = 86 \text{ kVp}.$$

To decrease exposure to the IR, multiply the kVp by 0.85 (original kVp − 15%):

$$75 \text{ kVp} \times 0.85 = 64 \text{ kVp}.$$

To maintain exposure to the IR, when increasing the kVp by 15% (kVp × 1.15), divide the original mAs by 2:

$$75 \text{ kVp} \times 1.15 = 86 \text{ kVp} \text{ and mAs/2}.$$

When decreasing the kVp by 15% (kVp × 0.85), multiply the mAs by 2:

$$75 \text{ kVp} \times 0.85 = 64 \text{ and mAs} \times 2.$$

 Radiation Protection Alert

kVp/mAs

Whenever possible, a higher kilovoltage and lower mAs should be used to reduce patient exposure. Increasing kilovoltage requires a lower mAs to maintain the desired exposure to the IR and decreases the radiation dose to the patient. For example, changing KVp from 75 to 86 when imaging a pelvis is a 15% increase and would require half the mAs needed for the original 75 kVp. Higher kVp increases the beam penetration, and therefore, less radiation is needed to achieve a desired exposure to the IR.

Kilovoltage Peak and Radiographic Contrast

Altering the penetrating power of the x-ray beam affects its absorption and transmission through the anatomic tissue being radiographed. Higher kVp increases the penetrating power of the x-ray beam and results in less absorption and more transmission in the anatomic tissues, which results in less variation in the x-ray intensities exiting the patient (lower subject contrast). As a result, images with lower contrast (more shades of gray) are produced (Figure 6-6). When a low kVp is used, the x-ray beam penetration is decreased, resulting in more absorption and less transmission, which results in greater variation in the x-ray intensities exiting the patient (higher subject contrast). A high-contrast (fewer shades of gray) radiographic image is produced (Figure 6-7).

 IMPORTANT RELATIONSHIP

kVp and Radiographic Contrast

A high kVp results in less absorption and more transmission in anatomic tissues, which results in less variation in the x-ray intensities exiting the patient (lower subject contrast), producing a low-contrast image. A low kVp results in more absorption and less x-ray transmission but with more variation in the x-ray intensities exiting the patient (higher subject contrast), producing a high-contrast image.

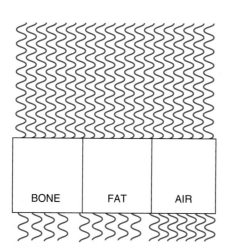

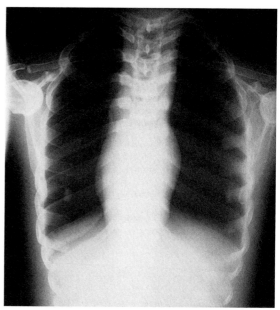

FIGURE 6-6 The kVp and exit-beam intensities. Higher kVp increases the penetrating power of the x-ray beam and results in less absorption and more transmission in the anatomic tissues, resulting in less variation in the x-ray intensities exiting the patient. As a result, images with lower contrast are produced.

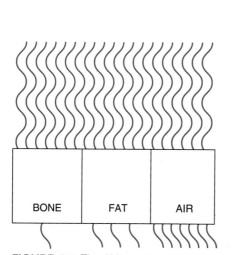

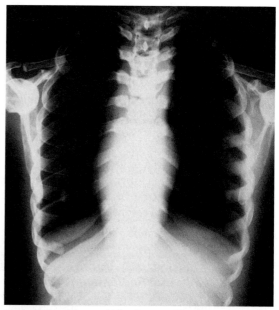

FIGURE 6-7 The kVp peak and exit-beam intensities. Lower kVp decreases the x-ray beam penetration, resulting in more absorption and less transmission, which results in greater variation in the x-ray intensities exiting the patient. As a result, images with higher contrast are produced.

In digital imaging, the kVp affects the variation in radiation intensities exiting the patient and image contrast; however, image brightness and contrast are primarily controlled during computer processing. When a low kVp is selected, the brightness and contrast are adjusted, but quantum noise may be visible. On the other hand, when a high kVp is selected, the image brightness and contrast are adjusted, but patient exposure may be increased. Although image contrast can be adjusted when using a high kVp, increased scatter radiation reaches the IR and may adversely affect image quality.

 IMPORTANT RELATIONSHIP

Kilovoltage and Digital Image Quality

Assuming that the body part has been adequately penetrated, changing the kVp affects the radiation exposure to the digital IR in a way similar to changing mAs; but unlike mAs, kVp also affects image contrast. However, image brightness and contrast are primarily controlled during computer processing.

Changing the kVp affects the beam's absorption and transmission as it interacts with anatomic tissue; however, using a higher kVp reduces the total number of interactions and increases the amount of x-rays transmitted. In these interactions, Compton scattering occurs more than x-ray absorption (photoelectric effect) and more scatter exits the patient. It is important to understand that in addition to kVp changing the subject contrast, it affects the amount of scatter reaching the IR and consequently, the radiographic contrast.

 IMPORTANT RELATIONSHIP

Kilovoltage, Scatter Radiation, and Radiographic Contrast

At higher kVp, more x-rays are transmitted with fewer overall interactions; however, a greater proportion of the interactions are from Compton scattering than x-ray absorption (photoelectric effect), which decreases the radiographic contrast. Decreasing the kVp will increase x-ray absorption and increase the number of interactions, but the proportion of Compton scattering will decrease compared to photoelectric interactions, increasing radiographic contrast.

The level of radiographic contrast desired—and therefore the kVp selected—depends on the type and composition of the anatomic tissue, the structures that must be visualized, and (to some extent) the type of IR. These factors make achieving a desired level of radiographic contrast more complex than achieving a desired level of exposure to the IR, especially for film-screen imaging. Radiographic film can be manufactured to display different levels of contrast. In addition to the type of film used, the selected kVp controls the level of contrast produced in the image.

For most anatomic regions, an accepted range of kVp provides an appropriate level of radiographic contrast. As long as the selected kVp is sufficient to penetrate the anatomic part, the kVp can be further manipulated to alter the radiographic contrast.

Radiographs are generally not repeated because of contrast errors. More often, the radiographer evaluates the level of contrast achieved to improve the contrast for additional radiographs or similar circumstances that arise with a different patient. If a repeat radiograph is necessary and kVp is to be adjusted either to increase or decrease the level of contrast, the 15% rule provides an acceptable method of adjustment. In addition, whenever a change of 15% is made in the kVp to maintain the exposure to the IR, the radiographer must adjust the mAs by a factor of 2. Note that a 15% change in kVp does not produce the same effect across the entire range of kVp used in radiography. A greater increase is needed for a high kVp (≥90) than for a low kVp (<70).

The selection of kVp alters its absorption and transmission through the anatomic part, regardless of the type of IR used; therefore, kVp must be wisely selected. Exposure techniques using higher kVp with lower mAs exposure techniques are recommended in digital imaging because contrast is primarily controlled during computer processing. Higher kVp and lower mAs values are not recommended as a general rule during film-screen imaging because of the contrast required to best visualize the anatomic structures.

SECONDARY FACTORS

Many secondary or influencing factors affect the amount of radiation reaching the IR and the image quality. It is important for the radiographer to understand their effects individually and in combination.

Focal Spot Size

On the control panel, the radiographer can select whether to use a small or large focal spot size. The physical dimensions of the focal spot on the anode target in x-ray tubes used in standard radiographic applications usually range from 0.5 to 1.2 mm. Small focal spot sizes are usually 0.5 or 0.6 mm, and large focal spot sizes are usually 1 or 1.2 mm. Focal spot size is determined by the filament size. When the radiographer selects a particular focal spot size, he/she is actually selecting a filament size that is energized during x-ray production. Focal spot size is an important consideration for the radiographer because it affects spatial resolution (Figure 6-8).

 IMPORTANT RELATIONSHIP

Focal Spot Size and Spatial Resolution

As focal spot size increases, unsharpness increases and spatial resolution decreases; as focal spot size decreases, unsharpness decreases and spatial resolution increases.

Generally, the smallest available focal spot size should be used for every exposure. However, exposure is limited for a small focal spot size. When a small focal spot is used, the heat created during the x-ray exposure is concentrated into a smaller area and could cause tube damage. The radiographer must weigh the importance of improved spatial resolution for a particular examination or anatomic part against the amount of radiation exposure used. Modern radiographic x-ray generators are equipped with safety circuits that prevent an exposure from being made if that exposure exceeds the tube loading capacity for the selected focal spot size. Repeated exposures made just under the limit over a long period can still jeopardize the life of the x-ray tube.

Source-to-Image-Receptor Distance

The distance between the radiation source and the IR, known as **source-to-image-receptor distance (SID)**, affects the amount of radiation reaching the patient. Because of the divergence of the x-ray beam, the intensity of the radiation varies at different distances.

This relationship between distance and x-ray beam intensity is best described by the **inverse-square law**. This law states that the intensity of an x-ray beam is inversely proportional to the square of the distance from the source. Because beam intensity varies as a function of the square

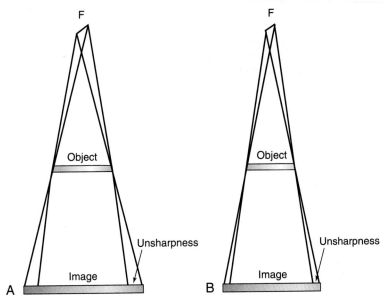

FIGURE 6-8 Focal spot size and spatial resolution. Focal spot size influences the amount of unsharpness recorded in the image. As focal spot size changes, so does the amount of unsharpness. **A,** Larger focal spot. **B,** Smaller focal spot.

of the distance, SID affects the quantity of radiation reaching the IR. As SID increases, the x-ray intensity becomes spread over a larger area, decreasing the overall intensity of the x-ray beam reaching the IR (Figure 6-9).

 IMPORTANT RELATIONSHIP

SID and X-ray Beam Intensity

As SID increases, the x-ray beam intensity becomes spread over a larger area. This decreases the overall intensity of the x-ray beam reaching the IR.

MATHEMATICAL APPLICATION

Inverse Square Law Formula

$$\frac{I_1}{I_2} = \frac{(D_2)^2}{(D_1)^2}$$

If the intensity of radiation at an SID of 40 in is equal to 400 mR, what is the intensity of radiation when the distance is increased to 72 in?

$$\frac{400 \text{ mR}}{X} = \frac{(72)^2}{(40)^2} \quad 400 \text{ mR} \times 1600 = 640,000 = 5184 \text{ X}; \quad \frac{640,000}{5184} = X; 123.5 \text{ mR} = X$$

Because increasing the SID decreases x-ray beam intensity, the mAs must be accordingly increased to maintain proper exposure to the IR. When the SID is decreased, the beam intensity increases; therefore, the mAs must be accordingly decreased to maintain proper exposure to the IR.

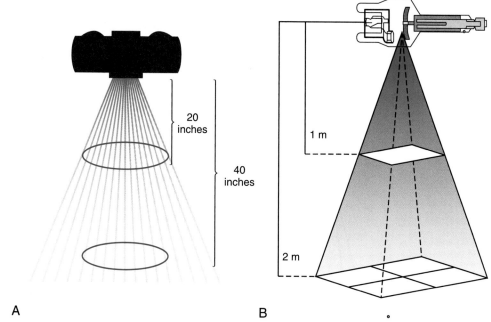

A   B

FIGURE 6-9 SID and radiation intensity. **A** and **B,** Changing SID and its effect on the intensity of the x-ray beam reaching the image receptor **(A)** and on the divergence of the beam **(B)**.

⚡ IMPORTANT RELATIONSHIP

SID and mAs

Increasing the SID requires the mAs to be increased to maintain exposure to the IR, and decreasing the SID requires a decrease in the mAs to maintain exposure to the IR.

Maintaining consistent radiation exposure to the IR when the SID is altered requires the mAs to be adjusted to compensate. The **mAs–distance compensation formula** provides a mathematical calculation for adjusting the mAs when changing the SID.

▶▶ MATHEMATICAL APPLICATION

mAs–Distance Compensation Formula

$$\frac{mAs_1}{mAs_2} \frac{(SID_1)^2}{(SID_2)^2}$$

Optimal exposure to the IR is achieved at an SID of 40 in using 25 mAs. The SID must be increased to 72 in. What adjustment of mAs is needed to maintain exposure to the IR?

$$\frac{25}{X} = \frac{(40)^2}{(72)^2} \;;\; 1600X = 129{,}600 \;;\; \frac{129{,}600}{1600} \;;\; X = 81 \; mAs_2$$

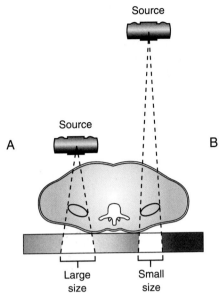

FIGURE 6-10 SID and size distortion. **A** and **B,** A long SID creates less magnification than a short SID. The image in **A** is larger than that in **B** because the object is closer to the source.

Standard distances are used in radiography to provide more consistency in radiographic quality. Most diagnostic radiography is performed at an SID of 40, 48, or 72 in. Certain circumstances, such as trauma or mobile radiography, do not permit the use of standard distances. In these circumstances, the radiographer must determine the change needed in the mAs to obtain a quality radiograph. When a 72 in (180 cm) SID cannot be used, adjusting the SID to 56 in (140 cm) requires half the mAs. When a 40 in (100 cm) SID cannot be used, adjusting the SID to 56 in (140 cm) requires twice the mAs. This quick method of calculating mAs changes should produce sufficient exposure to the IR.

In addition to altering the intensity of radiation, SID affects image distortion and spatial resolution regardless of the type of IR. As the distance between the source and the IR increases, the diverging x-rays become more perpendicular to the object being radiographed and thus reduce the size distortion produced on the radiograph (Figure 6-10).

> ### IMPORTANT RELATIONSHIP
> #### SID, Size Distortion, and Spatial Resolution
>
> As SID increases, size distortion (magnification) decreases and spatial resolution increases; as SID decreases, size distortion (magnification) increases and spatial resolution decreases.

Standard distances for SID are used in radiography to accommodate equipment limitations. Except for chest and cervical spine radiography, a 40 in (100 cm) or 48 in (120 cm) SID is standard. A larger 72 in (180 cm) SID, such as that used for chest imaging, decreases the magnification of the heart and records its size more accurately.

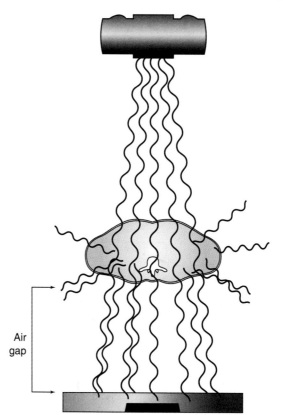

Air
gap

FIGURE 6-11 OID and air gap. The distance created between the object and the image receptor reduces the amount of scattered radiation reaching the image receptor.

Object-to-Image-Receptor Distance

When distance is created between the object being radiographed and the IR, known as **object-to-image-receptor distance (OID)**, a decrease in beam intensity may result. As the exit radiation continues to diverge, less overall intensity of the x-ray beam reaches the IR. Decreasing the exposure to the IR may require an increase in the mAs to compensate.

When sufficient distance between the object and IR exists, an air gap is created, also preventing the scatter radiation from striking the IR (Figure 6-11). Whenever the amount of scatter radiation reaching the IR is reduced, the radiographic contrast is increased. This effect on contrast is more visible for anatomic areas that produce a high percentage of scatter radiation exiting the patient. Reducing the scattered radiation reaching the IR by increasing the OID has a greater effect on contrast for film-screen IRs compared with digital IRs.

In addition to affecting the intensity of radiation reaching the IR, the OID affects the amount of image distortion and spatial resolution. Optimal spatial resolution is achieved when the OID is zero. However, this OID cannot realistically be achieved in radiographic imaging because there is always some distance created between the area of interest and the IR. As the exit beam leaves the patient, it continues to diverge. When distance is created between the area of interest and the IR, the diverging exit beam records the anatomic part with increased size distortion or magnification (Figure 6-12).

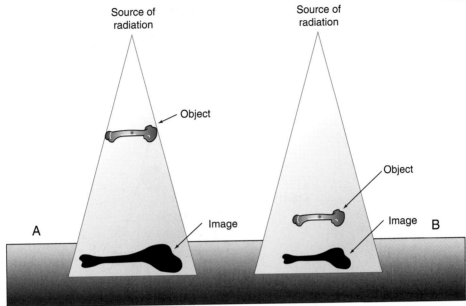

FIGURE 6-12 OID and size distortion. **A** and **B,** A long OID creates more magnification than a short OID. The image in **A** is larger than that in **B** because the object is farther from the image receptor.

IMPORTANT RELATIONSHIP

OID, Size Distortion, and Spatial Resolution

Increasing the OID increases magnification and decreases the spatial resolution, whereas decreasing the OID decreases magnification and increases the spatial resolution.

OID is a factor that affects the intensity of radiation reaching the IR, image contrast, magnification, and spatial resolution. The distance between the area of interest and the IR has the greatest effect on the amount of size distortion. The radiographer must position the area of interest as close to the IR as possible to minimize the distortion. Although the OID necessary to adversely affect image quality has not been standardized, the radiographer should minimize the OID whenever possible. In certain situations, it is difficult to minimize OID because of factors or conditions beyond the radiographer's control. In these situations, size distortion can still be reduced by increasing the SID.

Calculating Magnification

To observe the effect of distance (SID and OID) on size distortion, it is necessary to consider the **magnification factor (MF)**. This factor indicates how much size distortion or magnification is demonstrated on a radiograph. The MF can be mathematically expressed by the following formula:

$$MF = SID \div SOD.$$

Source-to-object distance (SOD) refers to the distance from the x-ray source (focal spot) to the object being radiographed. SOD can be mathematically expressed as follows:

$$SOD = SID - OID.$$

SOD is demonstrated in Figure 6-13.

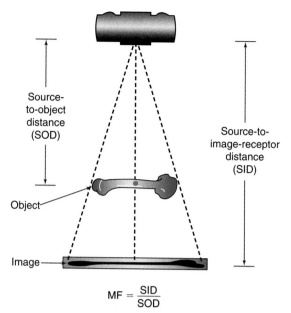

$$MF = \frac{SID}{SOD}$$

FIGURE 6-13 SOD. The SOD is the distance between the source of the x-ray and the object being radiographed.

An MF of 1 indicates no magnification, meaning that the image size matches the true object size. True object size on a radiograph is impossible to achieve because some magnification exists on every radiograph. MF values greater than 1 can be expressed as percentages of magnification. For example, an MF of 1.15 indicates that the image size is 15% larger than the object size.

⟫ MATHEMATICAL APPLICATION

Magnification Factor

An anteroposterior projection (AP) of the knee is produced with a SID of 40 in and an OID of 3 in (SOD is equal to 37 in). What is the MF?

$$SOD = SID - OID, \quad MF = \frac{40}{37}; \quad MF = 1.081,$$
$$37 = 40 - 3$$

In the case of the Mathematical Application for MF, an MF of 1.081 means that the image size is 8.1% larger than the true object size. It should be noted that the MF computed here is a minimum. A 3 in OID implies that the posterior surface of a patient's knee was 3 in away from the IR for an anteroposterior (AP) projection. Anatomy that is anterior to the posterior surface of the knee, such as the patella, is farther away from the IR and is magnified even more.

It may be helpful to know the measurement of the true object size in comparison with its size on a radiographic image. Once the MF is known, the object size can be determined. This requires the use of another formula:

$$Object\ size = \frac{Image\ size}{MF}.$$

MATHEMATICAL APPLICATION

Determining Object Size

On an AP image of a knee taken with an SID of 40 in and an OID of 3 in (SOD = 37 in), the size of a lesion measures 0.5 in in diameter on the radiograph. The MF has been determined to be 1.081. What is the object size of this lesion?

$$\frac{40}{37} = 1.081 \text{ MF} \quad \text{Object size} = \frac{0.5 \text{ inch}}{1.081}$$

The object size is 0.463 in.

If the sizes of both the object and the image are known, then the percentage of magnification of the object can be calculated by the following formula:

$$\text{Object \% of Magnification} = \frac{\text{Image size} - \text{Object size}}{\text{Object size}} \times 100.$$

 MATHEMATICAL APPLICATION

Determining Object % of Magnification

A lesion on the radiographic image measures 1.16 cm and the lesion's (object's) true size measures 1.06 cm. What is the object % of magnification?

$$\text{Object \% of magnification} = \frac{1.16 - 1.06}{1.06 \text{cm}} \times 100$$

$$\frac{0.10}{1.06} = 0.09434 \times 100 = 9.43\% \text{ object magnification}$$

Perhaps the most practical use of these formulas is to observe how changing the SID and OID affects the image size. Size distortion or magnification can be increased by decreasing the SID or increasing the OID. This increase in magnification can be mathematically demonstrated using the MF, and then calculating the change in the size of the object on the radiographic image. Any time magnification is increased, spatial resolution decreases.

Central Ray Alignment

Shape distortion of the anatomic area of interest can occur from inaccurate central ray (CR) alignment of the tube, the part being radiographed, or the IR. Any misalignment of the CR among these three factors alters the shape of the part recorded on the image.

For example, Figure 6-14 demonstrates shape distortion when the anatomic part and the IR are misaligned. In addition, shape distortion can occur if the CR of the primary beam is not directed to enter or exit the anatomy as required for the particular projection or position (off centring). This shape distortion occurs because the path of individual photons in the primary beam becomes more divergent as the distance increases from the CR. The radiographer must properly control alignment of the tube, part, and IR, and he/she must properly direct the CR to minimize shape distortion. In addition to creating shape distortion, CR angulation and misalignment of the tube, part, and IR could affect the exposure to the IR. For example, when the CR is angled, the

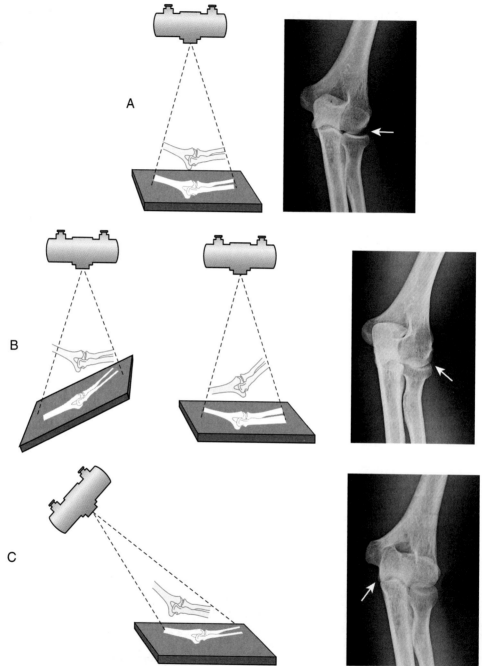

FIGURE 6-14 A, Proper alignment among the x-ray tube, part, and image receptor. Image **A** is a quality image with minimal distortion. Note the proper alignment of the radial head with the capitulum in the image. **B,** Improper alignment among the x-ray tube, part, and image receptor. The illustration on the left shows the image receptor misaligned to the part, and the one on the right shows the part not parallel to the image receptor. Image **B** has a distorted shape due to misalignment of the part and image receptor. Note the improper alignment of the radial head with the capitulum in the image. **C,** Improper alignment among the x-ray tube, part, and image receptor. Image **C** has shape distortion due to the central ray not being perpendicular to the part. Note the elongation of the olecranon process.

distance between the source of the radiation and the IR is increased. Generally, when the CR is angled, the SID is accordingly decreased to maintain exposure to the IR. If misalignment occurs among the tube, part, or IR, the distance between the source of radiation and the IR or the part and the IR could be increased or decreased. This change could affect the amount of exposure to the IR and the mAs may need adjustment.

Grids

A radiographic grid is a device that is placed between the anatomic area of interest and the IR to absorb scatter radiation exiting the patient. Limiting the amount of scatter radiation that reaches the IR improves the quality of the image. Much of the scatter radiation exiting the patient does not reach the IR when absorbed by a grid (Figure 6-15). The effect of less scatter, or unwanted exposure, on the image is to increase the radiographic contrast (Figure 6-16).

 IMPORTANT RELATIONSHIP

Grids, Scatter, and Contrast

Placing a grid between the anatomic area of interest and the IR absorbs scatter radiation exiting the patient and increases radiographic contrast.

The more efficient a grid is in absorbing scatter, the greater is its effect on radiographic contrast. Grids also absorb a certain amount of the transmitted radiation exiting the patient and therefore reduce the amount of radiation reaching the IR.

 IMPORTANT RELATIONSHIP

Grids and Image Receptor Exposure

Adding, removing, or changing a grid requires an adjustment in mAs to maintain radiation exposure to the IR.

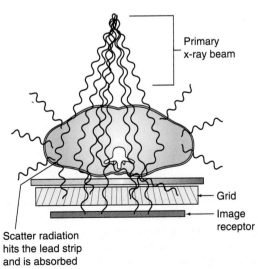

Primary x-ray beam

Grid

Image receptor

Scatter radiation hits the lead strip and is absorbed

FIGURE 6-15 Grids and scatter absorption. When a grid is used, much of the scatter radiation toward the image receptor is absorbed.

When grids are used, the mAs must be adjusted to maintain exposure to the IR. In addition, the more efficient a grid is in absorbing scatter, the greater is the increase in mAs. The grid conversion formula is a mathematical formula for adjusting the mAs for changes in the type of grid.

When a grid is added, the radiographer must multiply the mAs by the correct grid conversion factor (Table 6-1) to compensate for the decrease in exposure. When a grid is removed, the mAs must be divided by the correct conversion grid factor to compensate for the increase in exposure. When the grid ratio is changed, the following formula should be used to adjust the exposure:

$$\frac{\text{mAs}_1}{\text{mAs}_2} = \frac{\text{Grid conversion factor}_1}{\text{Grid conversion factor}_2}.$$

Grid construction and efficiency are discussed in greater detail in Chapter 7.

 MATHEMATICAL APPLICATION

Adjusting mAs for Changes in the Grid

A quality radiograph is obtained using 5 mAs at 70 kVp without using a grid. What new mAs is needed when adding a 12:1 grid to maintain the same exposure to the IR?

$$\frac{5\text{mAs}}{X} = \frac{1}{5}; 1X = 25; X = 25 \text{ mAs}.$$

The new mAs produces an exposure comparable with the IR.

! Radiation Protection Alert

Grid Selection

Decisions regarding the use of a grid and grid ratio should be made by balancing image quality and patient protection. To keep patient exposure as low as possible, grids should be used only when appropriate, and the grid ratio should be the lowest that would provide sufficient contrast improvement.

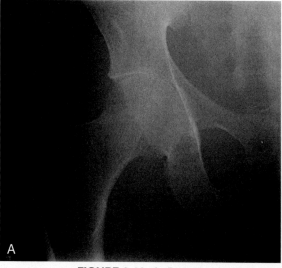 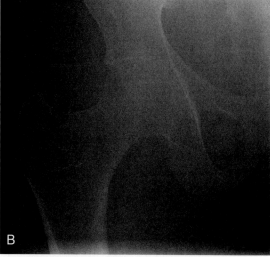

FIGURE 6-16 A, Radiograph obtained using a grid. **B,** Radiograph obtained without a grid.

TABLE 6-1 Grid Conversion Chart	
Grid Ratios	**Grid Conversion Factor (GCF)**
No grid	1
5:1	2
6:1	3
8:1	4
12:1	5
16:1	6

Beam Restriction

Any change in the size of the x-ray field alters the amount of tissue irradiated. A larger field size (decreasing collimation) increases the amount of tissue irradiated, causing more scatter radiation to be produced, thus increasing the amount of radiation reaching the IR. The increased amount of scatter reaching the IR results in less radiographic contrast. Conversely, a smaller field size (increasing collimation) reduces the amount of tissue irradiated, the amount of scatter radiation produced, and the amount of radiation reaching the IR. The decreased amount of scatter radiation reaching the IR results in higher radiographic contrast but requires an increase in the mAs. The effect of collimation is greater when imaging large anatomic areas, performing examinations without a grid, and using a high kVp.

 IMPORTANT RELATIONSHIP

Beam Restriction and Image Receptor Exposure

Changes in beam restriction alter the amount of tissue irradiated and therefore affect the amount of exposure to the IR. The effect of collimation is greater when imaging large anatomic areas, performing examinations without a grid, and using a high kVp.

! **Radiation Protection Alert**

Beam Restriction

In performing a radiographic examination, the radiographer should be aware of the anatomic area of interest and limit the x-ray field size to just beyond this area. Collimating to the appropriate field size is a basic method for protecting patients from unnecessary exposure.

Generator Output

Exposure techniques and radiation output depend on the type of generator used. Generators with more efficient output, such as three-phase or high-frequency units, require lower exposure technique settings to produce an image comparable with single-phase units. The radiographer must be aware of the generator output when using different types of equipment, especially when performing examinations in different departments. For example, imaging a knee using a single-phase generator requires more mAs than imaging a knee using a three-phase generator. In addition, x-ray generators must be periodically calibrated to ensure that they are producing consistent radiation output.

Tube Filtration

Small variations in the amount of tube filtration should not have any effect on radiographic quality. Variability of the x-ray tube filtration should be checked as a part of routine quality control checks on the radiographic equipment. X-ray tubes with excessive or insufficient filtration may affect image quality. Increasing the amount of tube filtration increases the ratio of higher-penetrating x-rays to lower-penetrating x-rays. As a result, the average energy of the x-ray beam has been increased and can increase the amount of scatter radiation reaching the IR. The increased x-ray energy (kVp) and scatter production decrease radiographic contrast. In addition, increasing the tube filtration will decrease the quantity of radiation reaching the patient and the IR. Insufficient tube filtration will increase the quantity of radiation and decreases the ratio of higher-penetrating x-rays to lower-penetrating x-rays. As a result, the average energy of the x-ray beam has been decreased, which can decrease the amount of scattered radiation reaching the IR. The decreased x-ray energy (kVp) and scatter production increase radiographic contrast. The amount of tube filtration should not vary greatly, and therefore, small changes would not have a visible effect on radiographic contrast.

 IMPORTANT RELATIONSHIP

Tube Filtration, Radiation Quantity, and Energy

Increasing tube filtration will decrease radiation quantity and increase the average energy of the x-ray beam. Decreasing tube filtration will increase radiation quantity and decrease the average energy of the x-ray beam.

Compensating Filters

When imaging an anatomic area that varies greatly in tissue thickness, a compensating filter can be placed in the primary beam to produce a more uniform exposure to the IR. The use of compensating filters requires an increase in the mAs to maintain the overall exposure to the IR. The amount of increase in the mAs depends on the thickness and type of compensating filter. In addition, the use of a compensating filter increases the exposure to the patient.

PATIENT FACTORS

Body Habitus

Body habitus refers to the general form or build of the body, including its size. It is important for the radiographer to consider body habitus when establishing exposure techniques. There are four types of body habitus: sthenic, hyposthenic, hypersthenic, and asthenic (Figure 6-17).

The sthenic body habitus accounts for approximately 50% of the adult population and is commonly called a *normal* or *average* build. The hyposthenic type accounts for approximately 35% of adults and refers to a similar type of body habitus as sthenic but with a tendency toward a more slender and taller build. Together, the sthenic and hyposthenic types of body habitus are, in terms of establishing radiographic techniques, classified as *normal* or *average* for adult population. These two types of body habitus account for approximately 85% of adults.

Hypersthenic and asthenic body habitus types are more extreme and are less common. The hypersthenic body habitus—a large, stocky build—accounts for only 5% of adults. These individuals have thicker part sizes compared with sthenic or hyposthenic individuals, so the exposure factors for their radiographic examinations are higher.

Asthenic refers to a very slender body habitus and accounts for only 10% of adults. Exposure factors for asthenic individuals are at the low end of technique charts because their respective part sizes are thinner than those of sthenic and hyposthenic individuals.

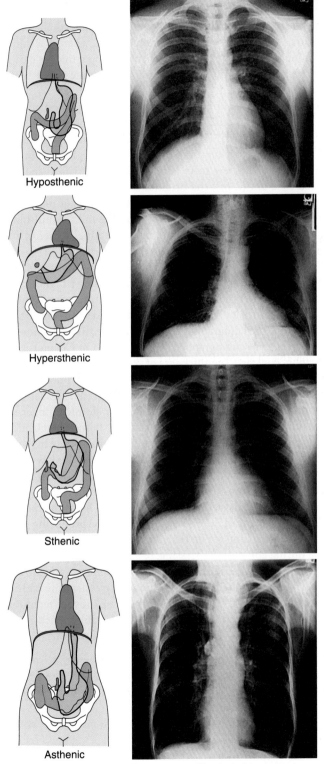

FIGURE 6-17 Four types of body habitus.

Part Thickness

The thickness of the anatomic part being imaged affects the amount of x-ray beam attenuation that occurs. A thick part absorbs more radiation, whereas a thin part transmits more radiation. Maintaining the exposure to the IR when imaging a thicker part requires the mAs to be accordingly increased. In addition, when a thinner anatomic part is being radiographed, the mAs must be accordingly decreased.

Because x-rays are exponentially attenuated, a general guideline is that for every change in part thickness of 4–5 cm (1.6–2 in), the radiographer should adjust the mAs by a factor of 2. For example, an optimal radiograph is obtained using 20 mAs on an anatomic part measuring 18 cm (7 in). The same anatomic part is radiographed in another patient and it measures 23 cm (9 in). What new mAs is needed to the expose the IR? Because the part thickness increased by 5 cm (2 in), the original mAs is multiplied by 2, yielding 40 mAs. If the same part in another patient measures 28 cm (11 in), what new mAs is needed? Because the part thickness increased by another 5 cm (2 in), the mAs is multiplied by 2, yielding 80 mAs. This mAs is four times greater than that for the original patient's anatomic part, which measured 10 cm (4 in) less.

As the thickness of a given type of anatomic tissue increases, the amount of scattered radiation increases and radiographic contrast decreases. Using a higher kVp for a thicker part only adds to the increase in scatter radiation. Increased scatter radiation would continue degrading the quality of the image because it creates fog, which decreases the contrast.

The amount of radiographic contrast achieved is also influenced by the composition of the anatomic part to be radiographed. As mentioned in Chapter 3, subject contrast is a category of radiographic contrast. The thickness of the tissue, atomic number, and cell compactness (tissue density) affect its absorption characteristics. The absorption characteristics of the anatomic tissue create the brightness levels produced on a radiograph. Tissues that have a higher atomic number absorb more radiation than tissues with a lower atomic number.

Anatomic structures having a wide range of tissue compositions, varying in parameters such as effective atomic number and tissue density, demonstrate high subject contrast. Anatomic structures consisting of a similar type of tissue demonstrate low subject contrast. The radiographer cannot control the composition of the anatomic part to be radiographed. Changing the kVp alters its absorption and transmission within anatomic tissues. Knowledge of the absorption characteristics of anatomic tissues and the effect of kVp helps the radiographer produce a desired level of radiographic contrast. The selection of kVp for producing a desired level of contrast is more critical when using film-screen IRs. Acquiring the image using digital IRs allows changes in image contrast during computer processing.

The quality of a radiographic image depends on a multitude of variables. Knowledge of these variables and their radiographic effect assists the radiographer in producing quality radiographs. Table 6-2 summarizes common exposure technique mathematical calculations. Table 6-3 is a chart demonstrating how the variables discussed in this chapter affect IR exposure and Table 6-4 is a chart demonstrating how the variables discussed in this chapter affect image quality.

TABLE 6-2 Exposure Technique Mathematical Calculations

Exposure Technique Factor	Relationship to Maintain Exposure to Image Receptor	Formula
mAs	↑ mA and ↓ second	mA × second = mAs
kVp: 15% Rule	↑ kVp and ↓ mAs	kVp × 1.15 and mAs/2 kVp × .85 and mAs × 2
mAs/Distance Compensation Formula	↑ SID and ↑ mAs	$\dfrac{mAs_1}{mAs_2} = \dfrac{(SID_1)^2}{(SID_2)^2}$
Grid Conversion Factor: No grid = 1 5:1 = 2 6:1 = 3 8:1 = 4 12:1 = 5 16:1 = 6	↑ Grid ratio and ↑ mAs	$\dfrac{mAs_1}{mAs_2} = \dfrac{GCF_1}{GCF_2}$
Patient Thickness	↑ Thickness and ↑ mAs	Every 4–5 cm change in thickness change mAs by a factor of 2

TABLE 6-3 Exposure Factors and Their Effects on the Primary and Remnant X-ray Beams

	Primary Beam Reaching Patient	Remnant Beam Reaching Image Receptor
mAs		
Increasing mAs	↑ Quantity	↑ Quantity
Decreasing mAs	↓ Quantity	↓ Quantity
kVp		
Increasing kVp	↑ Quantity and quality	↑ Quantity and quality
Decreasing kVp	↓ Quantity and quality	↓ Quantity and quality
Focal Spot Size		
Smaller focal spot size	No effect	No effect
Larger focal spot size	No effect	No effect
SID		
Increasing SID	↓ Quantity	↓ Quantity
Decreasing SID	↑ Quantity	↑ Quantity
OID		
Increasing OID	No effect	↓ Quantity and scatter
Decreasing OID	No effect	↑ Quantity and scatter
Central Ray (CR) Angle		
Increase CR Angle*	↓ Quantity	↓ Quantity
Grid		
Increasing grid ratio	No effect	↓ Quantity and scatter
Decreasing grid ratio	No effect	↑ Quantity and scatter

Continued

TABLE 6-3 Exposure Factors and Their Effects on the Primary and Remnant X-ray Beams—cont'd

	Primary Beam Reaching Patient	Remnant Beam Reaching Image Receptor
Beam Restriction		
Increasing collimation	↓ Quantity	↓ Quantity and scatter
Decreasing collimation	↑ Quantity	↑ Quantity and scatter
Generator Output		
Single-phase generator	↓ Quantity and quality	↓ Quantity and quality
High-frequency generator	↑ Quantity and quality	↑ Quantity and quality
Tube Filtration		
Adding Filtration	↓ Quantity and ↑ average energy	↓ Quantity and ↑ average energy
Removing Filtration	↑ Quantity and ↓ average energy	↑ Quantity and ↓ average energy
Compensating Filter		
Adding a compensating filter	↓ Quantity	↓ Quantity
Part Thickness		
Increasing part thickness	No effect	↓ Quantity
Decreasing part thickness	No effect	↑ Quantity

*without a decrease in SID

TABLE 6-4 Exposure Technique Factors and Image Quality

INDIVIDUAL FACTOR CHANGE WITHOUT EXPOSURE TECHNIQUE COMPENSATION AND RESULTS IN A DIAGNOSTIC RADIOGRAPH

Exposure Factor	IR Exposure	Density (Film Only)	Contrast*	Spatial Resolution	Distortion
mAs					
Increase	Increase	Increase	No effect	No effect	No effect
Decrease	Decrease	Decrease	No effect	No effect	No effect
kVp					
Increase	Increase	Increase	Decrease	No effect	No effect
Decrease	Decrease	Decrease	Increase	No effect	No effect
Focal Spot Size					
Increase	No effect	No effect	No effect	Decrease	No effect
Decrease	No effect	No effect	No effect	Increase	No effect
SID					
Increase	Decrease	Decrease	No effect	Increase	- Magnification
Decrease	Increase	Increase	No effect	Decrease	+ Magnification
OID					
Increase	Decrease	Decrease	Increase**	Decrease	+ Magnification
Central Ray Angle					
Increase	Decrease***	Decrease***	No effect	Decrease	+ Shape Distortion

TABLE 6-4   Exposure Technique Factors and Image Quality—cont'd

INDIVIDUAL FACTOR CHANGE WITHOUT EXPOSURE TECHNIQUE COMPENSATION AND RESULTS IN A DIAGNOSTIC RADIOGRAPH

Exposure Factor	IR Exposure	Density (Film Only)	Contrast*	Spatial Resolution	Distortion
Grid use					
Add grid	Decrease	Decrease	Increase	No effect	No effect
Remove grid	Increase	Increase	Decrease	No effect	No effect
Collimation					
Increase	Decrease	Decrease	Increase	No effect	No effect
Decrease	Increase	Increase	Decrease	No effect	No effect
Tube Filtration					
Excessive	Decrease	Decrease	Decrease	No effect	No effect
Insufficient	Increase	Increase	Increase	No effect	No effect
Patient Thickness					
Increase	Decrease	Decrease	Decrease	Decrease	+ Magnification
Decrease	Increase	Increase	Increase	Increase	- Magnification

*Increase is higher contrast and decrease is lower contrast.
**Increase (higher) contrast because of less scatter reaching image rector, effect dependent on anatomic region, thickness, and amount of OID.
***Without a decrease in SID.

CHAPTER SUMMARY

- The product of milliamperage and exposure time (mAs) is directly proportional to the quantity of x-rays produced and exposure to the IR.
- Milliamperage and exposure time have an inverse relationship to maintain exposure to the IR.
- The kVp changes the penetrating power of the x-ray beam and has a direct effect on exposure to the IR.
- Changing the kVp by 15% has the same effect on exposure to the IR as changing the mAs by a factor of 2.
- A numerical value or exposure indicator is displayed on the processed digital image that indicates the level of x-ray exposure received (incident exposure) on the IR.
- The kVp has an inverse relationship with radiographic contrast: a high kVp creates an image with low contrast and a low kVp creates an image with high contrast.
- Radiation exposure to a film-screen IR affects the level of density and contrast, whereas brightness and contrast are primarily controlled by computer processing in digital imaging.
- Focal spot size affects only spatial resolution. A smaller focal spot size increases spatial resolution.
- SID has an inverse squared relationship with the intensity of radiation reaching the patient and the IR.
- Increasing OID decreases exposure to the IR.
- Decreasing SID and increasing OID increases size distortion (magnification) and decreases spatial resolution.
- Grids absorb the scatter exiting the patient and increase radiographic contrast.
- Beam restriction affects the amount of tissue irradiated, scatter produced, and exposure to the IR.

- Changes in SID, grids, and patient thickness require a change in mAs to maintain the exposure to the IR.
- Generators with more efficient output, such as three-phase or high-frequency generators, require lower exposure techniques to produce the same exposure to the IR as a single-phase generator.
- Excessive or insufficient tube filtration will affect the exposure to the image receptor and contrast.
- Exposure factors may need to be modified for body habitus and part thickness.

REVIEW QUESTIONS

1. Which of the following is accurate regarding the relationship between milliamperage (mA) and exposure time to maintain the exposure to the image receptor?
   A. Directly proportional
   B. Direct
   C. Inverse
   D. Inversely proportional

2. A radiographic film image has excessive density. Which of the following is the best for correcting the exposure error?
   A. Decrease kVp by 50%
   B. Increase mAs by 15%
   C. Decrease mAs by 50%
   D. Decrease mAs by 15%

3. What exposure factor affects both the quality and the quantity of the x-ray beam?
   A. kVp
   B. SID
   C. mA
   D. Focal spot size

4. Which of the following is *not* affected by kilovoltage?
   A. Compton interactions
   B. Spatial resolution
   C. Film density
   D. Radiation quantity

5. Increasing the mAs has _____ effect on brightness displayed in digital imaging.
   A. a direct
   B. an indirect
   C. an inverse
   D. no

6. Which of the following would maintain radiation exposure to the image receptor when the kilovoltage is decreased by 15%?
   A. Increase mAs by 15%
   B. Increase mAs by 50%
   C. Double the mAs
   D. Halve the mAs

7. A quality image is produced using 70 kVp and 25 mAs at a 40 in SID. What calculated change in the exposure technique is necessary to maintain radiation exposure to the image receptor when the SID is increased to 56 in?
   A. 60 kVp at 25 mAs
   B. 70 kVp at 12.5 mAs

C. 70 kVp at 50 mAs
D. 60 kVp at 50 mAs

8. Without exposure technique compensation, increasing the OID by 4 in for a knee film image would
   (1) increase magnification
   (2) decrease density
   (3) increase contrast
   A. 1 and 2 only
   B. 1 and 3 only
   C. 2 and 3 only
   D. 1, 2, and 3

9. A quality image is produced using 80 kVp at 10 mAs with a 6:1 ratio grid. Calculate the change in exposure technique to maintain radiation exposure to the image receptor when changing to a 12:1 ratio grid.
   A. 80 kVp at 17 mAs
   B. 68 kVp at 20 mAs
   C. 80 kVp at 6 mAs
   D. 92 kVp at 5 mAs

10. Which of the following factors does *not* affect spatial resolution?
    A. Focal spot size
    B. SID
    C. OID
    D. Grid

11. Which of the following factors does *not* affect the radiation exposure to the image receptor?
    A. Collimation
    B. Focal spot size
    C. Compensating filters
    D. Body habitus

12. What exposure factor change is recommended to maintain radiation exposure to the image receptor when increasing the patient thickness by 5 cm?
    A. Double the kVp
    B. Double the mAs
    C. Decrease kVp by 15%
    D. Increase mAs by 15%

7

Scatter Control

CHAPTER OUTLINE

Scatter Radiation
Beam Restriction
**Beam Restriction and Scatter
    Radiation**
    Collimation and Contrast
    Compensating for
        Collimation
**Types of Beam-Restricting
    Devices**
    Aperture Diaphragms

Cones and Cylinders
Collimators
Automatic Collimators
Radiographic Grids
Grid Construction
Grid Pattern
Grid Focus
Types of Grids
Grid Performance
Grid Cutoff

Moiré Effect
Grid Usage
Radiation Protection
Air Gap Technique
**Scatter Control and Digital
    Imaging**
Shielding Accessories

OBJECTIVES

After completing this chapter, the reader will be able to perform the following:

1. Define all the key terms in this chapter.
2. State all the important relationships in this chapter.
3. Explain how scatter radiation affects radiographic images.
4. State the purpose of beam-restricting devices.
5. Describe each type of beam-restricting device.
6. State the purpose of automatic collimators or positive beam-limiting devices.
7. Describe the purpose of a radiographic grid.
8. Describe the construction of grids, including the different types of grid pattern, dimensions, and grid focus.
9. Calculate grid ratio.
10. List the various types of stationary grids and describe the function and purpose of a moving grid.
11. Demonstrate the use of the grid conversion formula.
12. Describe the different types of grid cutoff errors that can occur and their radiographic appearance.
13. Identify the factors to be considered in using a grid.
14. Recognize how beam restriction and the use of grids affect patient radiation exposure.
15. Explain the air gap technique and describe its use.

KEY TERMS

air gap technique
aperture diaphragm
automatic collimator
beam-restricting device
beam restriction

Bucky
Bucky factor
collimation
collimator
cone

convergent line
convergent point
crossed grid
cross-hatched grid
cylinder

KEY TERMS—cont'd

focal distance	grid cutoff	long dimension
focal range	grid focus	Moiré effect
focused grid	grid frequency	nonfocused grid
grid	grid pattern	parallel grid
grid cap	grid ratio	positive beam-limiting device
grid cassette	interspace material	short dimension
grid conversion factor	linear grid	wafer grid

Controlling the amount of scatter radiation produced in a patient and ultimately reaching the image receptor (IR) is essential for creating a good-quality image. Scatter radiation is detrimental to radiographic quality because it adds unwanted exposure (fog) to the image without adding any patient information.

Digital IRs are more sensitive to lower-energy levels of radiation such as scatter, which results in increased fog in the image. Additionally, scatter radiation decreases radiographic contrast for both digital and film-screen images. Increased scatter radiation, either produced within the patient or the higher-energy scatter exiting the patient, affects the exposure to the patient and anyone within close proximity. The radiographer must act to minimize the amount of scatter radiation reaching the IR.

Beam-restricting devices and radiographic grids are tools that the radiographer can use to limit the amount of such scatter radiation. Beam-restricting devices decrease the x-ray-beam field size and the amount of tissue irradiated, thereby reducing the amount of scatter radiation produced. Radiographic grids are used to improve radiographic image quality by absorbing scatter radiation exiting the patient, thereby reducing the amount of scatter reaching the IR. It should be noted that grids do nothing to prevent scatter *production*; they merely reduce the amount of scatter reaching the IR.

SCATTER RADIATION

Scatter radiation, as described in Chapter 3, is primarily the result of Compton interactions, in which an incoming x-ray photon loses energy and changes direction. Two major factors affect the amount and energy of scatter radiation exiting the patient: kilovoltage peak (kVp) and the volume of irradiated tissue. The volume of irradiated tissue depends on the thickness of the part and the x-ray-beam field size. Increasing the volume of irradiated tissue results in increased scatter production. In addition, using a higher kVp increases x-ray transmission and reduces its overall absorption (photoelectric interactions); however, higher kVp increases the percentage of Compton interactions and the energy of scatter radiation exiting the patient. Using higher kVp or increasing the volume of irradiated tissue results in increased scatter radiation reaching the IR.

 IMPORTANT RELATIONSHIP

kVp and Scatter

The amount and energy of scatter radiation exiting the patient depends, in part, on the kVp selected. Examinations using higher kVp produce a greater proportion of higher-energy scattered x-rays compared with examinations using low kVp.

IMPORTANT RELATIONSHIP

X-ray-Beam Field Size, Thickness of the Part, and Scatter

The larger the x-ray-beam field size, the greater the amount of scatter radiation produced. The thicker the part being imaged, the greater the amount of scatter radiation produced.

 IMPORTANT RELATIONSHIP

Volume of Tissue Irradiated and Scatter

The volume of tissue irradiated is affected by both the part thickness and the x-ray-beam field size. Therefore, the greater the volume of tissue irradiated, because of either or both factors, the greater the amount of scatter radiation produced.

BEAM RESTRICTION

It is the responsibility of the radiographer to limit the x-ray-beam field size to the anatomic area of interest. **Beam restriction** serves two purposes: limiting patient exposure and reducing the amount of scatter radiation produced within the patient.

The unrestricted primary beam is cone-shaped and projects a round field onto the patient and IR (Figure 7-1). If not restricted in some way, the primary beam goes beyond the boundaries of the IR, resulting in unnecessary patient exposure. Any time the x-ray field extends beyond the anatomic area of interest, the patient receives unnecessary exposure. Limiting the x-ray-beam field size is accomplished with a **beam-restricting device**. Located just below the x-ray tube housing, the beam-restricting device changes the shape and size of the primary beam.

The terms **beam restriction** and **collimation** are used interchangeably; they refer to a decrease in the size of the projected radiation field. The term *collimation* is used more often than the term *beam restriction* because collimators are the most popular type of beam-restricting device. Increasing collimation means decreasing the field size, and decreasing collimation means increasing the field size.

 IMPORTANT RELATIONSHIP

Beam Restriction and Patient Dose

As beam restriction or collimation increases, the field size and patient dose decrease. As beam restriction or collimation decreases, the field size and patient dose increase.

 Radiation Protection Alert

Appropriate Beam Restriction

In performing a radiographic examination, the radiographer should be aware of the anatomic area of interest and limit the x-ray field size to just beyond this area. Collimating to the appropriate field size is a basic method for protecting patients from unnecessary exposure.

BEAM RESTRICTION AND SCATTER RADIATION

In addition to decreasing the patient dose, beam-restricting devices reduce the amount of scatter radiation produced within the patient, reducing the amount of scatter to which the IR is exposed, thereby increasing the radiographic contrast. The relationship between collimation (field size) and the quantity of scatter radiation is illustrated in Figure 7-2. As previously stated, collimation means decreasing the size of the projected field; hence, increasing collimation means decreasing field size, and decreasing collimation means increasing field size.

 IMPORTANT RELATIONSHIP

Collimation and Scatter Radiation

As collimation increases, the field size and quantity of scatter radiation decrease; as collimation decreases, the field size and quantity of scatter radiation increase.

Collimation and Contrast

Because collimation decreases the x-ray-beam field size, less scatter radiation is produced within the patient, and hence, less scatter radiation reaches the IR. As described in Chapter 3, this affects the radiographic contrast.

 IMPORTANT RELATIONSHIP

Collimation and Radiographic Contrast

As collimation increases, the quantity of scatter radiation decreases and radiographic contrast increases; as collimation decreases, the quantity of scatter radiation increases and radiographic contrast decreases.

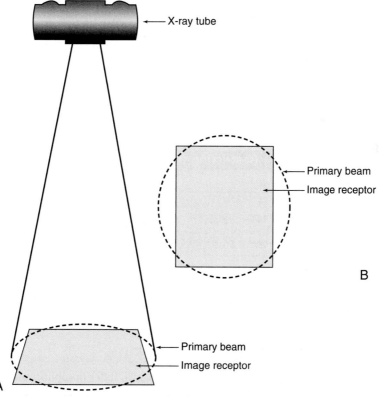

FIGURE 7-1 The unrestricted primary beam is cone-shaped, projecting a circular field. **A,** Side view. **B,** View from above.

Compensating for Collimation

Increasing the collimation decreases the volume of tissue irradiated, the amount of scatter radiation produced, the number of photons that strike the patient, and the number of x-ray photons that reach the IR to produce the latent image. As a result, the exposure-technique factors may need to be increased when increasing collimation to maintain exposure to the IR.

> **IMPORTANT RELATIONSHIP**
> ### Collimation and Exposure to the Image Receptor
> As collimation increases, exposure to the IR decreases; as collimation decreases, exposure to the IR increases.

It has been recommended that significant collimation requires the milliamperage/second (mAs) to be increased by 30% to 50% to compensate for the decrease in IR exposure.

Important relationships regarding the restriction of the primary beam are summarized in Table 7-1.

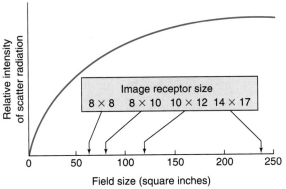

FIGURE 7-2 As field size increases, the relative quantity of scattered radiation increases.

TABLE 7-1	Restricting the Primary Beam
Increased Factor	**Result**
Collimation	Patient dose *decreases*
	Scatter radiation *decreases*
	Radiographic contrast *increases*
	Exposure to image receptor *decreases*
Field size	Patient dose *increases*
	Scatter radiation *increases*
	Radiographic contrast *decreases*
	Exposure to image receptor *increases*

TYPES OF BEAM-RESTRICTING DEVICES

Several types of beam-restricting devices, which differ in sophistication and utility, are available. Most beam-restricting devices are made of metal or a combination of metals that readily absorb x-rays.

Aperture Diaphragms

The simplest type of beam-restricting device is the aperture diaphragm. An **aperture diaphragm** is a flat piece of lead (diaphragm) that contains a hole (aperture). Commercially made aperture diaphragms are available (Figure 7-3), or hospitals can make their own for purposes specific to a radiographic unit. Aperture diaphragms are easy to use; they are placed directly below the x-ray tube window. An aperture diaphragm can be made by cutting rubberized lead into the size needed to create the diaphragm and cutting a hole of the appropriate shape and size into the center to create the aperture.

Although the size and shape of the aperture can be changed, the aperture cannot be adjusted from the designed size, and therefore, the projected field size is not adjustable. In addition, because of the aperture's proximity to the radiation source (focal spot), a large area of unsharpness surrounds the radiographic image (Figure 7-4). Although aperture diaphragms are still used in some applications, their use is not as widespread as other types of beam-restricting devices.

Cones and Cylinders

Cones and cylinders are shaped differently (Figure 7-5), but they have many similar attributes. A **cone** or **cylinder** is essentially an aperture diaphragm that has an extended flange attached to it. The flange can vary in length and can be shaped as either a cone or a cylinder. The flange can also be made to telescope, increasing its total length (Figure 7-6). Similar to aperture diaphragms, cones and cylinders are easy to use. They slide onto the tube, directly below the window. Cones and cylinders limit the unsharpness surrounding radiographic images more than aperture diaphragms do, with cylinders accomplishing this task slightly better than cones (Figure 7-7). However, they are limited in terms of available sizes, and they are not interchangeable among tube housings. Cones have a particular disadvantage compared with cylinders: if the angle of the flange of the cone is greater than the angle of divergence of the primary beam, the base plate or aperture diaphragm of the cone is the only metal actually restricting the primary beam. Therefore,

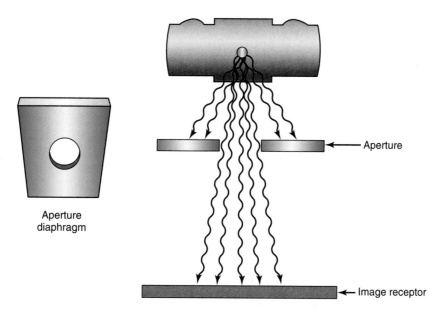

Aperture diaphragm

Aperture

Image receptor

FIGURE 7-3 Commercially made aperture diaphragm.

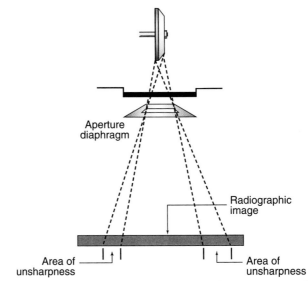

FIGURE 7-4 Radiographic image unsharpness using an aperture diaphragm.

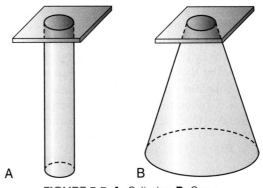

FIGURE 7-5 A, Cylinder. **B,** Cone.

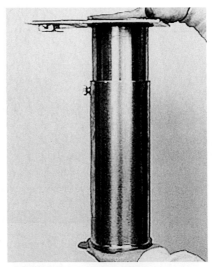

FIGURE 7-6 Telescoping cylinder.

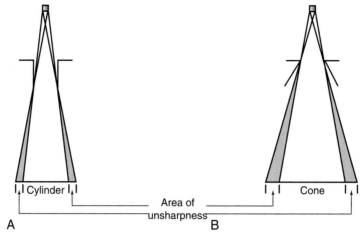

FIGURE 7-7 A cylinder **(A)** is better at limiting unsharpness than a cone **(B)**.

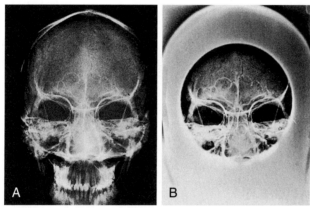

FIGURE 7-8 Radiograph of the frontal and maxillary sinuses not using a cone **(A)** and using a cone **(B)**.

cylinders generally are more useful than cones. Cones and cylinders are almost always made to produce a circular projected field, and they can be advantageously used for particular radiographic procedures (Figure 7-8).

Collimators

The most sophisticated, useful, and accepted type of beam-restricting device for radiography is the **collimator**. Beam restriction accomplished with the use of a collimator is referred to as *collimation*. The terms *collimation* and *beam restriction* are used interchangeably.

A collimator has two or three sets of lead shutters (Figure 7-9). Located immediately below the tube window, the entrance shutters limit the x-ray beam much as the aperture diaphragm would. One or more sets of adjustable lead shutters are located 3–7 in (8–18 cm) below the tube. These shutters consist of longitudinal and lateral leaves or blades, each with its own control. This design makes the collimator adjustable in terms of its ability to produce projected fields of varying sizes. The field shape produced by a collimator is always rectangular or square, unless an

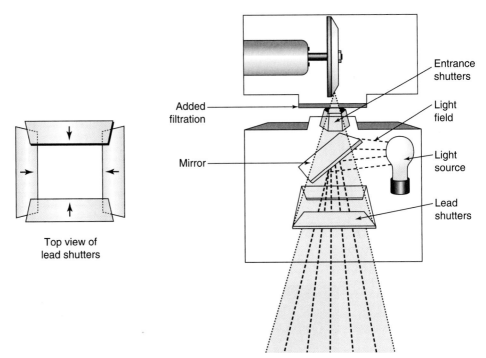

FIGURE 7-9 Collimators have two sets of lead shutters that are used to change the size and shape of the primary beam.

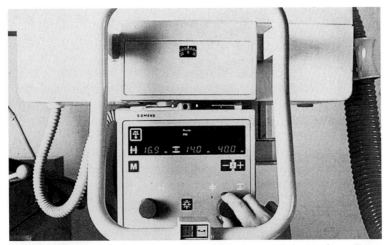

FIGURE 7-10 The x-ray field measurement guide on the front of a collimator.

aperture diaphragm, cone, or cylinder is slid in below the collimator. Collimators are equipped with a white light source and a mirror to project a light field onto the patient. This light is intended to accurately indicate where the primary x-ray beam will be projected during exposure. In case of failure of this light, an x-ray field measurement guide (Figure 7-10) is present on the front of the collimator. This guide indicates the projected field size on the basis of the adjusted size of the

---

BOX 7-1   Quality-Control Check: Collimator and Beam Alignment

- Lack of congruence of the x-ray field light and the exposure field and misalignment of the light and Bucky tray may affect the quality of the radiograph. In addition, if the x-ray central ray is not perpendicular to the table and Bucky tray, radiographic quality may be compromised. A collimator and beam alignment test tool template and cylinder can be easily radiographed and evaluated for proper alignment.
- Collimator misalignment should be less than 2% of the SID used, and the perpendicularity of the x-ray central ray must be misaligned by no more than 1°.

---

collimator opening at particular source-to-image-receptor distances (SIDs). This guide helps to ensure that the radiographer does not open the collimator to produce a field that is larger than the IR. Another problem that may occur is the lack of accuracy of the light field. The mirror that reflects the light down toward the patient or the light bulb itself could be slightly out of position, projecting a light field that inaccurately indicates where the primary beam will be projected. There is a means of testing the accuracy of this light field and the location of the center of the projected beam (Box 7-1).

A plastic template with crosshairs is affixed to the bottom of the collimator to indicate where the center of the primary beam—the central ray—will be directed. This template is of great assistance to the radiographer in accurately centering the x-ray field to the patient.

Automatic Collimators

An **automatic collimator**, also called a **positive beam-limiting device**, automatically limits the size and shape of the primary beam to the size and shape of the IR. For many years, automatic collimators were required by the U.S. federal law on all new radiographic installations. This law has since been rescinded, and automatic collimators are no longer a requirement on any radiographic equipment. However, they are still widely used. Automatic collimators mechanically adjust the primary beam size and shape to those of the IR when the IR is placed in the Bucky tray, which is located just below the tabletop. Automatic collimation makes it difficult for the radiographer to increase the size of the primary beam to a field larger than that of the IR, which would result in increasing the patient's radiation exposure. Positive beam-limiting devices were seen as a way to protect patients from overexposure to radiation; however, it should be noted that automatic collimators have an override mechanism that allows the radiographer to disengage this feature.

! Radiation Protection Alert

Limit Field Size to Image Receptor Size

Whether or not automatic collimation is being used, the radiographer should always be sure that the size of the x-ray field is the same as or less than the size of the IR except for digital flat-panel detectors. When using a digital flat-panel detector, the x-ray field size should be restricted to the anatomic area of interest. These digital IRs are typically of a similar size, and, in many instances, larger than the anatomic area of interest. Therefore, it is even more crucial for the radiographer to appropriately collimate for the imaging procedure so that the patient is not unnecessarily exposed to radiation.

RADIOGRAPHIC GRIDS

The radiographic grid was invented in 1913 by Gustave Bucky and continues to be the most effective means for limiting the amount of scatter radiation that reaches the IR. Approximately 1/4 in thick and ranging from 8 × 10 in (20 × 25 cm) to 17 × 17 in (43 × 43 cm), a **grid** is a device consisting of very thin lead strips with radiolucent interspaces intended to absorb scatter radiation emitted from the patient. Placed between the patient and the IR, grids are invaluable in the practice of radiography. They work well to improve radiographic contrast; however, they possess certain drawbacks. As discussed later in this chapter, using a grid requires additional mAs, resulting in a higher patient dose. Therefore, grids are typically used only when the anatomic part is 10 cm (4 in) or greater in thickness, and more than 60 kVp is needed for the examination.

As scatter radiation leaves the patient, a significant amount is directed toward the IR. As previously stated, scatter radiation is detrimental to image quality because it adds unwanted exposure to the IR without adding any radiographic information. Scatter radiation decreases radiographic contrast. Ideally, grids would absorb, or clean up, all scattered photons directed toward the IR and would allow all transmitted photons emitted from the patient to pass to the IR. Unfortunately, this does not happen (Figure 7-11). When used properly, however, grids can greatly increase the contrast of the radiographic image.

 IMPORTANT RELATIONSHIP

Scatter Radiation and Image Quality

Scatter radiation adds unwanted exposure to the IR and decreases image quality.

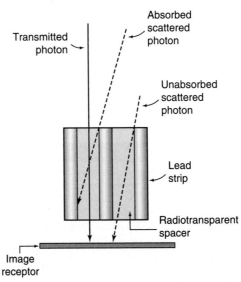

FIGURE 7-11 Ideally, grids would absorb all scattered radiation and allow all transmitted photons to reach the image receptor (IR). In reality, however, some scattered photons pass through to the IR and some transmitted photons are absorbed.

Grid Construction

Grids contain thin lead strips or lines that have a precise height, thickness, and space between them. Radiolucent **interspace material** separates the lead lines. Interspace material typically is made of aluminum. The lead lines and interspace material of the grid are covered by an aluminum front and back panel.

Grid construction can be described by grid frequency and grid ratio. **Grid frequency** expresses the number of lead lines per unit length, in inches, centimeters, or both. Grid frequencies can range in value from 25 to 80 lines/cm (63 to 200 lines/in). A typical value for grid frequency might be 40 lines/cm (100 lines/in). Another way of describing grid construction is by its grid ratio. **Grid ratio** is defined as the ratio of the height of the lead strips to the distance between them (Figure 7-12). Grid ratio can also be mathematically expressed as follows:

$$\text{Grid ratio} = h/D,$$

where h is the height of the lead strips and D is the distance between them.

 MATHEMATICAL APPLICATION

Calculating Grid Ratio

What is the grid ratio when the lead strips are 2.4 mm high and separated by 0.2 mm?

$$\text{Grid ratio} = h/D$$
$$\text{Grid ratio} = \frac{2.4}{0.2} = 12 \text{ or } 12:1$$

Grid ratios range from 4:1 to 16:1. High-ratio grids remove, or clean up, more scatter radiation than lower-ratio grids having the same grid frequency, thereby further increasing radiographic contrast.

There is a relationship among grid ratio, grid frequency, and the amount of lead content (measured in mass per unit area). Increasing the grid ratio for the same grid frequency increases the amount of lead content and therefore increases scatter absorption.

IMPORTANT RELATIONSHIP

Grid Ratio and Radiographic Contrast

As the grid ratio increases for the same grid frequency, scatter cleanup improves and radiographic contrast increases; as grid ratio decreases for the same grid frequency, scatter cleanup becomes less effective and radiographic contrast decreases.

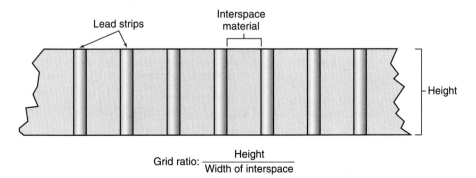

FIGURE 7-12 Grid ratio is the ratio of the height of the lead strips to the distance between them.

Information about a grid's construction is contained on a label placed on the tube side of the grid. This label usually states the type of interspace material used, grid frequency, grid ratio, grid size, and information about the range of SIDs that can be used with the grid. The radiographer should read this information before using the grid because these factors influence grid performance, exposure technique selection, grid alignment, and image quality.

Grid Pattern

Grid pattern refers to the linear pattern of the lead lines of a grid. Two types of grid patterns exist: linear and crossed or cross-hatched. A **linear grid** has lead lines that run in only one direction (Figure 7-13). Linear grids are the most popular grid pattern because they allow angulation of the x-ray tube along the length of the lead lines. A **crossed grid** or **cross-hatched grid** has lead lines that run at right angles to one another (Figure 7-14). Crossed grids remove more scattered photons than linear grids because they contain more lead strips, oriented in two directions. However, applications are limited with a crossed grid because the x-ray tube cannot be angled in any direction without producing grid cutoff (i.e., absorption of the transmitted x-rays). Grid cutoff is undesirable and is discussed later in this chapter.

Grid Focus

Grid focus refers to the orientation of the lead lines relative to one another. A **parallel grid** or **nonfocused grid** has lead lines that run parallel to one another (Figure 7-15). Parallel

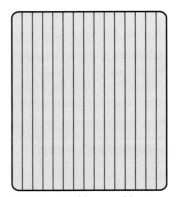

FIGURE 7-13 Linear grid pattern.

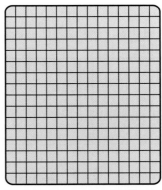

FIGURE 7-14 Crossed or cross-hatched grid pattern.

grids are used primarily in fluoroscopy and mobile imaging. A **focused grid** has lead lines that are angled, or canted, to approximately match the angle of divergence of the primary beam (Figure 7-16). The advantage of focused grids compared with parallel grids is that focused grids allow more transmitted photons to reach the IR. As seen in Figure 7-17, transmitted photons are more likely to pass through a focused grid to reach the IR than they are to pass through a parallel grid.

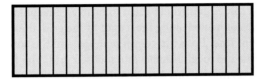

FIGURE 7-15 Parallel, or nonfocused, type of grid.

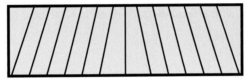

FIGURE 7-16 Focused type of grid.

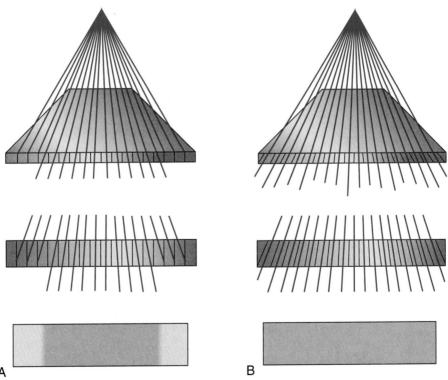

A   B

FIGURE 7-17 Comparison of transmitted photons passing through a parallel grid **(A)** and a focused grid **(B)**.

IMPORTANT RELATIONSHIP

Focused versus Parallel Grids

Focused grids have lead lines that are angled to approximately match the divergence of the primary beam. Thus, focused grids allow more transmitted photons to reach the IR than parallel grids.

As seen in Figure 7-18, if imaginary lines were drawn from each of the lead lines in a linearly focused grid, these lines would meet to form an imaginary point called the **convergent point**. If points were connected along the length of the grid, they would form an imaginary line called the **convergent line**. Both the convergent line and the convergent point are important because they determine the focal distance of a focused grid. The **focal distance** (sometimes referred to as *grid radius*) is the distance between the grid and the convergent line or point, and it is important because it is used to determine the focal range of a focused grid. The **focal range** is the recommended range of SIDs that can be used with a focused grid. The convergent line or point always falls within the focal range (Figure 7-19). For example, a common focal range is 36–42 in (90–105 cm), with a focal distance of 40 in (100 cm). Another common focal range is 66–74

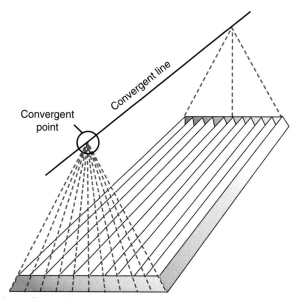

FIGURE 7-18 Imaginary lines drawn above a linear focused grid from each lead strip meet to form a convergent point; the points form a convergent line.

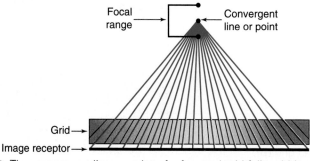

FIGURE 7-19 The convergent line or point of a focused grid falls within a focal range.

in (165–185 cm), with a focal distance of 72 in (180 cm). Because the lead lines in a parallel grid are not angled, they have a focal range extending from a minimum SID to infinity.

Types of Grids

Grids are available for use by the radiographer in several forms and can be stationary or moving. Stationary, nonmoving grids include the wafer grid, grid cassette, and grid cap. A **wafer grid** matches the size of the cassette and is used by placing it on top of the IR. Wafer grids typically are taped to the IR to prevent them from sliding during the radiographic procedure. A **grid cassette** is an IR that has a grid permanently mounted on its front surface. A **grid cap** contains a permanently mounted grid and allows the IR to slide in behind it; this is useful because the grid is secure and many IRs can be interchanged behind the grid before processing the image.

Stationary and Reciprocating Grids

When grids are stationary, it is possible to examine them closely and see the grid lines on the radiographic image. Slightly moving the grid during the x-ray exposure blurs the grid lines (motion unsharpness), rendering them less visible.

Moving or reciprocating grids are part of the **Bucky**, more accurately called the *Potter–Bucky diaphragm*. Located directly below the radiographic tabletop, the grid is found just above the tray that holds the IR. Grid motion is electrically controlled by the x-ray exposure switch. The grid moves slightly back and forth in a lateral direction over the IR during the entire exposure. These grids typically have dimensions of 17 × 17 in (43 × 43 cm) so that a 14 × 17 in (35 × 43 cm) IR can be positioned under the grid either lengthwise or crosswise, depending on the examination requirements.

Long-Dimension versus Short-Dimension Grids

Linear grids can be constructed with either long dimension or short dimension. A **long-dimension** linear grid has lead strips running parallel to its long axis, whereas a **short-dimension** linear grid has lead strips running perpendicular to its long axis (Figure 7-20).

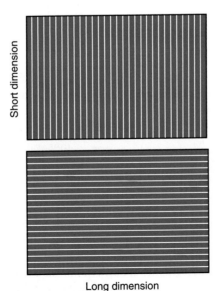

FIGURE 7-20 A long-dimension grid has lead strips running parallel to the long axis of the grid. A short-dimension grid has lead strips running perpendicular to the long axis of the grid.

For example, a 14 × 17 in (35 × 43 cm) long-dimension grid has 17 in (43 cm) long lead strips, whereas a short-dimension grid has 14 in (35 cm) long lead strips. A short-dimension grid may be useful for examinations where it is difficult to correctly center the central ray for the long-dimension grid.

Grid Performance

The purpose of using grids in radiography is to increase radiographic contrast. In addition to improving contrast by cleaning up scatter, grids reduce the total amount of x-rays reaching the IR. The better the grid is at absorbing scattered photons, such as with a higher-ratio grid, the fewer the photons reach the IR. To compensate for this reduction, additional mAs must be used to maintain exposure to the IR. The **grid conversion factor** (GCF), or **Bucky factor**, can be used to determine the required adjustment in mAs when changing from using a grid to nongrid (or vice versa) or for changing to grids with different grid ratios.

The GCF can be mathematically expressed as follows:

$$GCF = \frac{\text{mAs with the grid}}{\text{mAs without the grid}}$$

 IMPORTANT RELATIONSHIP

Grid Ratio and Exposure to Image Receptor

As the grid ratio increases, exposure to the IR decreases; as the grid ratio decreases, exposure to the IR increases.

Table 7-2 presents specific grid ratios and grid conversion factors. When a grid is added to the IR, mAs must be increased by the factor indicated to maintain the same number of x-ray photons reaching the IR. This calculation requires multiplication by the GCF for the particular grid ratio.

 MATHEMATICAL APPLICATION

Adding a Grid

If a radiographer produced a shoulder radiograph with nongrid exposure using 3 mAs and then wanted to use a 12:1 ratio grid, what mAs should be used to produce the same exposure to the IR?
  Nongrid exposure = 3 mAs
  GCF (for 12:1 grid) = 5 (from Table 7-2)

$$GCF = \frac{\text{mAs with the grid}}{\text{mAs without the grid}}$$

$$5 = \frac{\text{mAs with the grid}}{3}$$

$$15 = \text{mAs with the grid}$$

When adding a 12:1 ratio grid, mAs must be increased by a factor of 5 (in this case to 15 mAs).

Likewise, if a radiographer chooses not to use a grid during a procedure but knows the appropriate mAs only for when a grid is used, the mAs must be decreased by the GCF. This calculation requires division by the GCF for the particular grid ratio.

TABLE 7-2 Grid Conversion Factor (GCF)/Bucky Factor	
Grid Ratio	**GCF/Bucky Factor**
No grid	1
5:1	2
6:1	3
8:1	4
12:1	5
16:1	6

▶▶ MATHEMATICAL APPLICATION

Removing a Grid

If a radiographer produced a knee radiograph using an 8:1 ratio grid and 10 mAs and on the next exposure wanted to use nongrid exposure, what mAs should be used to produce the same exposure to the IR?

Grid exposure = 10 mAs
GCF (for 8:1 grid) = 4 (from Table 7-2)

$$GCF = \frac{mAs \text{ with the grid}}{mAs \text{ without the grid}}$$

$$4 = \frac{10 \text{ mAs}}{mAs \text{ without the grid}}$$

$$2.5 = mAs \text{ without the grid}$$

When removing an 8:1 ratio grid, mAs must be decreased by a factor of 4 (in this case to 2.5 mAs).

The GCF is also useful when changing between grids with different grid ratios. When changing from one grid ratio to another, the following formula should be used to adjust the mAs:

$$\frac{mAs_1}{mAs_2} = \frac{GCF_1}{GCF_2}$$

▶▶ MATHEMATICAL APPLICATION

Decreasing the Grid Ratio

If a radiographer used 40 mAs with a 12:1 ratio grid, what mAs should be used with a 6:1 ratio grid to produce the same exposure to the IR?

Exposure 1: 40 mAs, 12:1 grid, GCF = 5
Exposure 2: _____ mAs, 6:1 grid, GCF = 3

$$\frac{mAs_1}{mAs_2} = \frac{GCF_1}{GCF_2}$$

$$\frac{40}{mAs_2} = \frac{5}{3}$$

$$mAs_2 = 24$$

Decreasing the grid ratio requires less mAs.

MATHEMATICAL APPLICATION

Increasing the Grid Ratio

If a radiographer performed a routine portable pelvic examination using 40 mAs with an 8:1 ratio grid, what mAs should be used if a 12:1 ratio grid is substituted?

Exposure 1: 40 mAs, 8:1 grid, GCF = 4

Exposure 2: _____ mAs, 12:1 grid, GCF = 5

$$\frac{mAs_1}{mAs_2} = \frac{GCF_1}{GCF_2}$$

$$\frac{40}{mAs_2} = \frac{4}{5}$$

$$mAs_2 = 50$$

Increasing the grid ratio requires additional mAs.

The increase in mAs required to maintain the exposure to the IR results in an increase in patient dose. This increase is significant, as the GCF numbers indicate. It is important to remember that patient dose is increased by the following factors:

1. Using a grid compared with not using a grid;
2. Using a higher-ratio grid.

 IMPORTANT RELATIONSHIP

Grid Ratio and Patient Dose

As the grid ratio increases, patient dose increases; as the grid ratio decreases, patient dose decreases.

 Radiation Protection Alert

Grid Selection

Decisions regarding the use of a grid and grid ratio should be made by balancing image quality and patient protection. In order to keep patient exposure as low as possible, grids should be used only when appropriate and the grid ratio selected should be the lowest capable of providing sufficient contrast improvement.

Grid Cutoff

In addition to the disadvantage of increased patient dose associated with grid use, another disadvantage is the possibility of grid cutoff. **Grid cutoff** refers to a decrease in the number of transmitted photons that reach the IR because of some misalignment of the grid. The primary radiographic effect of grid cutoff is a further reduction in the number of photons reaching the IR. Grid cutoff often requires the radiographer to repeat the radiograph, increasing patient dose yet again. Grid ratio has a significant impact on grid cutoff, with higher grid ratios resulting in more potential cutoff.

Types of Grid Cutoff Errors

Grid cutoff can occur as a result of four types of errors in grid use. To reduce or eliminate grid cutoff, the radiographer must have a thorough understanding of the importance of proper grid alignment in relation to the IR and x-ray tube.

Upside-Down Focused. Upside-down focused grid cutoff occurs when a focused grid is placed upside-down on the IR, resulting in the grid lines going opposite the angle of divergence of the x-ray beam. Radiographically, there is significant loss of exposure along the edges of the image (Figure 7-21). Photons easily pass through the center of the grid because the lead lines are perpendicular to the IR surface. Lead lines that are more peripheral to the center have steeper angles and absorb the transmitted photons. Upside-down focused grid error is easily avoided because every focused grid should have a label indicating "Tube Side." This side of the grid should always face the tube, away from the IR.

 IMPORTANT RELATIONSHIP

Upside-Down Focused Grids and Grid Cutoff

Placing a focused grid upside-down on the IR causes the lateral edges of the IR to be highly underexposed.

Off-Level. Off-level grid cutoff results when the x-ray beam is angled across the lead strips. It is the most common type of cutoff and can occur from either the tube or the grid being angled (Figure 7-22). Off-level grid cutoff can often be seen with mobile radiographic studies or horizontal beam examinations and appears as a loss of exposure across the entire IR. This type of grid cutoff is the only type that occurs with both focused and parallel grids.

 IMPORTANT RELATIONSHIP

Off-Level Error and Grid Cutoff

Angling the x-ray tube across the grid lines or angling the grid itself during exposure produces an overall decrease in exposure to the image receptor.

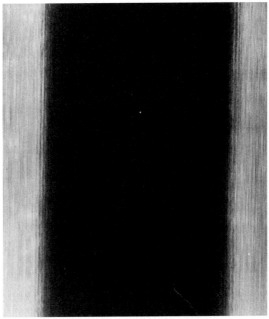

FIGURE 7-21 Radiograph produced with an upside-down focused grid.

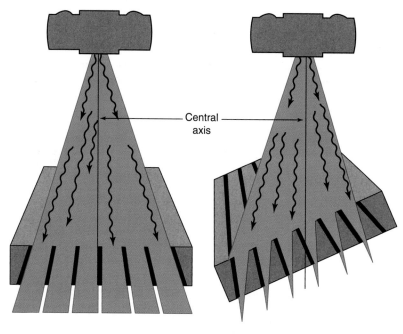

Proper position   Off-level

FIGURE 7-22 An off-level grid can cause grid cutoff.

Off-Center. Also called *lateral decentering*, off-center grid cutoff occurs when the central ray of the x-ray beam is not aligned from side to side with the center of a focused grid. Because of the arrangement of the lead lines of the focused grid, the divergence of the primary beam does not match the angle of these lead strips when not centered (Figure 7-23). Off-center grid cutoff may appear as an overall loss of exposure to the IR (Figure 7-24).

 IMPORTANT RELATIONSHIP

Off-Center Error and Grid Cutoff

If the center of the x-ray beam is not aligned from side to side with the center of a focused grid, grid cutoff occurs.

Off-Focus. Off-focus grid cutoff occurs when using an SID outside the recommended focal range. Grid cutoff occurs if the SID is less than or greater than the focal range. Radiographically, both appear as a loss of exposure at the periphery of the image (Figure 7-25).

 IMPORTANT RELATIONSHIP

Off-Focus Error and Grid Cutoff

Using an SID outside the focal range creates a loss of exposure at the periphery of the radiograph.

Grid Errors

A radiographic image with suboptimal exposure can be the result of many factors, one of which is grid cutoff. Before assuming that an underexposed image is due to technique factors and then re-exposing the patient, the radiographer should evaluate grid alignment. If misalignment is the cause of the underexposure, the patient can be protected from re-exposure with a technique factor adjustment.

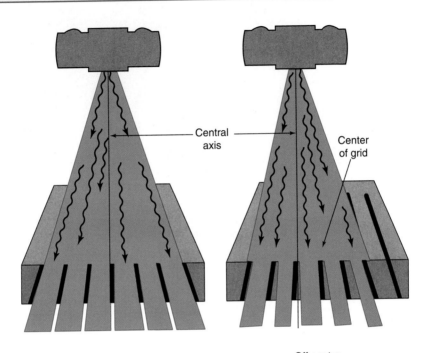

Proper position   Off-center

FIGURE 7-23 Centering to one side of a focused grid can cause off-center grid cutoff.

FIGURE 7-24 Radiograph demonstrating off-center grid cutoff.

FIGURE 7-25 Radiograph demonstrating off-focus grid cutoff.

TABLE 7-3 **Radiographic Grids**	
Increased Factor	**Result**
Grid ratio*	Contrast *increases*
	Patient dose *increases*
	The likelihood of grid cutoff *increases*

*mAs adjusted to maintain exposure to IR.

Table 7-3 summarizes important relationships regarding the use of radiographic grids.

Moiré Effect

The **Moiré effect** or zebra pattern is an artifact that can occur when a stationary grid is used during computed radiography (CR) imaging (Figure 7-26). If the grid frequency is similar to the laser scanning frequency during CR image processing, a zebra pattern can result on the digital image. The use of a higher grid frequency or a moving grid with CR digital imaging eliminates this type of grid error. In addition, if a grid cassette is placed in a Bucky, imaging the double grids creates a zebra pattern on the radiograph.

Grid Usage

The radiographer needs to consider numerous factors when deciding the type of grid, if any, to be used for an examination. Although quite efficient at preventing scatter radiation from reaching the IR, grids are not appropriate for all examinations. When appropriate, selection of a grid involves consideration of contrast improvement, patient dose, and the likelihood of grid cutoff. Radiographers typically choose between parallel and focused grids, high- and low-ratio grids, grids with different focal ranges, and whether to use a grid at all.

As indicated earlier, the choice of whether to use a grid is based on the kVp necessary for the examination and the thickness of the anatomic part being examined. Parts 10 cm (4 in) or larger, together with kVp values higher than 60, produce enough scatter to necessitate the use

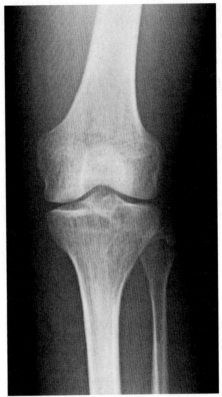

FIGURE 7-26 Moiré effect. Radiograph demonstrating the zebra pattern as a result of the Moiré effect.

of a grid. The next question is which grid to use. There is no single best grid for all situations. A 16:1 focused grid provides excellent contrast improvement, but the patient's dose is high, and the radiographer must ensure that the grid and x-ray tube are perfectly aligned to prevent grid cutoff. The 5:1 parallel grid does a mediocre job of scatter cleanup, especially at kVp values greater than 80. However, the patient dose is significantly lower, and the radiographer need not be concerned with the cutoff caused by being off-center, the SID used, or having the grid upside-down. Selection between grids with different focal ranges depends on the radiographic examination. Supine abdomen studies should use a grid that includes 40 in (100 cm) in the focal range; upright chest studies should have grids that include 72 in (180 cm). In general, most radiographic rooms use a 10:1 or 12:1 focused grid, which provides a compromise between contrast improvement and patient dose. Stationary grids, for mobile examinations in particular, may have a lower ratio, be a parallel type, or both to allow the radiographer greater positioning latitude.

Grids differ from one another in performance, especially in the areas of grid ratio and focal distance. Before using a grid, the radiographer must determine the grid ratio so that the appropriate exposure factors can be selected. Also, the radiographer must be aware of the focal range of focused grids so that an appropriate SID is selected.

Box 7-2 lists the attributes of the grid typically used in radiography. Box 7-3 summarizes grid errors and their radiographic effects. Box 7-4 provides information on quality-control checks for grid uniformity and alignment.

BOX 7-2   Typical Grid

- Is linear instead of crossed
- Is focused instead of parallel
- Is of mid-ratio (8:1 to 12:1)
- Has a focal range that includes an SID of 40 in (100 cm) or 72 (180 cm) in

---

BOX 7-3   Grid Cut-off Errors and Their Radiographic Effects

Grid Error	Radiographic Effect
Upside-Down Focused Grid: Placing a focused grid upside down on the IR	Significant underexposure to the lateral edges of the IR
Off-Level Error: Angling the x-ray tube across the grid lines or angling the grid itself during exposure	Decrease in radiation exposure to the IR
Off-Center Error: The center of the x-ray beam is not aligned from side to side with the center of a focused grid	Decrease in radiation exposure to the IR
Off-Focus Error: Using an SID outside the focal range	A loss of exposure at the periphery of the IR

IR, Image receptor; *SID,* source-to-image-receptor distance.

BOX 7-4   Quality-Control Check: Grid Uniformity and Alignment

- Nonuniformity of a grid (lack of uniform lead strips) may create artifacts on the image. Grid uniformity can be easily evaluated by imaging a grid and measuring optical densities throughout the image. Optical density readings should be within ±0.10 for proper uniformity.
- Misalignment of a focused grid (off-center) can reduce exposure to the IR as a result of grid cutoff. A grid alignment tool made of radiopaque material with cut-out holes in a line can be imaged to evaluate correct alignment of the grid with the x-ray field. A properly aligned grid would produce a greater center hole optical density than the optical densities of the side holes.

Radiation Protection

Limiting the size of the x-ray field to the anatomic area of interest will decrease scatter production and reduce patient exposure. Although the mAs may be increased to compensate for decreasing the size of the x-ray field, the tissues located closest to the lateral edge or outside the collimated x-ray beam will receive the least amount of radiation exposure. Those tissues that lie inside the collimated edge of the x-ray beam will receive the greatest amount of radiation exposure. Collimating to the anatomic area of interest is an important radiation protection practice that should be routinely performed.

The use of grids requires an increase in mAs to maintain exposure to the image receptor. As a result, patient radiation exposure is increased when using grids. The higher the grid ratio, the greater the mAs needed to maintain exposure to the image receptor, and therefore, patient radiation exposure is increased. Limiting the use of grids or using a grid with a lower grid ratio will decrease the radiation exposure to the patient.

AIR GAP TECHNIQUE

Although the radiographer may use the grid most often to prevent scatter from reaching the IR, the grid is not the only available tool. The air gap technique, although limited in its usefulness, provides another method for limiting the scatter reaching the IR. The **air gap technique** is based on the simple concept that much of the scatter will miss the IR if there is increased distance between the patient and the IR (increased object-to-image-receptor distance [OID]) (Figure 7-27). The greater the gap, the greater the reduction in scatter reaching the IR. Similar to a grid, contrast is increased, the number of photons reaching the IR is reduced because less scatter reaches the IR, and the mAs must be increased to compensate. There may be slightly less exposure because a grid absorbs some of the transmitted photons (grid cutoff), whereas the air gap technique does not.

The air gap technique is limited in its usefulness because the necessary OID results in decreased spatial resolution. To overcome this increase in unsharpness, an increase in SID is required, which may not always be feasible.

 IMPORTANT RELATIONSHIP

Air Gap Technique and Scatter Control

The air gap technique is an alternative to using a grid to control the scatter reaching the IR. By moving the IR away from the patient, more scatter radiation will miss the IR. The greater the gap, the lesser the scatter reaches the IR.

Scatter control is important when using digital or film-screen imaging systems. Reducing the amount of scatter produced through beam restriction, reducing the amount of scatter reaching the IR by using a grid, avoiding grid cutoff errors, and making appropriate exposure adjustments as needed help to produce quality radiographic images.

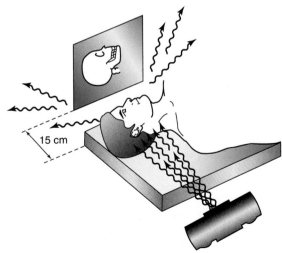

FIGURE 7-27 The air gap technique used in magnification radiography of the lateral skull.

SCATTER CONTROL AND DIGITAL IMAGING

Computer processing during digital imaging will produce an image with appropriate brightness. If the amount of x-ray exposure reaching the IR is low, computer processing will function to produce the appropriate brightness, which may result in an image with increased quantum noise. This can occur with all forms of grid cutoff or if the mAs is not increased to compensate for adding a grid or changing to a higher-ratio grid. Excessive noise in a digital image is one of the primary reasons for repeating the image.

If the digital IR receives too much exposure, computer processing produces appropriate brightness; however, image contrast is decreased because of excessive scatter. This may occur when a grid is removed and mAs is not decreased or by not making adjustments in mAs when a change is made to a lower-ratio grid.

Grid errors during digital imaging can easily be masked by computer processing. The radiographer should evaluate the exposure indicator value along with the overall quality of the digital image to determine whether any exposure errors exist.

SHIELDING ACCESSORIES

Efforts to control the amount of scatter radiation produced within the patient and reaching the IR are important considerations during radiography. Restricting the size of the x-ray beam to the anatomic area of interest reduces the radiation exposure to the patient and improves image quality. There are situations in which it is beneficial to use shielding devices to absorb the scatter radiation exiting the patient; placing a lead shield on the x-ray table close to the edge of the area of interest absorbs scatter exiting the patient that could degrade image quality. The lateral lumbar spine projection and the lateral spot are projections in which a significant amount of scatter exits the patient. Placing a lead shield behind the patient's lower back absorbs the scatter and reduces the amount striking the IR (Figure 7-28). It is important to note that placing a lead shield on the table to limit the scatter radiation reaching the IR does not reduce the exposure to the patient.

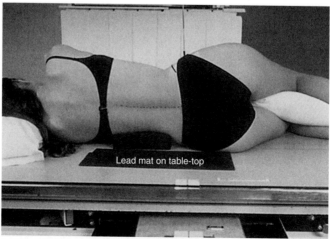

Lead mat on table-top

FIGURE 7-28 Shielding Accessory. Lead shield placed to absorb scatter radiation from the patient.

Because the patient is the greatest source of scatter radiation, any individual remaining in the radiographic room during an exposure must wear a lead apron. This, together with standing as far from the patient as possible, decreases the amount of occupational exposure to scatter radiation.

It is the radiographer's responsibility to reduce the amount of scatter radiation produced and reaching the IR. Reducing the amount of scatter produced through beam restriction and the amount reaching the IR using a grid, avoiding grid cutoff errors, and making appropriate exposure adjustments as needed help to produce good-quality radiographic images.

CHAPTER SUMMARY

- Scatter radiation, the result of Compton interactions, is detrimental to radiographic image quality. Excessive scatter results in additional unwanted exposure and reduced contrast.
- The effect of scatter radiation can be reduced by limiting the amount produced and by absorbing the scatter before it reaches the IR.
- The amount of scatter produced increases as the volume of irradiated tissue increases, and the proportion and energy of scatter exiting the patient increase as kVp increases.
- Beam restriction limits the area exposed to radiation, the patient dose, and the amount of scatter produced in the patient. Aperture diaphragms, cones and cylinders, and collimators are types of beam restrictors.
- Radiographic grids are devices placed between the patient and the IR to absorb scatter radiation. Consisting of a series of lead strips and radiolucent interspaces, grids allow transmitted radiation to pass through while scatter radiation is absorbed.
- Grid designs include linear parallel, focused parallel, crossed, short dimension, and long dimension, each with advantages and disadvantages.
- The use of a grid in a radiographic examination results in fewer photons reaching the IR. The grid conversion (or Bucky) factor is used to calculate the exposure needed when grids are used.
- Adding a grid will require an increase in mAs to maintain exposure to the IR, therefore increasing radiation exposure to the patient.
- Grid errors, producing grid cutoff, include using an upside-down focused grid and errors caused by off-level, off-center, and off-focus equipment alignment.
- The use and type of a grid depends on the thickness of the part, kVp, patient dose, contrast improvement, and likelihood of grid errors.
- The air gap technique is another method, although seldom used, for reducing the amount of scatter reaching the IR.
- Grid errors during digital imaging can easily be masked by computer processing.

REVIEW QUESTIONS

1. The projected shape of the unrestricted primary beam is _____.
   A. square
   B. rectangular
   C. circular
   D. elliptical
2. A purpose of beam-restricting devices is to _____ by changing the size and shape of the primary beam.
   A. increase patient dose
   B. decrease scatter radiation produced

    C. increase exposure to the image receptor

    D. decrease image contrast

3. The most effective type of beam-restricting device is the _____.

    A. cone

    B. aperture diaphragm

    C. cylinder

    D. collimator

4. Of the beam-restricting devices listed in question 3, which two are most similar to one another?

    A. A and B

    B. A and C

    C. B and C

    D. B and D

5. The purpose of automatic collimation is to ensure that _____.

    A. the quantity of scatter production is minimal

    B. the field size does not exceed the image receptor size

    C. maximal spatial resolution and contrast are achieved

    D. exposure to the image receptor is maintained

6. When making a significant increase in collimation, _____.

    A. mAs should be increased

    B. kVp should be increased

    C. mAs should be decreased

    D. kVp should be decreased

7. Which one of the following increases as collimation increases?

    A. Patient exposure

    B. Scatter production

    C. Fog

    D. Contrast

8. Which of the following statements is true for positive beam-limiting devices?

    A. They are required on all radiographic installations.

    B. They are required on all new radiographic installations.

    C. They have never been required on radiographic installations.

    D. They were once required on new radiographic installations.

9. The purpose of a grid in radiography is to _____.

    A. increase exposure to the image receptor

    B. increase image contrast

    C. decrease patient dose

    D. increase spatial resolution

10. Grid ratio is defined as the ratio of the _____.

    A. height of the lead strips to the distance between them

    B. width of the lead strips to their height

    C. number of lead strips to their width

    D. width of the lead strips to the width of the interspace material

11. Compared with parallel grids, focused grids _____.

    A. have a greater grid frequency and lead content

    B. can be used with either side facing the tube

    C. have a wider range of grid ratios and frequencies

    D. allow more transmitted photons to reach the image receptor

12. With which one of the following grids would a convergent line be formed if imaginary lines from its grid lines were drawn in space above it?
    A. Linear focused
    B. Crossed focused
    C. Linear parallel
    D. Crossed parallel
13. If 15 mAs is used to produce a particular level of exposure to the image receptor without a grid, what value of mAs would be needed to produce that same level of exposure using a 16:1 grid?
    A. 45
    B. 60
    C. 90
    D. 105
14. With exposure technique compensation, which of the following would result in the greatest radiation exposure to the patient?
    A. 14 × 17 x-ray field size
    B. Air gap technique
    C. Cylinder beam restrictor
    D. 12:1 grid ratio
15. Off-focus grid cutoff occurs by using an SID that is not _____.
    A. within the focal range of the grid
    B. equal to the focal distance of the grid
    C. at the level of the convergent line of the grid
    D. at the level of the convergent point of the grid
16. The type of motion most often used for moving grids today is _____.
    A. longitudinal
    B. reciprocating
    C. circular
    D. single stroke
17. A grid should be used whenever the anatomic part size exceeds _____.
    A. 3 cm
    B. 6 cm
    C. 10 cm
    D. 12 cm
18. The air gap technique uses an increased _____ instead of a grid.
    A. kVp
    B. mAs
    C. SID
    D. OID

8

Exposure Technique Selection

CHAPTER OUTLINE

Automatic Exposure Control
Radiation Detectors
mAs Readout
kVp and mA Selections
Minimum Response Time
Backup Time
Density Adjustment
Alignment and Positioning
    Considerations
Compensating Issues

**Anatomically Programmed
    Technique**
Exposure Technique Charts
Conditions
Types of Technique Charts
Exposure Technique Chart
    Development
Special Considerations
Pediatric Patients
Geriatric Patients

Bariatric Patients
Projections and Positions
Casts and Splints
Pathologic Conditions
Soft Tissue
Contrast Media

OBJECTIVES

After completing this chapter, the reader will be able to perform the following:

1. Define all the key terms in this chapter.
2. State all the important relationships in this chapter.
3. State the purpose of automatic exposure control (AEC) in radiography.
4. Differentiate among the types of radiation detectors used in AEC systems.
5. Recognize how detector size and configuration affect the response of an AEC device.
6. Explain how alignment and positioning affect the response of an AEC device.
7. Discuss patient and exposure technique factors and their effects on the response of an AEC device.
8. Analyze unacceptable images produced using AEC and identify possible causes.
9. Describe the patient radiation protection issues associated with AEC.
10. State the importance of calibration of the AEC system to the type of image receptor used.
11. Define anatomically programmed techniques.
12. Differentiate between the types of exposure technique charts.
13. State exposure technique modifications for the following considerations: pediatric, geriatric, and bariatric patients and varying projections and positions, soft tissue, casts and splints, contrast media, and pathological conditions.

KEY TERMS

anatomically programmed
    techniques
automatic exposure control
    (AEC)
backup time

calipers
comparative anatomy
contrast medium
density controls
detectors

exposure technique charts
extrapolated
fixed kVp/variable mAs
    technique chart
ionization chamber

KEY TERMS—cont'd

ion chamber	optimal kVp	variable kVp/fixed mAs
mAs readout	photomultiplier tube	technique chart
minimum response time	phototimer	

The radiographer is responsible for selecting exposure factor techniques to produce quality radiographs for a wide variety of equipment and patients. There are many thousands of possible combinations of kVp, mA, SID, exposure time, image receptors (IRs), and grid ratios. When patients of various sizes and with various pathological conditions are considered, the selection of proper exposure factors becomes a formidable task. Tools are available to assist the radiographer in selecting appropriate exposure techniques: automatic exposure control (AEC) devices, anatomically programmed techniques, and exposure technique charts. Knowledge about the performance of these tools and their operation assists the radiographer in producing quality radiographic images.

AUTOMATIC EXPOSURE CONTROL

An AEC system is a tool available on most modern radiographic units to assist the radiographer in determining the amount of radiation exposure to produce a quality image. **Automatic exposure control (AEC)** is a system used to consistently control the amount of radiation reaching the IR by terminating the length of exposure. AEC systems also are called *automatic exposure devices,* and sometimes they are erroneously referred to as *phototiming.* When using AEC systems, the radiographer must still use individual discretion to select an appropriate kVp, mA, IR, and grid. However, the AEC device determines the exposure time (and total exposure) that is used.

 IMPORTANT RELATIONSHIP

Principle of Automatic Exposure Control Operation

> Once a predetermined amount of radiation is transmitted through a patient, the x-ray exposure is terminated. This determines the exposure time and therefore the total amount of radiation exposure to the IR.

AEC systems are excellent at producing consistent levels of exposure when used properly; however, the radiographer must also be aware of the limitations of using an AEC system in patient positioning and centering, detector size and selection, collimation, and IR variation.

Radiation Detectors

All AEC devices work by the same principle of operation: radiation is transmitted through the patient and converted into an electrical signal, terminating the exposure time; this occurs when a predetermined amount of radiation has been detected, as indicated by the charge of the electrical signal produced. The predetermined level of radiation that must be achieved before exposure termination is calibrated by service personnel to meet the departmental standards of image quality.

The difference in AEC systems lies in the type of device that is used to convert radiation into electricity. Two types of AEC systems have been used: phototimers and ionization chambers. Phototimers represent the first generation of AEC systems used in radiography, and it is from this type of system that the term *phototiming* has evolved. *Phototiming* specifically refers to the use of an AEC device that uses photomultiplier tubes or photodiodes, even though these systems

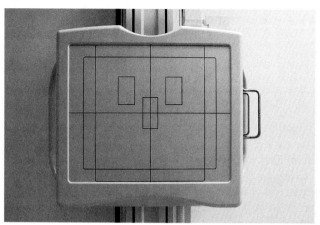

FIGURE 8-1 The size and arrangement of the three AEC detectors are clear on this upright chest unit.

are uncommon today. Therefore, the use of the term *phototiming* is usually incorrect. The more common type of AEC system uses ionization chambers. Regardless of the specific type of AEC system used, almost all systems use a set of three radiation-measuring detectors, arranged in a specific manner (Figure 8-1). The radiographer selects the configuration of these devices, determining which one (or more) of the three actually measures radiation exposure reaching the IR. These devices are variously referred to as *sensors*, *chambers*, *cells*, or *detectors*. These radiation-measuring devices are referred to here for the remainder of the discussion as **detectors**.

IMPORTANT RELATIONSHIP
Radiation-Measuring Devices

Detectors are the AEC devices that measure the amount of radiation transmitted. The radiographer selects the combination of the three detectors to use.

Phototimers

Phototimers use a fluorescent (light-producing) screen and a device that converts light into electricity. A **photomultiplier tube** is an electronic device that converts visible light energy into electrical energy. A photodiode is a solid-state device that performs the same function. Phototimer AEC devices are considered as exit-type devices because the detectors are positioned behind the IR (Figure 8-2) so that radiation must exit the IR before it is measured by the detectors. Light paddles, coated with a fluorescent material, serve as the detectors; radiation interacts with these paddles, producing visible light. This light is transmitted to remote photomultiplier tubes or photodiodes that convert it into electricity. The timer is tripped, and the radiographic exposure is terminated when a sufficiently large charge has been received. This electrical charge is in proportion to the radiation to which the light paddles have been exposed. Phototimers have largely been replaced with ionization chamber systems.

Ionization Chamber Systems

An **ionization chamber**, or **ion chamber**, is a hollow cell that contains air and is connected to the timer circuit via an electrical wire. Ionization chamber AEC devices are considered to be entrance-type devices because the detectors are positioned in front of the IR (Figure 8-3) so that radiation can interact with the detectors just before interacting with the IR. When the ionization chamber

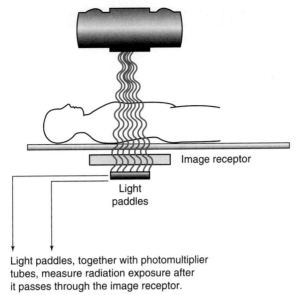

Light paddles, together with photomultiplier
tubes, measure radiation exposure after
it passes through the image receptor.

FIGURE 8-2 The phototimer AEC system has the light paddles (detectors) located directly below the IR. This is an exit-type device in that the x-rays must exit the IR before they are measured by the detectors.

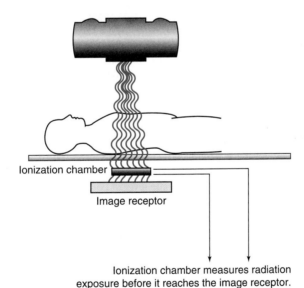

Ionization chamber measures radiation
exposure before it reaches the image receptor.

FIGURE 8-3 The ionization chamber AEC system has the detectors located directly in front of the IR. This system is termed *entrance-type* because the x-ray exposure is measured just before entering the IR.

is exposed to radiation from a radiographic exposure, the air inside the chamber becomes ionized, creating an electrical charge. This charge travels along the wire to the timer circuit. The timer is tripped, and the radiographic exposure is terminated when a sufficiently large charge has been received. This electrical charge is in proportion to the radiation to which the ionization chamber has been exposed. Compared with phototimers, ion chambers are less sophisticated and less accurate, but they are less prone to failure. Most AEC systems today use ionization chambers.

IMPORTANT RELATIONSHIP

Function of the Ionization Chamber

The ionization chamber interacts with exit radiation before it reaches the IR. Air in the chamber is ionized, and an electrical charge proportional to the amount of radiation is created.

mAs Readout

When a radiographic study is performed using an AEC device, the total amount of radiation (mAs) required to produce the appropriate exposure to the IR is determined by the system. Many radiographic units include an **mAs readout** display, where the actual amount of mAs used for that image is displayed immediately after the exposure, sometimes for only a few seconds. It is critical for the radiographer to take note of this information when it is available. Knowledge of the mAs readout has numerous advantages. It allows the radiographer to become more familiar with manual exposure technique factors. If the image is suboptimal, knowing the mAs readout provides a basis from which the radiographer can make exposure adjustments by switching to a manual technique. There may be studies with different positions where AEC and the manual technique are combined because of difficulty with accurate centering. For example, knowing the mAs readout for the anteroposterior (AP) lumbar spine gives the radiographer an option to switch to manual techniques for the oblique exposures, making technique adjustments based on reliable mAs information.

 IMPORTANT RELATIONSHIP

Automatic Exposure Control and mAs Readout

If the radiographic unit has an mAs readout display, the radiographer should take note of the reading after an exposure is made. This information can be invaluable.

kVp and mA Selections

AEC controls only the quantity of radiation reaching the IR and has no effect on other image characteristics, such as contrast. The kVp for a particular examination should be selected as it would be for that examination, regardless of whether an AEC device is used. The radiographer must select the kVp level that provides an appropriate level of contrast and is at least the minimum kVp needed to penetrate the part under examination. Although contrast can be computer manipulated in digital imaging, the kVp should still be selected to best visualize the area of interest. In addition, the higher the kVp value used, the shorter the exposure time needed by the AEC device. Because high kVp radiation is more penetrating (reducing the total amount of x-ray exposure to the patient because more x-ray photons exit the patient) and the detectors are measuring the quantity of radiation, the preset amount of radiation exposure is reached sooner with a higher kVp.

 IMPORTANT RELATIONSHIP

kVp and Automatic Exposure Control Response

The radiographer must set the kVp as needed to ensure adequate penetration while producing the appropriate level of contrast. The kVp selected determines the length of exposure time when using AEC. A low kVp requires more exposure time to reach the predetermined amount of exposure. A high kVp decreases the exposure time to reach the predetermined amount of exposure and reduces the overall radiation exposure to the patient.

> **❗ Radiation Protection Alert**
>
> ### *Kilovoltage Selection*
>
> Using a higher kVp with AEC decreases the exposure time and the overall mAs needed to produce a diagnostic image, significantly reducing patient exposure. The kVp selected for an examination should produce the desired image contrast for the part examined while being as high as possible to minimize the patient's radiation exposure.

When the radiographer uses a control panel that allows the mA and time to be set independently, he/she should select the mA value as it would be for that particular examination, regardless of whether an AEC device is used. The mA value selected will affect the exposure time needed by the AEC device. Therefore, if the radiographer wants to decrease the exposure time for a particular examination, he/she may easily do so by increasing the mA value. For a given procedure, increasing the mA on the control panel decreases the exposure time, and decreasing the mA selected on the control panel increases the exposure time.

> **IMPORTANT RELATIONSHIP**
>
> ### *mA and Automatic Exposure Control Response*
>
> If the radiographer can set the mA when using AEC, it will affect the time of exposure for a given procedure. Increasing the mA decreases the exposure time to reach the predetermined amount of exposure. Decreasing the mA increases the exposure time to reach the predetermined amount of exposure.

Minimum Response Time

The term **minimum response time** refers to the shortest exposure time that the system can produce. Minimum response time (1 ms with modern AEC systems) is usually longer with AEC systems than with other types of radiographic timers (i.e., other types of radiographic timers usually are able to produce shorter exposure times than AEC devices). This can be a problem with some segments of the patient population, such as pediatric or uncooperative patients. Typically, the radiographer increases the mA so that the time of exposure terminates more quickly. If the minimum response time is longer than the amount of time needed to terminate the preset exposure, it results in an increased amount of radiation reaching the IR. With pediatric patients and other patients who cannot or will not cooperate with the radiographer by holding still or holding their breath during the exposure, AEC devices may not be the technology of choice.

Backup Time

Backup time refers to the maximum length of time for which the x-ray exposure will continue when using an AEC system. The backup time may be set by the radiographer or automatically controlled by the radiographic unit. It may be set as backup exposure time or as backup mAs (the product of mA and exposure time). The backup time acts as a safety mechanism when an AEC system fails or the equipment is not used properly. In either case, the backup time protects the patient from receiving unnecessary exposure and protects the x-ray tube from reaching or exceeding its heat-loading capacity. If the backup time is automatically controlled, it should terminate at a maximum of 600 mAs.

IMPORTANT RELATIONSHIP

Function of Backup Time

Backup time, the maximum exposure time allowed during an AEC examination, serves as a safety mechanism when AEC is not used properly or is not functioning properly.

The backup time might be reached as a result of operator oversight when an AEC examination, such as a chest x-ray, is conducted at the upright Bucky and the radiographer has set the control panel for a table Bucky. The table detectors are forced to wait for an excessively long time to measure enough radiation to terminate the exposure. The backup time is reached and the exposure is terminated, limiting patient exposure and preventing the tube from overloading. However, newer x-ray units with AEC include a sensor in the Bucky tray for the IR and do not allow an exposure to activate if the table Bucky detectors are selected but the x-ray tube is centered to the upright Bucky.

When controlled by the radiographer, the backup time should be set high enough to exceed the exposure needed but low enough to protect the patient from excessive exposure in case of a problem. Setting the backup time at 150% - 200% of the expected exposure time is appropriate.

 IMPORTANT RELATIONSHIP

Setting Backup Time

Backup time should be set to 150%–200% of the expected exposure time. This allows the properly used AEC system to appropriately terminate the exposure but protects the patient and tube from excessive exposure if a problem occurs.

! **Radiation Protection Alert**

Monitoring Backup Time

To minimize patient exposure, the backup time should be neither too long nor too short. Backup time that is too short results in the exposure being stopped prematurely, and the image may need to be repeated because of poor image quality. Backup time that is too long results in the patient receiving unnecessary radiation if a problem occurs and the exposure does not end until the backup time is reached. In addition, the image may have to be repeated because of poor image quality.

Density Adjustment

AEC devices are equipped with **density controls** that allow the radiographer to adjust the amount of preset radiation detection values. These are generally in the form of buttons on the control panel that are numbered −2, −1, +1, and +2. The actual numbers presented on density controls vary, but each button changes exposure time by a certain predetermined amount or increment expressed as a percentage. A common increment is 25%, meaning that the predetermined exposure level needed to terminate the timer can be either increased or decreased from normal in one increment (+25% or −25%) or two increments (+50% or −50%). Manufacturers usually provide information for their equipment on how these density controls should be used. Common sense and practical experience should also serve as guidelines for the radiographer. Routinely using plus or minus density settings to produce an acceptable radiograph indicates that a problem exists, possibly a problem with the AEC device.

Alignment and Positioning Considerations

Detector Selection

Selection of the detectors to be used for a particular examination is critical when using an AEC system. AEC systems with multiple detectors typically allow the radiographer to select any combination of one, two, or all three detectors. The selected detectors actively measure radiation during exposure, and the electrical signals are averaged. Typically, the detector that receives the greatest amount of exposure has the greatest impact on the total exposure.

Measuring radiation that passes through the anatomic area of interest is important. The general guideline is to select the detectors that would be superimposed by the anatomic structures that are of greatest interest and need to be visualized on the radiograph. Failure to use proper detectors could result in either underexposure or overexposure to the IR. In the case of a posteroanterior (PA) chest radiograph, the area of radiographic interest includes the lungs and heart; therefore, one or two outside detectors should be selected to place the detectors directly beneath the critical anatomic area. If the center detector were mistakenly selected, the anatomy superimposing this detector includes the thoracic spine. If the exposure is made, the resultant image shows sufficient exposure in the spine, with the lungs overexposed (Figure 8-4). In the manual that accompanies a radiographic unit, the AEC device manufacturer provides recommendations for which detectors to use for specific examinations. In addition, recommendations for detector combination can be found in many radiographic procedure textbooks.

Many radiographic units have AEC devices in both a table Bucky and an upright Bucky. If more than one Bucky per radiographic unit uses AEC, the radiographer must be certain to select the correct Bucky before making an exposure. Failure to do so may result in the patient and IR being exposed to excessive radiation. If the backup time is reached, the exposure is prematurely terminated and a repeat radiographic study may need to be done, increasing patient dose.

A similar problem can occur in some systems when not using a Bucky, such as with cross-table, tabletop or stretcher, or wheelchair studies. If the AEC system is activated with these types of examinations, an unusually long exposure results because the detectors are not being exposed to radiation. Again, the backup time will likely be reached, and the patient's dose will be excessive. Some radiographic units are designed so that an exposure does not occur if the AEC device has been selected and there is no IR detected in the Bucky.

 IMPORTANT RELATIONSHIP

Detector Selection

The combination of detectors affects the amount of exposure reaching the IR. If the area of radiographic interest is not directly over the selected detectors, that area will likely be overexposed or underexposed. When performing a radiographic study where the IR is located outside the Bucky, the AEC system should be deactivated and a manual technique should be used.

Patient Centering

Proper centering of the part being examined is crucial when using an AEC system. The anatomic area of interest must be properly centered over the detectors that the radiographer has selected; improper centering of the part over the selected detectors may underexpose or overexpose the IR. For example, when an AEC device is used for a lateral lumbar spine image, if the central ray is too far posterior and the center detector is selected (as appropriate), the soft tissue superimposes the detector rather than the spine. In this case, the soft tissue behind the spine demonstrates sufficient exposure, but the spine itself is underexposed (Figure 8-5).

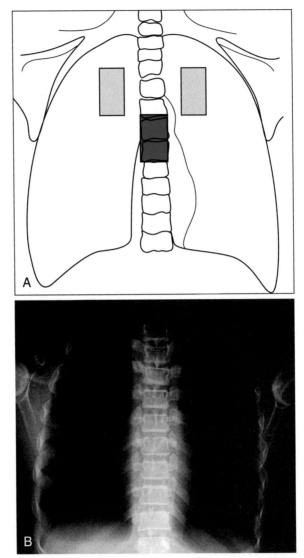

FIGURE 8-4 Selecting the detectors to be located directly under the critical anatomic area may make the difference between a diagnostic image and an unacceptable image. The PA chest should be imaged using both outside detectors to locate them directly under the lung tissue. **A,** This diagram shows that the center detector was inappropriately selected for the PA chest image, placing the thoracic spine directly over the detector. **B,** The resulting chest radiograph demonstrates the diagnostic density in the area of the spine, but the lungs are notably overexposed.

IMPORTANT RELATIONSHIP

Patient Centering

Accurate centering of the area of interest over the detectors is critical to ensure proper exposure to the IR. If the area of interest is not properly centered to the detectors, overexposure or underexposure may occur.

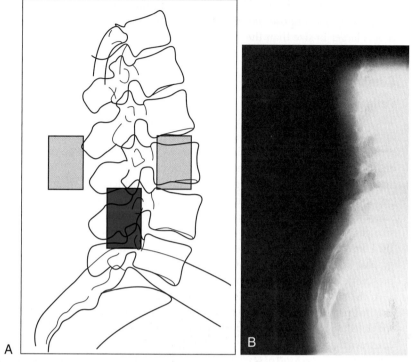

FIGURE 8-5 Centering the key anatomic area directly over the AEC detector is critical in producing diagnostic radiographs. Whatever anatomic area is located over the detector has diagnostic exposure. **A,** With the center detector selected, the centering for this lateral lumbar spine image is posterior to the lumbar vertebral bodies. The lamina, spinous processes, and soft tissue cover the detector. **B,** The resulting radiograph demonstrates the appropriate density just posterior to the vertebral bodies, but the bodies themselves are underexposed. This radiograph is unacceptable because of inaccurate centering, resulting in underexposure of the anatomy of interest.

Inaccurate centering is probably the most common cause of suboptimal film-screen images when AEC is used. When the anatomy of interest is not centered directly over the detector, the image is underexposed or overexposed, possibly requiring the image to be repeated and the patient to receive more radiation than necessary.

If a digital IR is underexposed or overexposed, the computer adjusts the exposure error, but the image quality, patient exposure, or both are compromised. Underexposure may result in the visibility of quantum noise, and overexposure increases patient exposure and may decrease contrast.

Detector Size

The size of the detectors manufactured within an AEC system is fixed and cannot be adjusted. Therefore, it is important for the radiographer to determine whether AEC should be used during the radiographic procedure. The radiographer must first determine whether the patient's anatomic area of interest can adequately cover the detector combination. For example, if the patient for a procedure is very small, such as a toddler, his/her chest may not adequately cover the outer two detectors. In this case, the patient's chest is smaller than the dimensions of the selected detectors. If a portion of the detector is directly exposed to the primary beam, the radiation exposure level necessary to terminate the exposure is reached almost immediately, resulting in underexposure of the area of interest.

It is critical for the radiographer to determine whether the anatomic area of interest can adequately superimpose the dimension of the detector combination. If the detector combination is larger in size than the area of interest, the use of a manual exposure technique would be necessitated.

Compensating Issues

Patient Considerations

The AEC system is designed to compensate for changes in patient thickness. If the area of interest is thicker because of an increase in the patient's size, the exposure time will lengthen in order to reach the preset exposure to the detectors. AEC systems that do not adequately compensate for changes in patient thickness may need to be calibrated.

Some patients may require greater technical consideration when AEC is used for radiographic procedures. Abdominal examinations using AEC can be compromised if a patient has an excessive amount of bowel gas. If a detector is superimposed by an area of the abdomen with excessive gas, the timer will prematurely terminate the exposure, resulting in underexposure to the IR. Likewise, destructive pathological conditions can cause underexposure of the area of radiographic interest. The presence of positive contrast media, an additive pathological condition, or a prosthetic device superimposing the detector can cause excessive exposure.

If the anatomic area directly over the detector does not represent the anatomic area of interest, inappropriate exposure to the IR may result. This can happen when the anatomic area over the detector contains a foreign object, a pocket of air, or contrast media. The radiographer must consider these circumstances individually and determine how to best image the patient or part. Using the density control buttons may work in some cases, whereas in others it may be necessary to recenter the patient or part. Sometimes, the best solution is a manual technique determined through use of a technique chart. AEC is not a replacement for a knowledgeable radiographer using critical thinking skills.

!   **Radiation Protection Alert**

Patient Variability

Factors related to the patient affect the time of exposure reaching the IR and ultimately the image quality; such factors include pathology, contrast media, foreign objects, and pockets of gas. Increases or decreases in patient thickness result in changes in the time of exposure if the AEC system is functioning properly.

Collimation

The size of the x-ray field is a factor when AEC systems are used because the additional scatter radiation produced by failure to accurately restrict the beam may cause the detector to prematurely terminate the exposure. The detector is unable to distinguish transmitted radiation from scattered radiation and, as always, ends the exposure when a preset amount of exposure has been reached. Because the detector is measuring both types of radiation exiting the patient, the timer is turned off too soon when scatter is excessive, resulting in underexposure of the area of interest.

In addition, if the x-ray field size is collimated too closely, the detector does not initially receive sufficient exposure and may prolong the exposure time, which could result in overexposure. The radiographer should open the collimator to the extent that the part being radiographed is appropriately imaged but not so much as to cause the AEC device to terminate the exposure before the area being imaged is properly exposed.

IMPORTANT RELATIONSHIP

Collimation and Automatic Exposure Control Response

Excessive or insufficient collimation may affect the amount of exposure reaching the IR. Insufficient collimation may result in excessive scatter reaching the detectors, causing the exposure time to terminate too quickly. Excessive collimation may result in an extremely long exposure time.

Image Receptor Variations

Different types of IRs cannot be interchanged easily once an AEC device is calibrated to terminate exposures at a preset level. When calibration is performed, it is done for a particular type of IR.

 IMPORTANT RELATIONSHIP

Type of Image Receptor and Automatic Exposure Control Response

The AEC system is calibrated based on the type of IR used. If an IR of a different type is used, the detectors will not sense the difference and the exposure time will terminate at the preset value, which may jeopardize image quality.

The AEC device cannot sense when the radiographer uses a different type of IR and instead produces an exposure based on the system for which it was calibrated, resulting in either too much or too little exposure for that IR.

Calibration

As with any radiographic unit, it is imperative that systematic equipment testing be performed to ensure proper system performance. Calibration and quality control testing are essential procedures to maintain the proper functioning of the AEC system (Box 8-1).

For an AEC device to function properly, the radiographic unit, including the type of IR, and the AEC device must be calibrated to meet departmental standards. When a radiographic unit with AEC is first installed, the AEC device is calibrated (and at intervals thereafter). The purpose of this calibration is to ensure that consistent and appropriate exposures to the IR are produced.

Failure to maintain regular calibration of the unit results in a lack of consistent and reproducible exposures to the detectors and could affect image quality. This situation ultimately leads to overexposure of the patient, poor efficiency of the imaging department, and the possibility of improper interpretation of radiographs.

The radiographer must use AEC accurately, regardless of the type of IR used. Failure to do so can result in overexposure of the patient to ionizing radiation or production of a poor-quality image. The visual cues of increased or decreased radiographic density present when using film-screen IRs that

BOX 8-1 Quality-Control Check: Automatic Exposure Control

- The AEC device should provide consistent optical densities for variations in exposure factors, patient thicknesses, and detector selection. Several aspects of the AEC performance can be monitored with a densitometer by imaging a homogeneous patient-equivalent phantom plus additional thickness plates.
- Consistency of exposures with varying mA, kVp, part thicknesses, and detector selection can be evaluated individually and in combination by imaging the phantom and measuring the resultant optical densities. Optical densities should be within ±0.2 for proper performance of the AEC device. In addition, reproducibility of exposures for a given set of exposure factors and selected detectors should result in optical densities within ±0.10.

are lacking in digital imaging. It cannot be overstated that when using digital IRs, the radiographer must be very conscientious about excessive radiation exposure to the patient. If a high amount of radiation reaches the digital IR, the image will probably appear diagnostic while the patient receives unnecessary exposure. During computer processing, image brightness can be adjusted following underexposure; however, there may be an increase in the visibility of quantum noise. The radiographer must monitor the exposure indicator as a means of detecting AEC malfunctions for digital IRs.

> ### ▧ IMPORTANT RELATIONSHIP
> #### *Digital Image Receptors and the Automatic Exposure Control Response*
>
> Because the visual cues of increased or decreased radiographic density when using film-screen IRs are lacking in digital imaging, the radiographer must be very conscientious about excessive radiation exposure to the patient.

Tables 8-1 and 8-2 clarify the relationship between exposure technique factors and AEC for digital IRs (see Table 8-1) and film-screen IRs (see Table 8-2).

ANATOMICALLY PROGRAMMED TECHNIQUE

Anatomically programmed technique refers to a system that allows the radiographer to select a particular button on the control panel that represents an anatomic area; a preprogrammed set of exposure factors is displayed and selected for use. The appearance of these controls varies depending on the unit (Figure 8-6), but the operation of all anatomically programmed systems is based on the same principle. Anatomically programmed techniques are controlled by an integrated circuit or computer chip programmed with exposure factors for different projections and positions of different anatomic parts. Once an anatomic part and projection or position has been selected, the radiographer can adjust the exposure factors that are displayed.

Anatomically programmed technique systems and AEC are not related in their functions, other than as systems for making exposures. However, these two different systems are commonly combined in radiographic units because of their similar dependence on integrated computer circuitry. Anatomically programmed techniques and AEC often are used in conjunction with one another. A radiographer can use an anatomically programmed technique to select a projection or position for a specific anatomic part and view the kVp, mA, and exposure time for a manual technique. When anatomically programmed techniques are used in conjunction with AEC on some radiographic units, the system not only selects and displays manual exposure factors but also selects and displays the AEC detectors to be used for a specific radiographic examination. For example, pressing the Lungs PA button results in selection of 120 kVp, the upright Bucky, and the two outside AEC detectors. As with AEC, the anatomically programmed technique is a system that automates some of the work of radiography. However, the individual judgment and discretion of the radiographer is still required to use the anatomically programmed technique system correctly for the production of diagnostic quality images.

> ### ⚠ Radiation Protection Alert
> #### *Anatomically Programmed Technique and Patient Exposure*
>
> When using a preprogrammed set of exposure factors, the radiographer must evaluate the appropriateness of the selected exposure technique factors. Adjustment of the preprogrammed exposure factors may be necessary for that patient or procedure.

TABLE 8-1   Digital Imaging and AEC

An upright PA chest examination performed using the following factors produces an optimal image:

Flat-panel detector	AEC with 2 outside detectors
120 kVp	upright Bucky
400 mA	0 (normal) density

Assuming all other factors remain the same, unless indicated, how would the following changes affect the response of the AEC device and image quality?

Change	Effect on Exposure Time	Effect on Brightness in Area of Interest	Explanation
CR image receptor	0	0	The AEC is calibrated to the flat-panel detector. The exposure ends when the exposure is sufficient for the IR, which is suboptimal for the CR image receptor. The computer maintains the brightness, but quantum noise is apparent because of underexposure of the imaging plate.
Center detector selected	↑	0	Because the thoracic spine lies over the center detector, the IR receives more exposure than is needed. The exposure indicator will reflect an increase in exposure to the image receptor. The computer maintains the brightness but the image contrast is decreased because of excessive scatter, and the patient is overexposed.
70 kVp	↑	0	The length of exposure to the IR will be increased, resulting in an increase in the actual mAs to maintain the exposure to the IR. However, the contrast is increased due to the lower kVp.
100 mA	↑	0	The length of exposure is increased to maintain exposure to the IR.
−2 density	↓	0	Changing the density selector changes the setting of the AEC so it turns off the exposure much sooner. The exposure indicator will reflect a decrease in exposure to the IR. The computer maintains the brightness, but quantum noise is apparent because of underexposure of the IR.
Selecting the table Bucky setting but still using the upright Bucky	↑	0	Excessive radiation reaches the imaging plate because the detectors in the table Bucky are unable to terminate the exposure. The exposure indicator will reflect an increase in exposure to the IR. The computer maintains the brightness but the image contrast is decreased because of excessive scatter, and the patient is overexposed.
Patient has cardiac pacemaker positioned over detector	↑	0	The detector that is behind the pacemaker takes a long time to turn the exposure off because the radiation has to pass through the pacemaker. The exposure indicator will reflect an increase in exposure to the IR. The computer maintains the brightness, but the image contrast is decreased because of excessive scatter, and the patient is overexposed.

TABLE 8-2   Film-Screen Radiography and AEC

An upright PA chest examination done using the following factors produces an optimal image:

400 speed film-screen system	AEC with 2 outside detectors
120 kVp	upright Bucky
400 mA	0 (normal) density

Assuming all other factors remain the same, how would the following changes affect the response of the AEC device and image quality?

Change	Effect on Exposure Time	Effect on Density in Area of Interest	Explanation
100 speed film-screen IR	0	↓	AEC is calibrated to the 400 speed film-screen system. The exposure ends when the exposure is sufficient for the 400 speed IR, which is not sufficient for the 100 speed IR.
Center detector selected	↑	↑	The exposure time is increased. Because the thoracic spine lies over the center detector, the spine has appropriate density, but the lungs have too much density.
70 kVp	↑	0	Changing the kVp does not affect the density, because AEC simply waits for the right number of photons to exit the patient. The exposure time will be increased and result in an increase in the actual mAs. However, the contrast is increased.
100 mA	↑	0	Changing the mA does not affect the density, because AEC simply waits for the right number of photons to exit the patient. However, the length of exposure is increased.
−2 density	↓	↓	Changing the density selector changes the setting of the AEC so that it turns off the exposure much sooner, resulting in a reduced density.
Selecting the table Bucky AEC device but still using the upright Bucky	↑	↑	The AEC device in the table Bucky is waiting for enough exit radiation to strike the detectors so that the exposure can be terminated. Because the x-ray beam is aimed at the upright Bucky, it is a very long exposure and results in increased density.
Patient has cardiac pacemaker positioned over detector	↑	↑	The detector that is behind the pacemaker takes a long time to terminate the exposure, because the radiation has to pass through the pacemaker. This results in increased density.

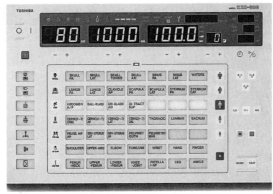

FIGURE 8-6 Anatomically programmed technique selections are displayed on this console. The radiographer can choose from PA lungs, lateral skull, knee, and hand among others. Each selection displays the preprogrammed technical factors that the radiographer can decide to use or adjust.

EXPOSURE TECHNIQUE CHARTS

Exposure technique charts are useful tools that assist the radiographer in selecting a manual exposure technique or when using AEC, regardless of the type of IR. Exposure technique charts are equally valuable for digital or film-screen IRs. **Exposure technique charts** are pre-established guidelines used by the radiographer to select standardized manual or AEC exposure factors for each type of radiographic examination. Technique charts standardize the selection of exposure factors for the typical patient so that the quality of radiographic images is consistent. Additional information, such as collimation, AEC detector selection, and patient shielding, can be included in the technique chart.

> **! Radiation Protection Alert**
>
> ### Exposure Technique Charts and Digital Imaging
>
> Exposure technique charts are just as important, if not more so, when using digital IRs. Underexposure or overexposure of a film-screen IR can result in a radiograph with decreased or increased density. Because image brightness is controlled by computer processing, the visual cues for overexposure or underexposure are missing. Exposure technique charts are an effective tool in selecting appropriate exposure techniques for a quality digital image.

For each radiographic procedure, the radiographer consults the technique chart for the recommended exposure variables—kVp, mAs, type of IR, grid, and SID. Based on the thickness of the anatomic part to be imaged, the radiographer selects the exposure factors presented in the technique chart. For example, if a patient is scheduled for a routine abdominal examination, the radiographer positions the patient and aligns the central ray to the patient and IR, measures the abdomen for a manual technique, and consults the chart for the predetermined standardized exposure variables.

Because many factors have an impact on the selection of appropriate exposure factors, technique charts are instrumental in the production of consistent quality radiographs, reduction in repeat radiographic studies, and reduction in patient exposure. The proper development and use of technique charts are keys to the selection of appropriate exposure factors.

IMPORTANT RELATIONSHIP

Exposure Technique Charts and Radiographic Quality

Exposure technique charts are just as important for digital imaging because digital systems have a wide dynamic range and can compensate for exposure technique errors. Technique charts should be developed and used with all types of radiographic imaging systems to maintain patient radiation exposure *as low as reasonably achievable* (ALARA).

Conditions

A technique chart presents the exposure factors that are to be used for a particular examination on the basis of the type of radiographic equipment. Technique charts help to ensure that consistent image quality is achieved throughout the entire radiology department; they also decrease the number of repeat radiographic studies needed and therefore decrease patient exposure.

Technique charts do not replace the critical thinking skills required of the radiographer. The radiographer must continue to use individual judgment and discretion in properly selecting exposure factors for each patient and type of examination. The primary task of the radiographer is to produce the highest-quality radiograph while delivering the least amount of radiation exposure. Technique charts are designed for an average or typical patient and do not account for unusual circumstances. Patient variability in terms of body build or physical condition or the presence of a pathological condition requires the radiographer to problem solve when selecting exposure factors. These atypical conditions require accurate patient assessment and appropriate exposure technique adjustment by the radiographer.

A technique chart should be established for each x-ray tube, even if a single generator is used for more than one tube. For example, if a radiographic room has two x-ray tubes, one for a radiographic table and one for an upright Bucky unit, each tube should have its own technique chart because of possible inherent differences in the radiation output produced by each tube. Furthermore, a portable radiographic unit must also have its own technique chart.

For technique charts to be effective tools in producing radiographs of consistent quality, departmental standards for radiographic quality should be established. In addition, the standardization of exposure factors and the use of accessory devices are needed. For example, an adult knee can be adequately radiographed with or without the use of a grid. Although both radiographs might be acceptable, departmental standards may specify that the knee be radiographed with the use of a grid. These types of decisions should be made before technique chart development takes place so that the departmental standards can be clarified. Technique charts are then constructed using these standards, to which radiographers should adhere.

For technique charts to be effective, the radiographic system should be operating properly. A good-quality control program for all radiographic equipment ensures monitoring of any variability in the performance of the equipment.

Accurate measurement of part thickness is a critical condition for the effective use of technique charts. The measured part thickness determines the selected kVp and mAs values for the radiographic examination. If the part is measured inaccurately, incorrect exposure factors may be selected. Measurement of part thickness must be standardized throughout the radiology department.

Calipers are devices that measure part thickness and should be readily accessible in every radiographic room (Figure 8-7). In addition, the technique chart should specify the exact location for measuring part thickness. Part measurement may be performed at the location of the central

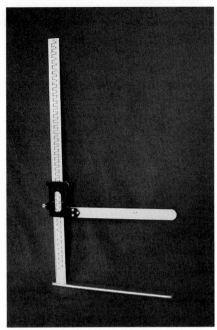

FIGURE 8-7 A caliper is used to measure part thickness.

ray midpoint or the thickest portion of the area to be radiographed. Errors in part thickness measurement are common mistakes made when one is consulting technique charts.

Because the range of exposures needed to produce a quality digital image is wider (wide exposure latitude), precise measurement of the anatomic part is not as critical. Although the technique charts discussed in this chapter use patient measurement to determine the exposure factors to be selected, categorizing the typical patient according to size (small, medium, and large) should be sufficient when using digital IRs.

Types of Technique Charts

Technique charts can vary widely in terms of their design, but they share some common characteristics. The primary exposure factors of kVp and mA and common accessory devices used, such as IRs of various types and grid ratios, are included regardless of the type of technique chart used. Two primary types of exposure technique charts exist: fixed kVp/variable mAs and variable kVp/fixed mAs. Each type of chart has different characteristics, and both have advantages and disadvantages.

Variable kVp/Fixed mAs Technique Chart

The **variable kVp/fixed mAs technique chart** is based on the concept that kVp can be increased as the anatomic part size increases. Specifically, the baseline kVp is increased by 2 for every 1 cm (0.4 in) increase in part thickness, whereas mAs is maintained (Table 8-3). The baseline kVp is the original kVp value predetermined for the anatomic area to be radiographed. The baseline kVp is then adjusted for changes in part thickness.

Accurate measurement of part thickness is critical to the effective use of this type of technique chart. Part thickness must be accurately measured to ensure that the 2 kVp adjustment is

TABLE 8-3   Variable kVp/Fixed mAs Technique Chart

Anatomic part: Knee
Projection: AP
Measuring point: Midpatella
SID: 40 in

IR: Flat panel
Tabletop/Bucky: Bucky
Grid ratio: 12:1
Focal spot size: Small

Cm	kVp	mAs
10	63	20
11	65	20
12	67	20
13	69	20
14	71	20
15	73	20
16	75	20
17	77	20
18	79	20

appropriately applied. The radiographer consults the technique chart and prepares the exposure factors specified for the type of radiographic examination (i.e., mAs, SID, grid use, and type of IR). The anatomic part is accurately measured, and the kVp is appropriately adjusted. For example, a standard exposure technique for a patient's knee measuring 10 cm (4 in) is 63 kVp at 10 mAs, flat-panel IR, and the use of a 12:1 table Bucky grid. A patient with a knee measuring 15 cm (6 in) would require a change only in the kVp from 63 to 73 (2 kVp change for every 1 cm [approximately 0.5 in] change in part thickness).

 IMPORTANT RELATIONSHIP

Variable kVp/Fixed mAs Technique Chart

The variable kVp chart adjusts the kVp for changes in part thickness while maintaining a fixed mAs.

Determination of the baseline kilovoltage for each anatomic area has not been standardized. Historically, various methods have been used to determine the baseline kVp value. The goal is to determine a kVp value that adequately penetrates the anatomic part when using a 2 kVp adjustment for every 1 cm (approximately 0.5 in) change in tissue thickness. The baseline kVp value can be experimentally determined with the use of radiographic phantoms (patient-equivalent devices).

Developing a variable kVp technique chart that can be used effectively throughout the kilovoltage range has proved to be problematic. In addition, technology advances in IRs may challenge the applicability of the variable kVp/fixed mAs-type technique chart.

In general, changing the kVp values for variations in part thickness may be ineffective throughout the entire range of radiographic examinations. A variable kVp/fixed mAs chart may be most effective with pediatric patients or when small extremities, such as hands, toes, and feet, are being imaged. At low kVp levels, small changes in kVp may be more effective than changing the mAs.

This type of chart has the advantage of being easy to formulate because making kVp changes to compensate for different part sizes is simple. However, because kVp is variable, radiographic contrast may also vary, and these types of charts tend to be less accurate for part-size extremes. In addition, adequate penetration of the part is not assured.

TABLE 8-4	Fixed kVp/Variable mAs Technique Chart	

Anatomic part: Knee
Projection: AP
Measuring point: Midpatella
SID: 40 in

IR: Flat panel
Tabletop/Bucky: Bucky
Grid ratio: 12:1
Focal spot size: Small

Cm	kVp	mAs
10–13	73	10
14–17	73	20
18–21	73	40

Fixed kVp/Variable mAs Technique Chart

The **fixed kVp/variable mAs technique chart** (Table 8-4) uses the concept of selecting an optimal kVp value that is required for the radiographic examination and adjusting the mAs for variations in part thickness. **Optimal kVp** can be described as the kVp value that is high enough to ensure penetration of the part but not too high to diminish radiographic contrast. For this type of chart, the optimal kVp value for each part is indicated and mAs is varied as a function of part thickness.

> ### IMPORTANT RELATIONSHIP
>
> *Fixed kVp/Variable mAs Technique Charts*
>
> Fixed kVp/variable mAs technique charts identify optimal kVp values and alter the mAs for variations in part thickness.

Optimal kVp values required for each anatomic area have not been standardized. Although charts identifying common kVp values for different anatomic areas can be found, experienced radiographers tend to develop their own optimal kVp values. The goal is to determine the kVp that penetrates the part without compromising radiographic contrast. Digital computer processing provides the opportunity to vary the image contrast displayed, and therefore, the optimal kVp determined for digital IRs could be higher than the kVp for film-screen IRs. Specifying the optimal kVp value used in a fixed kVp/variable mAs technique chart encourages all radiographers to adhere to the departmental standards.

Once optimal kVp values are established, fixed kVp/variable mAs technique charts alter the mAs for variations in the thickness of the anatomic part. Because x-rays are attenuated exponentially, a general guideline is that for every 4–5 cm (1.6–2 in) change in part thickness, the mAs should be adjusted by a factor of 2. Using the previous example for a patient's knee measuring 10 cm (4 in) and an optimal kVp, the exposure technique would be 63 kVp at 10 mAs, flat-panel IR with a 12:1 table Bucky grid. A patient with a knee measuring 15 cm (6 in) would require a change only in the mAs from 10 to 20 (a 5 cm [2 in] increase in part thickness requires a doubling of the mAs).

Accurate measurement of the anatomic part is important but is less critical compared with the precision needed with variable kVp charts. An advantage of fixed kVp/variable mAs technique charts is that patient groups can be formed for around 4–5 cm (1.6–2 in) changes. Patient thickness groups can be created instead of listing thickness changes in increments of 1 cm (approximately 0.5 in).

The fixed kVp/variable mAs technique chart has the advantages of easier use, more consistency in the production of quality radiographs, greater assurance of adequate penetration of all anatomic parts, uniform radiographic contrast, and increased accuracy with extreme variation in the size of the anatomic part.

Exposure Technique Chart Development

Radiographers can develop effective technique charts that assist in exposure technique selection. The steps involved in technique chart development are similar, regardless of the design of the technique chart. The primary tools needed are radiographic phantoms, calipers for accurate measurement, and a calculator. Once optimal radiographs are produced using these phantoms, exposure techniques can be **extrapolated** (mathematically estimated) for imaging other similar anatomic areas.

A critical component in technique chart development is to determine the minimal kVp value that adequately penetrates the anatomic part being radiographed. One available method is to use the concept of **comparative anatomy**, which can assist the radiographer in determining minimal kVp values. This concept states that different parts of the same size can be radiographed by use of the same exposure factors, provided that the minimal kVp value needed to penetrate the part is used in each case. For example, a radiographer knows what exposure factors to use with a particular radiographic unit for a knee that measures 10 cm (4 in) for the AP projection, but he/she now needs to radiograph a shoulder; the radiographer measures the shoulder for the AP projection and determines that it measures 10 cm (4 in). The radiographer does not have a technique for a shoulder for this radiographic unit. The concept of comparative anatomy states that the shoulder in this case can be successfully radiographed using the same technique that the radiographer has used for the 10 cm (4 in) knee as long as the minimal kVp to penetrate the part has been used for the shoulder or knee.

The stages for development of exposure technique charts are similar, regardless of the type of chart (Box 8-2). Patient-equivalent phantoms for sample anatomic areas provide a means for establishing standardized exposure factors. Using the concept of comparative anatomy assists the radiographer in extrapolating exposure techniques for similar anatomic areas. After the initial development of an exposure technique chart, the chart must be tested for accuracy and revised if necessary.

Poor radiographic quality may result when the exposure technique chart is not used properly. Radiographers need to problem solve by evaluating the numerous exposure variables that could have contributed to a poor-quality radiograph before assuming that the chart is ineffective.

A commitment by management and staff to use exposure technique charts is critical to the consistent production of quality radiographs. Well-developed technique charts are of little use if radiographers choose not to consult them.

BOX 8-2   How to Develop an Exposure Technique Chart

1. Select a kVp value appropriate to the anatomic area to be radiographed. Determine the mAs value that produces the desired exposure to the IR.
2. Using a patient-equivalent phantom, produce several radiographs by varying the kVp and mAs values. Use the general rules for exposure technique adjustment (i.e., the 15% rule). Exposures to the IR should be similar.
3. Evaluate the quality of the radiographs, and eliminate those deemed unacceptable.
4. Of the remaining acceptable radiographs, select those having a kVp value appropriate for the type of technique chart desired and according to departmental standards.
5. Extrapolate the exposure techniques (variable kVp or variable mAs) for changes in part thickness.
6. Use the concept of comparative anatomy to develop technique charts for similar anatomic areas.
7. Test the technique chart for accuracy, and revise if needed.

SPECIAL CONSIDERATIONS

Appropriate exposure factor selection and its modification for variability in the patient are critical to the production of a quality radiograph. The radiographer must be able to recognize a multitude of patient and equipment variables and have a thorough understanding of how these variables affect the resulting radiograph to make adjustments to produce a quality image.

Pediatric Patients

Pediatric patients are a technical challenge for radiographers for many reasons. Because of their smaller size, they require lower kVp and mAs values compared with adults.

Pediatric chest radiography requires the technologist to choose fast exposure times to stop diaphragm motion in patients who cannot or will not voluntarily suspend their breathing. A fast exposure time may eliminate the possibility of using AEC systems for pediatric chest radiography. Owing to their small size, the pediatric patient may not adequately cover the AEC detectors, and therefore, a manual exposure technique should be used.

Exposure factors used for the adult skull can be used for pediatric patients aged 6 years and older, because the bone density of these children has developed to an adult level. However, exposure factors must be modified for patients younger than 6 years. It is recommended for the radiographer to decrease the kVp by at least 15% to compensate for this lack of bone density. In addition, one should limit the use of grids whenever possible. Radiographic examination of all other parts of pediatric patients' anatomy requires an adjustment in exposure techniques.

Because pediatric patients are more sensitive to ionizing radiation and have a longer life span than adults, it is even more critical to monitor the exposure indicator during digital imaging in an effort to minimize unnecessary radiation exposure.

Geriatric Patients

Aging patients may experience physical changes such as limitations in hearing, vision, and balance. Additionally, their skin is thinner and more easily torn or bruised. Psychological changes in the mental state of geriatric patients may impact their ability to follow instructions during imaging procedures. The radiographer should be prepared to provide enhanced patient care in terms of additional time for the imaging procedure, sensitivity to patient comfort by using a table pad, positioning sponges, blankets for warmth, and attention to the safety of geriatric patients during transport on and off of the table and positioning during the procedure.

Exposure techniques may need to be decreased for patients who appear thin and frail. Tissues may be lower in subject contrast and therefore require decreased kVp, which results in higher image contrast. In an effort to eliminate motion, it is recommended for the radiographer to accordingly adjust the mA and exposure time.

Bariatric Patients

Imaging patients who are categorized as obese are more commonplace in radiology. Bariatric surgery is becoming more routine and therefore imaging procedures may be needed both prior to and post surgery. Bariatric patients bring unique challenges in terms of their weight and body diameter.

Important issues to consider when imaging bariatric patients include the table weight limit and the size (aperture) diameter of fluoroscopic imaging equipment. Bariatric patients need an increase in both kVp and mAs values to produce diagnostic images. In addition, the use of a grid is important to reduce the scatter radiation from reaching the image receptor, which would decrease image contrast. Depending on the imaging procedure performed, bariatric patients may need to be imaged in quadrants owing to the size limitation of the image receptor.

Projections and Positions

Different radiographic projections and patient positions of the same anatomic part often require modification of exposure factors. For example, an oblique position of the lumbar spine requires more exposure than an AP projection because of an increase in the amount of tissue through which the primary beam must pass. However, an oblique ankle radiograph requires slightly less exposure than the AP for comparable exposure to the IR.

General guidelines, based on variations in radiographic projection or patient position, can be followed to change exposure factors. When compared with an AP projection, an increase or a decrease in the amount of tissue should determine any changes in exposure factors for oblique and lateral patient positions.

Casts and Splints

Casts and splints can be produced from materials that attenuate x-rays differently. Selecting appropriate exposure factors can be challenging because of the wide variety of materials used for these devices. The radiographer should pay close attention to both the type of material and how the cast or splint is used.

Casts

Casts can be made of either fiberglass or plaster. Fiberglass generally requires no change in exposure factors from the values used for the same anatomic part without a cast.

Plaster presents a problem in terms of exposure factors. Plaster casts require an increase in exposure factors compared with that needed to radiograph the same part without a cast. However, the method and amount of increase in exposure have not been standardized.

Exposure factor adjustments for cast materials may be based on the part thickness using a technique chart. For example, if an AP ankle measured through the CR is 4 in (10 cm) without the cast and 8 in (20 cm) with the cast, the radiographer simply increases the exposure technique to that of an ankle measuring 8 in (20 cm) to obtain an acceptable radiograph.

Splints

Splints present less of a challenge for the determination of appropriate exposure factors than casts. Inflatable (air) and fiberglass splints do not require any increase in exposure. Wood, aluminum, and solid plastic splints may require that exposure factors be increased but only if they are in the path of the primary beam. For example, if two pieces of wood are bound to the sides of a lower leg, no increase in exposure is necessary for an AP projection because the splint is not in the path of the primary beam and does not interfere with the radiographic image. Using the same example, if a lateral projection is produced, the splint is in the path of the primary beam and interferes with the radiographic imaging of the part. An increase in the exposure technique is required to produce a properly exposed radiograph.

Pathologic Conditions

Pathological conditions that can alter the absorption characteristics of the anatomic part being examined are divided into two categories. *Additive diseases* are diseases or conditions that increase the absorption characteristics of the part, making the part more difficult to penetrate. *Destructive diseases* are diseases or conditions that decrease the absorption characteristics of the part, making the part less difficult to penetrate. Table 8-5 lists additive and destructive diseases. Generally, it is necessary to increase the kVp when radiographing parts that have been affected by additive diseases and to decrease the kVp when radiographing parts affected by destructive diseases.

TABLE 8-5   **Common Additive and Destructive Diseases and Conditions by Anatomic Area**

Additive Conditions	Destructive Conditions
Abdomen	
Aortic aneurysm	Bowel obstruction
Ascites	Free air
Cirrhosis	
Hypertrophy of some organs (e.g., splenomegaly)	
Chest	
Atelectasis	Emphysema
Congestive heart failure	Pneumothorax
Malignancy	
Pleural effusion	
Pneumonia	
Skeleton	
Hydrocephalus	Gout
Metastases (osteoblastic)	Metastases (osteolytic)
Osteochondroma (exostoses)	Multiple myeloma
Paget's disease (late stage)	Paget's disease (early stage)
Osteoporosis	
Nonspecific Sites	
Abscess	Atrophy
Edema	Emaciation
Sclerosis	Malnutrition

However, it is not necessary to compensate for all additive and destructive diseases. It is often desirable to image diseases with exposure factors that would normally be used for a specific anatomic part so that the effect of that disease on that part can be clearly visualized.

When it is necessary or desirable to compensate for additive or destructive diseases or conditions, it is best to make changes in the kVp. Changing the kVp is fundamentally correct because the kVp affects the penetrating ability of the primary beam, and it is the penetrability of the anatomic part that is affected by these particular diseases and conditions. It is impossible to state an exact amount or percentage by which the kVp should be changed, because the state or severity of the disease or condition differs with each patient; however, a minimum change of 15% in kVp is recommended. There are some instances in which a change in mAs may be more appropriate to the type of pathological condition. For example, if the anatomic area has a significant increase in gas, such as in bowel obstruction, a large decrease in mAs is best.

Soft Tissue

Objects such as small pieces of wood, glass, or swallowed bones are difficult to radiographically visualize using the normal exposure factors for a particular anatomic part. Several situations in which a soft tissue technique may be needed are visualization of the larynx in a young child with croup, possible foreign body obstruction in the throat, and foreign body location in the extremities (Figure 8-8). Exposure factors must be altered to demonstrate these soft tissues for film-screen imaging. When the area of interest requires less density to visualize the soft tissue, the mAs

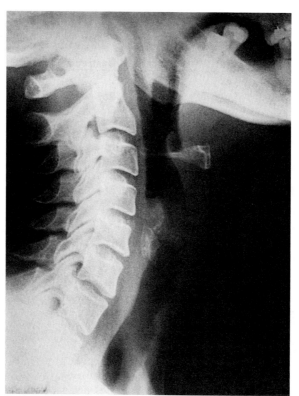

FIGURE 8-8 Soft tissue imaging. Lateral soft tissue neck radiograph.

should be decreased accordingly. Digital imaging systems allow the visualization of soft tissues without changing the exposure technique.

Contrast Media

A contrast medium (also called *contrast agent*) is used when imaging anatomic tissues that have low subject contrast. A **contrast medium** is a substance that can be instilled into the body by injection or ingestion. The type of contrast medium used changes the absorption characteristics of the tissues by either increasing or decreasing the attenuation of the x-ray beam. Positive contrast agents, such as barium and iodine, have a high atomic number and absorb more x-rays (increase attenuation) than the surrounding tissue (Figure 8-9). Negative contrast agents, such as air, decrease the attenuation of the x-ray beam and transmit more radiation than the surrounding tissue (Figure 8-10). Positive contrast agents produce more brightness than the adjacent tissues; negative contrast agents produce less brightness than the adjacent tissues.

Although negative contrast agents decrease the attenuation characteristics of the part being examined, their use does not require a change in exposure factors. Negative contrast agents can also be used in conjunction with positive contrast agents. Positive contrast media studies require an increase in exposure factors compared with imaging the same part without a positive contrast medium.

The use of a contrast agent is an effective method of increasing the radiographic contrast when imaging areas of low subject contrast.

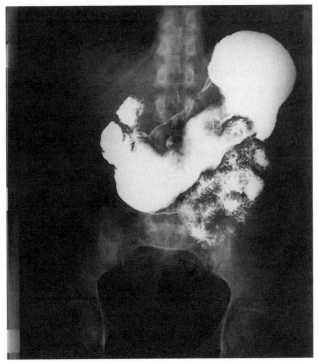

FIGURE 8-9 Positive contrast agents. Radiograph showing increased brightness because of the increase in x-ray beam attenuation by use of a positive contrast agent.

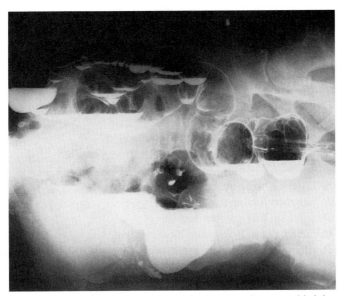

FIGURE 8-10 Negative contrast agents. Radiograph showing decreased brightness because of the decrease in x-ray beam attenuation by use of a negative contrast agent.

CHAPTER SUMMARY

- AEC systems are designed to produce optimal radiation exposure to the IR to produce a quality image.
- AEC uses detectors (typically ionization type) that measure the amount of radiation exiting the patient and terminate the exposure when it reaches a preset amount; this amount corresponds to the amount of radiation needed to produce diagnostic image quality.
- The kVp selected must penetrate the part and produce the desired scale of contrast. Increasing or decreasing the kVp causes the exposure time to be decreased or increased accordingly.
- Changing the mA, when available, causes the exposure time to be decreased or increased accordingly.
- In order for AEC to work accurately, the x-ray beam must be centered precisely to the anatomic area of interest, the correct detectors must be selected and the anatomic part must cover the dimension of the detectors.
- The mAs readout displayed informs the radiographer of the total radiation exposure used for the procedure.
- Other AEC features can be manipulated or used: density selectors allow increased or decreased exposure to the IR; backup time (or mAs) provides a safety mechanism that prevents the exposure from exceeding a set amount; and the mAs readout displays exactly how much mAs was used to produce the image.
- Limitations of AEC systems include that they typically allow only one type of IR and that the minimum response time may be longer than the exposure needed.
- Anatomically programmed technique is another exposure system that allows the selection of a specific body part and position, resulting in display of preprogrammed exposure factors. These may include AEC information.
- Exposure technique charts standardize the selection of exposure factors for a typical patient so that the quality of radiographic images is consistent.
- The variable kVp/fixed mAs technique chart is based on the concept that kVp can be increased as the anatomic part size increases. The baseline kVp is adjusted for changes in part thickness.
- The fixed kVp/variable mAs technique chart uses the concept of selecting an optimal kVp value that is required for the radiographic examination and adjusting the mAs for variations in part thickness.
- Exposure factors may need to be modified for pediatric, geriatric, and bariatric patients and varying projections and positions, casts and splints, pathological conditions, soft tissue, and contrast media.

REVIEW QUESTIONS

1. AEC devices work by measuring _____.
   A. radiation leaving the tube
   B. radiation that exits the patient
   C. radiation that is absorbed by the patient
   D. attenuation of primary radiation by the patient
2. How many detectors are typically found in an AEC system?
   A. One
   B. Two
   C. Three
   D. Four

3. Minimum response time refers to _____.
   A. the proper exposure time needed for an optimal exposure when an AEC device is used
   B. exposure time minus the amount of time the AEC detectors spend measuring the radiation
   C. the difference in exposure times between AEC systems and electronic timers
   D. the shortest exposure time possible when an AEC device is used
4. Which of the following statements about using AEC during digital imaging is true?
   A. Adjusting the mA value affects image brightness.
   B. Adjusting the kVp value affects image brightness.
   C. Adjusting the backup time affects image brightness.
   D. Adjusting the density controls affects the exposure to the IR.
5. Which one of the following statements comparing ionization chamber AEC systems with phototimers is true?
   A. Ionization chamber systems are accurately called *phototimers.*
   B. Ionization chamber systems measure radiation before it interacts with the image receptor.
   C. Phototimers are more modern.
   D. Phototimers measure radiation before it interacts with the image receptor.
6. The purpose of the backup timer is to _____.
   A. ensure a diagnostic exposure each time AEC is used
   B. produce consistent levels of exposure on all radiographs
   C. determine the exposure time that is used
   D. limit unnecessary x-ray exposure
7. What happens if AEC is activated for a stretcher chest study?
   A. An inappropriately short exposure occurs.
   B. An inappropriately long exposure occurs.
   C. An appropriate exposure probably occurs.
   D. Underexposure of the radiograph occurs.
8. The purpose of anatomically programmed techniques is to _____.
   A. present the radiographer with a preselected set of exposure factors
   B. override AEC when the radiographer has made a mistake in its use
   C. determine which AEC detectors should be used for a particular examination
   D. prevent overexposure and underexposure of radiographs, which sometimes happen when AEC is used
9. Which statement concerning both AEC and anatomically programmed techniques is true?
   A. The skilled use of both requires less knowledge of exposure factors on the part of the radiographer.
   B. The use of both requires the radiographer to be less responsible for accurate centering of the anatomic part.
   C. The individual judgment and discretion of the radiographer is still necessary when using these systems.
   D. The tasks involved with practicing radiography generally are made more difficult with these systems.
10. When using AEC with digital imaging systems, assuming all other factors are correct, selecting the center chamber on a PA chest image results in _____.
    A. decreased exposure in the lung area
    B. increased exposure in the lung area
    C. appropriate exposure in the lung area
    D. increased quantum noise in the image

11. When using AEC with digital imaging systems, assuming all other factors are correct, selecting the minus 2 density on a PA chest image results in _____.
    A. increased quantum noise
    B. increased brightness in the lung area
    C. appropriate brightness in the lung area
    D. A and C

12. Using a film-screen system and AEC, a chest in the lateral position is imaged with 70 kVp instead of the typical 120 kVp. Compared with an optimal lateral chest image, this image would have _____.
    A. increased density
    B. decreased density
    C. increased contrast
    D. decreased contrast

13. What type of exposure technique system uses a fixed mAs regardless of part thickness?
    A. Fixed kVp
    B. Variable kVp
    C. Manual
    D. AEC

14. A primary goal of an exposure technique chart is to _____.
    A. extend the life of the x-ray tube
    B. improve the radiographer's accuracy
    C. produce quality images consistently
    D. increase the patient work flow

15. Which of the following is an important condition required for technique charts to be effective?
    A. Equipment must be calibrated to perform properly.
    B. One technique chart should be used for all radiographic units.
    C. All technologists should use the same mAs setting.
    D. The chart should not be revised once it has been used.

16. Instilling a negative contrast agent in the gastrointestinal tract has what effect in the area of interest on the digital image?
    A. Increased brightness
    B. Decreased contrast
    C. Decreased brightness
    D. No effect

CHAPTER OUTLINE

Criteria for Image Evaluation
   Brightness or Density
   Contrast
   Spatial Resolution or
      Recorded Detail
   Distortion

   Quantum Noise
   Exposure Indicator
   Image Artifacts
Exposure Technique Factors
   Image Quality
   Image Evaluation

Image Analysis

OBJECTIVES

After completing this chapter, the reader will be able to perform the following:

1. Define the attributes of a good-quality radiographic image.
2. Identify exposure factors and their radiographic effects.
3. Identify factors that contribute to poor image quality.
4. Recognize exposure factor errors and their effect on the exposure indicator.
5. Identify factors that could contribute to quantum noise and artifacts.
6. Given a poor-quality image, identify the factors contributing to its effect.
7. Given exposure factors, explain their contribution to poor image quality.
8. Calculate exposure technique factors to improve image quality.

The previous chapters discussed how a radiographic image is formed; attributes describing the quality of the image; exposure technique factors; and methods of acquiring, processing, and displaying an image. The focus of this chapter is to apply the knowledge previously gained in evaluating image quality and develop problem-solving skills related to exposure technique factors. Criteria used for image evaluation or attributes of image quality are briefly reviewed. The remaining sections provide students the opportunity to evaluate image quality and problem solve to identify factors contributing to poor image quality and strategies for improvement.

CRITERIA FOR IMAGE EVALUATION

A quality radiographic image accurately represents the anatomic area of interest, and its information is well visualized for diagnosis. The *visibility* of the anatomic structures and the *accuracy* of their recorded structural lines (sharpness) determine the overall quality of the radiographic image. Visibility of the recorded detail refers to the *brightness* or *density* of the image along with image contrast; the accuracy of the structural lines is achieved by maximizing *spatial resolution* or *recorded detail* and minimizing *distortion*. Visibility of the recorded detail is achieved by the proper balance of image brightness or density and contrast.

Brightness or Density

Brightness and *density* refer to the same image quality attribute but are defined differently. *Brightness* is defined as the amount of luminance (light emission) of a display monitor. *Density* is defined as the amount of overall blackness on the processed image. An area of increased brightness, if viewed on the computer monitor, shows decreased density on a film image. An area of decreased brightness visualized on a computer monitor has increased density on a film image.

A radiograph must have sufficient brightness or density to visualize the anatomic structures of interest (Figure 9-1). A radiograph that is too light has excessive brightness or insufficient density to visualize the structures of the anatomic part under examination. Conversely, a radiograph that is too dark has insufficient brightness or excessive density, and the anatomic part cannot be well visualized (Figure 9-2). The radiographer must evaluate the overall brightness or density on the image to determine whether it is sufficient to visualize the anatomic area of interest. He/she then decides whether the radiograph is diagnostic or unacceptable.

Contrast

In addition to sufficient brightness or density, the radiograph must exhibit differences in the adjacent brightness levels or densities in order to differentiate among the anatomic tissues. Because of these differences in brightness or density (i.e., contrast), the anatomic tissues are

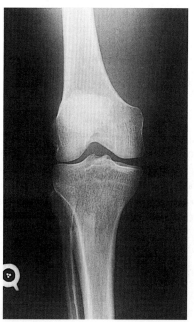

FIGURE 9-1 Radiograph demonstrating sufficient density.

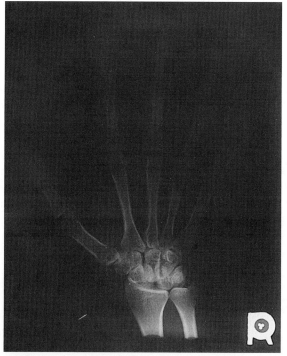

FIGURE 9-2 Radiograph demonstrating excessive density.

easily differentiated. Tissues that attenuate the x-ray beam similarly are more difficult to visualize because the brightness or densities are too alike to differentiate.

The level of radiographic contrast desired in an image is determined by the composition of the anatomic tissue to be radiographed and the amount of information needed to visualize the tissue for an accurate diagnosis. For example, the level of contrast desired in a chest image is different from that required in an image of an extremity.

Radiographic contrast or *image contrast* is a term used in both digital and film-screen imaging to describe the variations in brightness and density. In digital imaging, the number of different shades of gray that can be stored and displayed by a computer system is termed *gray scale*. Because the digital image is processed and reconstructed in the computer as digital data, its contrast can be altered.

Radiographic film images are typically described by their scale of contrast or the range of densities visible. A film image with few densities but great differences among them is said to have high contrast (Figure 9-3). This is also described as *short-scale contrast*. A radiograph with a large number of densities but few differences among them is said to have low contrast (Figure 9-4). This is also described as *long-scale contrast*. Figure 9-5 shows images with high (short-scale) contrast and low (long-scale) contrast.

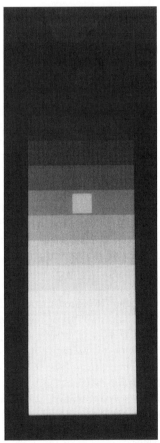

FIGURE 9-3 High-contrast (short-scale) image showing fewer gray levels and greater differences between individual densities.

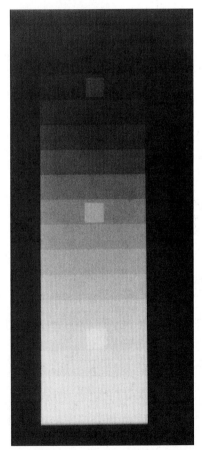

FIGURE 9-4 Low-contrast (long-scale) image showing many gray levels and few differences between individual densities.

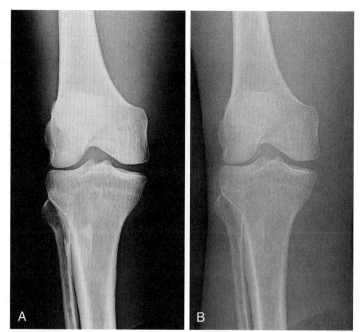

FIGURE 9-5 A, Radiograph demonstrating high contrast. **B,** Radiograph demonstrating low contrast.

Spatial Resolution or Recorded Detail

The quality of a radiographic image depends on both the visibility and the accuracy of the anatomic structural lines recorded (sharpness). Adequate visualization of the anatomic area of interest (brightness/density and contrast) is just one component of radiographic quality. To produce a quality radiograph, the anatomic details must be recorded accurately and with the greatest amount of sharpness.

The ability of a radiographic image to demonstrate sharp lines determines the quality of the spatial resolution or recorded detail. The imaging process makes it impossible to produce a radiographic image without a certain degree of unsharpness. A radiographic image that has greater spatial resolution or recorded detail minimizes the unsharpness of the anatomic structural lines. Figure 9-6 shows an image with decreased recorded detail because of motion unsharpness.

Distortion

Distortion results from the radiographic misrepresentation of either the size (magnification) or the shape of the anatomic part. When the part is distorted, spatial resolution or recorded detail is also reduced.

Radiographic images of objects are always magnified in relation to the true object size. The source-to-image-receptor distance (SID) and object-to-image-receptor distance (OID) play important roles in minimizing the size distortion of the radiographic image.

When producing images of three-dimensional objects, some size distortion always occurs as a result of OID. The parts of the object that are far away from the IR are radiographically represented with more size distortion than those that are close to the IR. Even if the object is in close contact with the IR, some part of the object is still far away from the IR than the other parts of the object. SID also influences the total amount of magnification on the image. As SID increases, size distortion (magnification) decreases; as SID decreases, size distortion (magnification) increases.

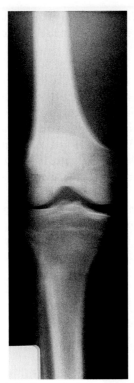

FIGURE 9-6 Radiograph demonstrating motion unsharpness.

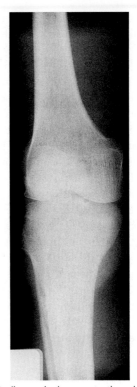

FIGURE 9-7 Radiograph demonstrating shape distortion.

In addition to size distortion, objects that are being imaged can be radiographically misrepresented by distortion of their shape. Shape distortion can radiographically appear in two different ways: elongation or foreshortening.

Shape distortion can occur from inaccurate central ray alignment of the tube, the part being radiographed, or the IR. Any misalignment of the central ray among these three factors—tube, part, or IR—alters the shape of the part recorded on the image (Figure 9-7).

The factors that determine the amount of image distortion are equally important for digital and film-screen imaging. Both SID and OID determine the magnification of the anatomic structures on the image. In addition, improper alignment of the central ray, anatomic part, IR, or a combination of these components distorts the shape of the part, whether obtained with a digital or a film-screen IR.

Quantum Noise

Image noise contributes no useful diagnostic information and serves only to detract from the quality of the image. Quantum noise is a concern in digital and film-screen imaging (quantum mottle) and is photon dependent. Quantum noise is visible as brightness or density fluctuations on the image. The fewer the photons reaching the IR to form the image, the greater the quantum noise visible on the digital image.

Although quantum noise (mottle) can be a problem for both digital and film-screen imaging, it is more likely in digital imaging. As previously discussed, the digital computer system can adjust for low or high x-ray exposures during image acquisition; when the x-ray exposure to the IR is too low (decreased number of photons), computer processing alters the appearance of the digital image to make the brightness acceptable, but the image displays increased quantum noise (Figure 9-8).

Exposure Indicator

An important feature of digital image processing is its ability to create an image with the appropriate amount of brightness (as described earlier), regardless of the exposure to the IR (within reason). As a result of the histogram analysis (described in Chapter 4), valuable information is provided to the radiographer regarding the exposure to the digital IR. The exposure indicator provides a numerical value indicating the level of radiation exposure to the digital IR. Box 9-1 lists common computed radiography (CR) exposure indicator values and their relationship to exposure intensity.

In CR, the exposure indicator value represents the exposure level to the imaging plate, and the values are vendor specific:

- Fuji and Konica use sensitivity (S) numbers, and the value is inversely related to the exposure to the plate. An S number of 200 is the result of 1 mR of exposure to the plate. An increase in the S number from 200 to 400 would indicate a decrease in exposure to the IR by half. Conversely, a decrease in the S number from 200 to 100 would indicate an increase in exposure to the IR by a factor of 2, or a doubling of the exposure.
- Carestream (Kodak) uses exposure index (EI) numbers; the value is directly related to the exposure to the plate, and the changes are logarithmic expressions. For example, a change in EI from 1500 to 1800, a difference of 300, is equal to a factor of 2 and represents twice as much exposure to the plate.

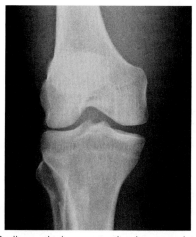

FIGURE 9-8 Radiograph demonstrating increased quantum noise.

BOX 9-1	**Computed Radiography Vendor-Specific Exposure Indicators**				
Vendor	**Exposure Indicator**	**Value = 1 mR exposure**	**2 × Exposure**	**½ Exposure**
Fuji and Konica	Sensitivity (S)	200	100	400
Carestream (Kodak)	Exposure index (EI)	2000	2300	1700
Agfa	Log median value (lgM)	2.5	2.8	2.2

- Agfa uses log median (lgM) numbers; the value is directly related to exposure to the plate, and the changes are logarithmic expressions. For example, a change in lgM from 2.5 to 2.8, a change of 0.3, is equal to a factor of 2 and represents twice as much exposure to the IR.

Optimal ranges of the exposure indicator values are not standardized but are rather vendor specific, and vary among the types of procedures, such as abdomen/chest versus extremity imaging. Direct radiography (DR) imaging systems also display an exposure indicator that varies according to the manufacturer's specifications. The radiographer should monitor the exposure indicator values as a guide for proper exposure techniques; if the exposure indicator value is within the acceptable range, adjustments can be made for contrast and brightness with postprocessing functions. However, if the exposure is outside the acceptable range, attempting to adjust the image data with postprocessing functions would not rectify improper receptor exposure and might result in noisy or suboptimal images that should not be submitted for interpretation. Overwriting the original image with a postprocessed replica at the radiographer's workstation may reduce the diagnostic and archival quality of the data; this is not recommended.

As a result of the variability among manufacturers' exposure indicators, the industry has recommended a universal standard exposure indicator. Although there are some variations between the standard exposure indicators, there is common terminology. The Deviation Index (DI) is a value that reflects the difference between the desired or target exposure to the IR and the actual exposure to the IR. A DI of 0 would indicate there is no difference between the desired EI and the actual EI. A DI that is above 0 indicates there is increased exposure to the IR, and a DI below 0 indicates there is decreased exposure to the IR. It is important to note that all EIs, even the recommended standard DI, have limitations. Variables such as collimation, kVp, and centering, may influence the EI and therefore the level of noise and image quality should be evaluated along with the EI or DI value. The radiographer needs to be knowledgeable about the EI value on the equipment she/he uses in digital imaging and how exposure techniques can be altered to correct for exposure errors. In addition, the Department standards should be followed for how over- and under-exposures are to be handled before repeating the image. For accurate computer processing of the latent image, the radiographer selects the appropriate anatomic part and projection. This step indicates which computer algorithm to use. If the radiographer selects a part other than the one imaged, a histogram analysis error may occur. In addition, any errors that occur, such as during data extraction from the IR or rescaling during computer processing, could affect the exposure indicator and provide a false value. It is important for radiographers not only to consider carefully the exposure indicator value but also to recognize its limitations.

Image Artifacts

An artifact is any unwanted image on a radiograph (Figure 9-9). Artifacts are detrimental to radiographs because they can make the visibility of anatomy, pathologic conditions, or patient identification information difficult or impossible. Moreover, they decrease the overall quality of radiographic images. Various methods are used to classify artifacts. Generally, artifacts can be classified as *plus-density* or *minus-density*. Plus-density artifacts are greater in density than the area of the image immediately surrounding them, whereas minus-density artifacts are lower in density than this area.

Although the causes of certain artifacts are the same regardless of the type of imaging system, others are specific to digital or film imaging. Artifacts from patient clothing and imaged items that are not a part of the area of interest are the same for both film and digital systems. The radiographer must be diligent in removing clothing or items that could obstruct visibility of the anatomic area of interest. Scatter radiation or fog and image noise have also been classified as radiographic artifacts, because they add unwanted information to the image.

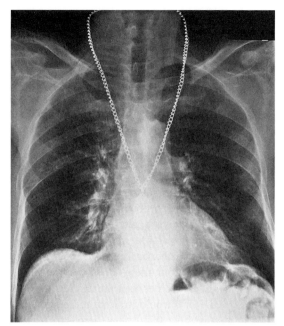

FIGURE 9-9 Radiograph demonstrating a patient artifact.

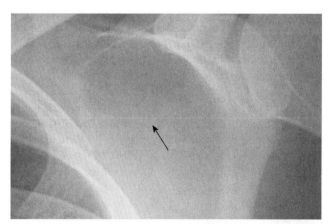

FIGURE 9-10 Radiograph demonstrating a CR reader light guide artifact.

Artifacts specific to film-screen imaging are typically a result of film storage, handling, and chemical processing. Digital image artifacts can be a result of errors during extraction of the latent image (Figure 9-10) from the IR or the performance of the electronic detectors.

EXPOSURE TECHNIQUE FACTORS

The following charts show how changes in exposure technique factors affect image quality. Because exposure technique factors affect the film image differently than the digital image, two charts are presented. Look for differences and similarities between exposure technique factors and their effect on digital and film image quality.

Image Quality

Digital Image Receptors

Factors	Exposure to IR	Brightness*	Contrast*†	Spatial Resolution	Distortion
mAs					
• Increase	Increase	No effect	No effect	No effect	No effect
• Decrease	Decrease	No effect	No effect	No effect	No effect
kVp					
• Increase	Increase	No effect	Decrease	No effect	No effect
• Decrease	Decrease	No effect	Increase	No effect	No effect
OID					
• Increase	Decrease	No effect	Increase‡	Decrease	Increase
SID					
• Increase	Decrease	No effect	No effect	Increase	Decrease
• Decrease	Increase	No effect	No effect	Decrease	Increase
Focal Spot Size					
• Increase	No effect	No effect	No effect	Decrease	No effect
• Decrease	No effect	No effect	No effect	Increase	No effect
Grid					
• Increase ratio	Decrease	No effect	Increase	No effect	No effect
• Decrease ratio	Increase	No effect	Decrease	No effect	No effect
Beam Restriction					
• Increase	Decrease	No effect	Increase	No effect	No effect
• Decrease	Increase	No effect	Decrease	No effect	No effect
Patient Thickness					
• Increase	Decrease	No effect	Decrease	Decrease	Increase
• Decrease	Increase	No effect	Increase	Increase	Decrease
Patient Motion					
	No effect	No effect	No effect	Decrease	No effect
Central Ray					
• Increase angle	Decrease	No effect	No effect	Decrease	Increase

*Brightness and contrast can be adjusted by the computer.
†Increase is higher contrast, and decrease is lower contrast.
‡Increased (higher) contrast because of less scatter reaching the IR; this effect is dependent on the anatomic region, thickness, and amount of OID.

Film-Screen Image Receptors

Factors	Exposure to IR	Density	Contrast[†]	Recorded Detail	Distortion
mAs					
• Increase	Increase	Increase	No effect*	No effect	No effect
• Decrease	Decrease	Decrease	No effect*	No effect	No effect
kVp					
• Increase	Increase	Increase	Decrease	No effect	No effect
• Decrease	Decrease	Decrease	Increase	No effect	No effect
OID					
• Increase	Decrease	Decrease	Increase[‡]	Decrease	Increase
SID					
• Increase	Decrease	Decrease	No effect	Increase	Decrease
• Decrease	Increase	Increase	No effect	Decrease	Increase
Focal Spot Size					
• Increase	No effect	No effect	No effect	Decrease	No effect
• Decrease	No effect	No effect	No effect	Increase	No effect
Grid					
• Increase ratio	Decrease	Decrease	Increase	No effect	No effect
• Decrease ratio	Increase	Increase	Decrease	No effect	No effect
Beam Restriction					
• Increase	Decrease	Decrease	Increase	No effect	No effect
• Decrease	Increase	Increase	Decrease	No effect	No effect
Film-Screen Speed					
• Increase	No effect	Increase	No effect	Decrease	No effect
• Decrease	No effect	Decrease	No effect	Increase	No effect
Patient Thickness					
• Increase	Decrease	Decrease	Decrease	Decrease	Increase
• Decrease	Increase	Increase	Increase	Increase	Decrease
Patient Motion	No effect	No effect	No effect	Decrease	No effect
Central Ray					
• Increase angle	Decrease	Decrease	No effect	Decrease	Increase

[†]Increase is higher contrast, and decrease is lower contrast.

*Contrast is not affected unless the density is insuffcient or excessive.

[‡]Increased (higher) contrast because of less scatter reaching IR; this effect is dependent on the anatomic region, thickness, and amount of OID.

❓ ACTIVITY 1

Image Quality
Digital
An optimal digital image of the hip was produced using the following exposure technique:

200 mA
50 ms
70 kVp
40 in SID
0.6 mm small focal spot

12:1 grid ratio
CR image receptor
8 × 12 in collimation
Patient thickness 10 cm
Minimal OID

Without compensation, the proposed changes are made one by one. On the following chart, indicate the effect, if any, that each change has on the brightness, contrast, and spatial resolution of the radiographic image.

1. If the exposure to the IR, contrast, or spatial resolution of the image is increased, mark a plus symbol (+) in the space provided.
2. If the exposure to the IR, contrast, or spatial resolution of the image is decreased, mark a minus symbol (−) in the space provided.
3. If the exposure to the IR, contrast, or spatial resolution of the image is unchanged, mark a 0 in the space provided.

Proposed individual change	Exposure to IR	Contrast	Spatial Resolution
85 kVp			
1.25 mm focal spot size			
45" SID			
50 mA @ 0.20 s			
Patient thickness 6 cm			
Remove grid			
Increase OID 4"			
14 × 17 in collimation			

ACTIVITY 2

Image Quality

Film-Screen

An optimal film radiograph of the pelvis was produced using the following exposure technique:

100 mA
0.5 s
70 kVp
40 in SID
1.25 mm large focal spot
92°F development temperature
90 s processing time

12:1 grid ratio
400 speed F/S
14 × 17 in collimation
Patient thickness 14 cm
Minimal OID

Without compensation, the proposed changes are made one by one. On the following chart, indicate the effect, if any, that each change has on the density, contrast, and recorded detail of the radiographic image.

1. If the radiographic density, contrast, or recorded detail of the image is increased, mark a + in the space provided.
2. If the radiographic density, contrast, or recorded detail of the image is decreased, mark a − in the space provided.
3. If the radiographic density, contrast, or recorded detail of the image is unchanged, mark a 0 in the space provided.

Proposed Change	Density	Contrast	Recorded Detail
Increase SID to 48"			
Use 200 mAs			
Increase kVp to 80			
Film-screen speed 200			
Increase patient thickness to 18 cm			
10 × 12 collimation			
Development temperature decreased			
Patient moves during exposure			
Angle tube 20°			
Change to 8:1 grid ratio			
Use 0.6 mm focal spot size			
Increase OID 3"			

? ACTIVITY 3

Image Quality Calculations
Mathematical Calculations

Exposure Technique Factor	Relationship Between Variables	Formula
mAs	↑ mA and ↓ second	mA × second = mAs
kVp 15% Rule	↑ kVp and ↓ mAs	kVp × 1.15 and mAs/2 kVp × 0.85 and mAs × 2
Inverse Square Law	↑ SID and ↓ Intensity	$\text{Intensity}_1 = (SID_2)^2$ $\text{Intensity}_2 = (SID_1)^2$
mAs/Distance Compensation Formula	↑ SID and ↑ mAs	$\dfrac{mAs_1 = (SID_1)^2}{mAs_2 = (SID_2)^2}$

Exposure Technique Factor	Relationship Between Variables	Formula
Grid Conversion Factor No grid = 1 5:1 = 2 6:1 = 3 8:1 = 4 12:1 = 5 16:1 = 6	↑ Grid ratio and ↑ mAs	$\dfrac{mAs_1 = GCF_1}{mAs_2 = GCF_2}$
Patient Thickness	↑ Thickness and ↑ mAs	Every 4–5 cm change in thickness changes mAs by a factor of 2
Film-Screen Speed	↑ Speed (RS) and ↓ mAs	$\dfrac{mAs_1 = RS_2}{mAs_2 = RS_1}$
Magnification Factor (MF)	↑ OID and ↓ SID and ↑ mag	$MF = \dfrac{SID}{SOD}$
	Image size = Object size × MF	$Object\ size = \dfrac{Image\ size}{MF}$

Solve for the missing variable or calculate the new exposure factor to maintain exposure to the IR as in the initial exposure technique. Show all calculations.

mAs

mA = 100
time = 0.25 s
mAs =

mA =
time = 100 ms
mAs = 50

mA = 50
time =
mAs = 15

15% Rule

Initial kVp = 70
Initial mAs = 10
New kVp = 70 + 15% =
New mAs =

Initial kVp = 80
Initial mAs = 100
New kVp = 80 − 15% =
New mAs =

Initial kVp = 75
Initial mAs = 35
New kVp = 75 + 2(15%) =
New mAs =

mAs–Distance Conversions

Initial mA = 100   Initial time = 0.5 s   Initial mAs = 125
Initial SID = 40 in   Initial SID = 60 in   Initial SID = 56 in
New SID = 72 in   New SID = 25 in   New SID = 40 in

New mA =   New time =   New mAs =

Grid Conversions

No grid, initial mAs = 10   12:1 grid, initial mAs = 50   5:1 grid, initial time = 0.05 s
Add 8:1 grid, new mAs =   6:1 grid, new mAs =   12:1 grid, new time =

Film-Screen Speed (F/S spd.)

Initial mAs = 25   Initial mAs = 10   Initial time = 0.25
Initial F/S spd = 200   Initial F/S spd = 600   Initial F/S spd = 100
New F/S spd = 400   New F/S Spd = 300   New F/S Spd = 50

New mAs =   New mAs =   New time =

Word Problems

1. A digital image of the hip was created using 75 kVp @ 5 mAs, a 12:1 grid, a 40 in SID, and a small focal spot size. The exposure indicator value denotes insufficient exposure to the IR and the image displays excessive noise. What adjustments to the exposure technique would improve the quality of the image if repeated?

2. During a fluoroscopic procedure, the radiation exposure is 50 mR at a distance of 100 cm from the radiation source. Calculate the radiation exposure at a distance of 150 cm.

3. A good-quality AP pelvis image was created in the radiology department using 80 kVp @ 15 mAs, a 40 in SID, and a 12:1 grid ratio. A request to image a similar-sized patient's pelvis with the mobile x-ray unit requires the SID to be increased to 48 in and the use of an 8:1 grid ratio. What adjustments in the exposure technique would provide a similar quality image?

4. A good-quality KUB image was created on a patient measuring 10 cm using 80 kVp @ 20 mAs, a 40 in SID, a 12:1 grid, and a large focal spot size. What adjustment in exposure technique would be required if the next patient requiring a KUB measured 15 cm?

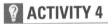 SAMPLE ACTIVITY

Image Quality Exposure Conversions

Calculate the new exposure factor required to maintain a similar exposure to the IR as in the initial exposure technique. Show all calculations.

Initial Exposure Technique

25 mAs

65 kVp   TO

No grid

40 in SID

New Exposure Technique

_____ mAs

75 kVp

6:1 grid

48 in SID

Calculations:

a. Increase from 65 to 75 kVp = 15% increase

b. Decrease mAs by 0.5 = 12.5 mAs

c. Add a 6:1 grid = increase mAs × 3 = 12.5 × 3 = 37.5 mAs

d. Increase SID from 40 in to 48 in = $\dfrac{37.5}{X} = \dfrac{40^2}{48^2}$; 1600X = 86,400; X = 54 mAs

e. The new mAs needed to maintain a similar exposure to the IR as the initial technique is 54

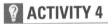 ACTIVITY 4

Image Quality Exposure Conversions

Calculate the new exposure factor required to maintain a similar exposure to the IR as in the initial exposure technique. Show all calculations.

Initial Digital Exposure Technique

100 mAs

80 kVp   TO

12:1 grid

56 in SID

New Digital Exposure Technique

_____ mAs

58 kVp

No grid

40 in SID

Calculations:

💡 ACTIVITY 5

Image Quality Exposure Conversions

Calculate the new exposure factor required to maintain a similar exposure to the IR as in the initial exposure technique. Show all calculations.

Initial Film-Screen Exposure Technique		**New Film-Screen Exposure Technique**
200 mA		____ mA
0.05 s		$^1\!/_5$ s
65 kVp	TO	75 kVp
6:1 grid		8:1 grid
40 in SID		56 in SID
400 F/S speed		100 F/S speed

Calculations:

Image Evaluation

The ability to recognize exposure technique errors and their resultant effect on the radiographic image is an important problem-solving skill. The following exercises provide you with an opportunity to apply the knowledge gained from previous chapters in identifying causes of poor-quality images for both digital and film-screen IRs.

💡 ACTIVITY 6

Image Evaluation

Matching

One of the four computed radiography (CR) images is good quality, whereas the others are the results of errors. Match each image with its corresponding statement:

1. Good-quality lateral skull image   _____

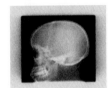
A.

2. Imaging plate placed upside down   _____

B.

3. Grid placed upside down on the imaging plate   _____

C.

4. Grid removed with mAs adjustment   _____

D.

ACTIVITY 7

Image Evaluation
Multiple Choice

Select the most likely exposure technique error responsible for the poor-quality image, and write your answer in the middle column:

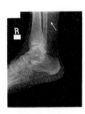
CR image

_____

A. Artifact from CR reader error
B. Excessive fog
C. Insufficient quantity of radiation reaching the IR
D. Upside-down imaging plate

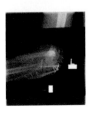
CR image

_____

A. Excessive quantity of radiation reaching the IR
B. Upside-down grid
C. Double exposure to the IR
D. Excessive quantum noise

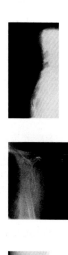

Film-screen AEC image

_____   A. Off-centering using AEC
B. Too high kVp
C. No grid
D. mA set too low

CR image

_____   A. Excessive quantity of radiation
exposure reaching the IR
B. Motion unsharpness
C. Excessive collimation
D. Insufficient quantity of radiation
reaching the IR

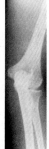

Film-screen image

_____   A. Excessive fog
B. Insufficient quantity of radiation
reaching the IR
C. Too high kVp
D. Excessive quantum noise

IMAGE ANALYSIS

The ability to evaluate image quality and problem solve for improvement involves several skills. The knowledge of how exposure factors affect image quality individually and in combination is the first step toward successful problem solving. In addition, the ability to accurately calculate exposure factor changes is necessary for improving image quality.

The following image quality exercises are opportunities to develop problem-solving skills by applying the knowledge learned from the previous chapters.

🔆 SAMPLE ACTIVITY

Image Analysis
Film Image Evaluation: Image Quality Analysis

Radiograph 1
kVp = 75
F/S speed = 400
mAs = 10
Grid ratio = 12:1
SID = 40 in
Focal spot = small
Optical density = 1.35

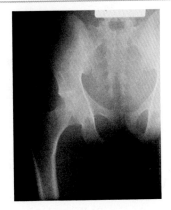

Radiograph 2
kVp = 86
F/S speed = 400
mAs = 2.5
Table top = no grid
SID = 45 in
Focal spot = large
Optical density = 2.03

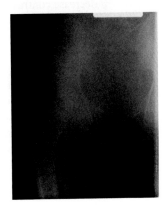

Evaluation:
- Visually compare Radiograph 1 and Radiograph 2, and comment on the quality of the density and contrast of Radiograph 2. State whether Radiograph 2 needs to be repeated and explain why.
- Evaluate each change in exposure factor, and discuss its appropriateness and how it affects the density or contrast (or both) of the image and patient exposure.
- Calculate the appropriate mAs value for each of the cumulative changes to determine why Radiograph 2 displays its level of density or contrast (or both).
- Identify the correct mAs value that should have been used for each of the exposure factor changes to maintain density as in Radiograph 1. Last, compare the actual mAs used in Radiograph 2 with the calculated mAs value that was needed to maintain density and contrast.

Calculate and Respond:
The kVp increased by 15% in Radiograph 2 and requires a decrease in mAs by a factor of 2:

$$\frac{10 \ mAs}{2} = 5 \ mAs$$

The grid was removed, and the mAs needs to decrease:

$$\frac{5\ mAs}{X} = \frac{5}{1}\ ;\ 5X = 5\ ;\ X = 1\ mAs$$

The SID was increased to 45 in in Radiograph 2 and requires an increase in mAs:

$$\frac{1\ mAs}{X} = \frac{(40)^2}{(45)^2}\ ;\ 1600X = 2{,}025\ ;\ X = 1.27\ mAs$$

- On comparing Radiograph 2 with Radiograph 1, there is increased density on Radiograph 2. In the area of interest, Radiograph 2 had an OD of 2.03, which is at the high end of the diagnostic range. This image would be considered unacceptable and needs to be repeated because visibility of the area of interest is too low for diagnosis.
- Radiograph 2 has an increase in kVp of 15% (75 to 86), which would increase the density and decrease contrast; therefore, a decrease in mAs by a factor of 2 would be needed to compensate. The mAs would need to be 5 instead of 10. A higher kVp in the hip region is not typically used with film because it would decrease contrast and increase the proportion of scatter reaching the film. However, using a higher kVp requires the mAs to be decreased, and this would reduce patient exposure.
- The grid was removed, which would decrease contrast because more scatter radiation would reach the film and density would be increased. Radiographic contrast would be decreased because of the excessive scatter reaching the film. The mAs would need to be decreased to compensate and should have been 1 instead of 5. A grid should be used with the hip because significant amounts of scatter will be produced and reach the film. However, removing the grid requires a decrease in mAs, and this would reduce patient exposure.
- The SID was increased to 45 in in Radiograph 2, which would reduce the exposure to the IR and result in decreased density. The mAs would need to be increased from 1 to 1.27 mAs. In addition to reducing the exposure to the IR, increasing the SID will decrease magnification of the anatomic part and increase the recorded detail.
- After all the changes in exposure factors, Radiograph 2 is too dark because 2.5 mAs was used instead of 1.27 mAs. In addition, the contrast was decreased by the increase in kVp and grid removal.

ACTIVITY 8

Image Analysis

Film Image Evaluation: Image Quality Analysis

Radiograph 1

kVp = 70

F/S speed = 400

mAs = 4

Grid ratio = 12:1

SID = 40 in

Focal spot = small

Optical density = 1.04

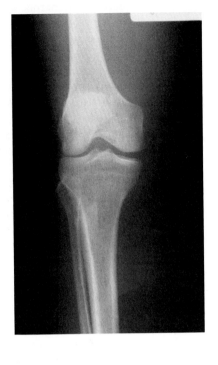

Radiograph 2

kVp = 60

F/S speed = 100

mAs = 6.3

Grid ratio = 6:1

SID = 34 in

Focal spot = large

Optical density = 0.30

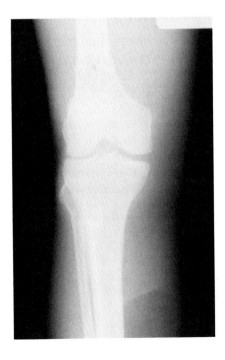

Evaluation:

- Visually compare Radiograph 1 and Radiograph 2, and comment on the quality of the density, contrast, and sharpness of Radiograph 2. State whether Radiograph 2 needs to be repeated and explain why.
- Evaluate each change in exposure factor, and discuss its appropriateness and how it affects the density, contrast, or sharpness (even if not apparent) of the image and patient exposure.
- Calculate the appropriate mAs value for each of the cumulative changes to determine why Radiograph 2 displays its level of density, contrast, and sharpness.
- Identify the correct mAs value that should have been used for each of the exposure factor changes in order to maintain density as in Radiograph 1. Last, compare the actual mAs used in Radiograph 2 with the calculated mAs value that was needed to maintain density and contrast. In addition, make other exposure factor recommendations to improve the quality of the image.

Calculate and Respond:

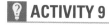

ACTIVITY 9

Image Analysis
Computed Radiography Image Evaluation (Recommended S number Between 100 and 300)

Radiograph 1
kVp = 81
mAs = 5
Focal spot = small
Grid ratio = 12:1
SID = 40 in
Central ray perpendicular
S number = 156

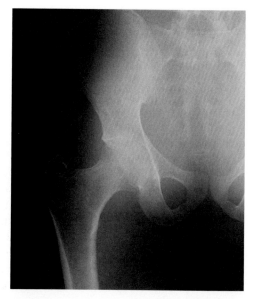

Radiograph 2
kVp = 59
mAs = 1.1
Focal spot = large
Table top = no grid
SID = 30 in
Central ray angled 20° caudad
S number = 620

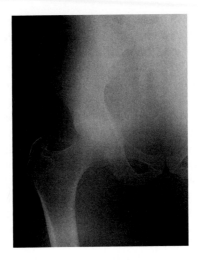

Evaluation:
- Visually compare Radiograph 1 and Radiograph 2, and comment on the quality of the contrast and spatial resolution of Radiograph 2. State whether Radiograph 2 should be repeated and explain why.
- Evaluate each change in exposure factor, and discuss its appropriateness and how it affects the exposure to the IR, contrast and/or spatial resolution (even if not apparent) of the image and patient exposure.
- Calculate the appropriate mAs value for each of the cumulative changes to determine why Radiograph 2 displays its level of contrast, spatial resolution, and S number.
- Identify the correct mAs value that should have been used for each of the exposure factor changes in order to maintain the quality as in Radiograph 1. Last, compare the actual mAs used in Radiograph 2 with the calculated mAs value that was needed to maintain sufficient exposure to the IR. In addition, make other exposure factor recommendations to improve the quality of the image.

Calculate and Respond:

CHAPTER SUMMARY

- The visibility of the anatomic structures and the accuracy of their recorded structural lines (sharpness) determine the overall quality of the radiographic image.
- *Visibility* of the recorded detail refers to the *brightness* or *density* of the image along with image contrast; the accuracy of the structural lines is achieved by maximizing the amount of *spatial resolution* or *recorded detail* and minimizing the amount of *distortion*.
- *Brightness* and *density* refer to the same image quality attribute but are defined differently. *Brightness* is defined as the amount of luminance (light emission) of a display monitor. *Density* is defined as the amount of overall blackness on the processed image.

- An area of increased brightness, if viewed on the computer monitor, shows decreased density on a film image. An area of decreased brightness visualized on a computer monitor has increased density on a film image.
- In addition to sufficient brightness or density, the radiograph must exhibit differences in the adjacent brightness levels or densities in order to differentiate among the anatomic tissues.
- In digital imaging, the number of different shades of gray that can be stored and displayed by a computer system is termed *gray scale*. Because the digital image is processed and reconstructed in the computer as digital data, its contrast can be altered.
- A film image with few densities but many differences among them is said to have high contrast. A radiograph with numerous densities but few differences among them is said to have low contrast.
- A radiographic image that has greater spatial resolution or recorded detail minimizes the amount of unsharpness of the anatomic structural lines.
- Distortion results from the radiographic misrepresentation of either the size (magnification) or the shape of the anatomic part. When the part is distorted, spatial resolution or recorded detail is also reduced.
- Quantum noise (mottle) is visible as brightness or density fluctuations on the image. The fewer the photons reaching the IR to form the image, the greater the quantum noise visible on the digital image.
- The exposure indicator provides a numerical value indicating the level of radiation exposure to the digital IR.
- Artifacts are detrimental to radiographs because they can make visibility of anatomy, a pathological condition, or patient identification information difficult or impossible.
- It is important for the radiographer to comprehend how exposure technique variables affect the radiation exposure to the IR and their individual and combined effects on the quality of digital and film-screen images.

REVIEW QUESTIONS

1. *Visibility* of the recorded detail refers to what image quality attribute?
   - **A.** Distortion
   - **B.** Spatial resolution
   - **C.** Brightness
   - **D.** A and B

2. *Accuracy* of the structural lines refers to what image quality attribute?
   - **A.** Distortion
   - **B.** Spatial resolution
   - **C.** Brightness
   - **D.** A and B

3. How would an area with increased density on the film image be described when viewed on a display monitor?
   - **A.** Decreased brightness
   - **B.** Increased contrast
   - **C.** Decreased spatial resolution
   - **D.** Increased brightness

4. Excessive radiation exposure to the IR would result in a digital image displayed with _____.
   - **A.** excessive brightness
   - **B.** acceptable brightness
   - **C.** insufficient brightness
   - **D.** increased quantum noise

5. Density fluctuations on a radiographic image could be a result of _____.
   A. artifacts
   B. distortion
   C. quantum mottle
   D. excessive exposure

6. Without exposure technique compensation, removing a grid would result in the film image displaying _____.
   (1) increased density
   (2) decreased recorded detail
   (3) decreased contrast
   A. 1 and 2 only
   B. 1 and 3 only
   C. 2 and 3 only
   D. 1, 2, and 3

7. Without exposure technique compensation, increasing the film-screen speed would result in the film image displaying _____.
   (1) increased density
   (2) decreased recorded detail
   (3) decreased contrast
   A. 1 and 2 only
   B. 1 and 3 only
   C. 2 and 3 only
   D. 1, 2, and 3

8. Without exposure technique compensation, increasing the SID would result in the digital image displaying _____.
   (1) decreased brightness
   (2) increased spatial resolution
   (3) decreased distortion
   A. 1 and 2 only
   B. 1 and 3 only
   C. 2 and 3 only
   D. 1, 2, and 3

9. The initial exposure technique for a good-quality radiograph is 15 mAs at 70 kVp, a 40 in (100 cm) SID, using an 8:1 grid ratio. If the grid is removed and the SID reduced to 36 in (90 cm), which of the following exposure techniques would best maintain the exposure to the IR?
   A. 3 mAs at 70 kVp
   B. 4.6 mAs at 70 kVp
   C. 7.5 mAs at 80 kVp
   D. 13.5 mAs at 70 kVp

10. Given an adequate exposure indicator value, the digital image of a hip is displayed with increased fog after the use of 20 mAs at 80 kVp without a grid. Which of the following exposure techniques would be best for improving the quality of the digital image?
    A. 40 mAs at 80 kVp, without a grid
    B. 10 mAs at 68 kVp, without a grid
    C. 20 mAs at 80 kVp and add a 12:1 ratio grid
    D. 50 mAs at 92 kVp and add a 12:1 ratio grid

10

Dynamic Imaging: Fluoroscopy

CHAPTER OUTLINE

Fluoroscopy
    Image Intensification
    Automatic Brightness Control
    Magnification Mode

    Viewing Systems
    Recording Systems
Mobile C-arm Units
Digital Fluoroscopy

Continuous Versus Pulsed
    Fluroscopy
Radiation Safety
Quality Control

OBJECTIVES

After completing this chapter, the reader will be able to perform the following:

1. Define all the key terms in this chapter.
2. State all the important relationships in this chapter.
3. Differentiate between fluoroscopic and radiographic imaging.
4. Recognize the unique features of an image-intensified fluoroscopic unit and explain how the image is created and viewed.
5. Explain the process of brightness gain and the conversion factor during image intensification.
6. Define *automatic brightness control* and state its function.
7. Explain how using the magnification mode affects image quality and patient exposure.
8. Identify common types of image degradation resulting from image-intensified fluoroscopy.
9. Differentiate among the types of television cameras used to convert the output phosphor image for viewing on a television monitor.
10. List the types of recording devices available for image-intensified fluoroscopy.
11. Compare and contrast features of image-intensified units from digital fluoroscopic units.
12. Differentiate between continuous and pulsed fluoroscopy and their impacts on patient radiation dose.
13. State radiation safety procedures used to reduce exposure to the patient and personnel.
14. Recognize the need for quality control on fluoroscopic units.

KEY TERMS

analog-to-digital converter (ADC)
automatic brightness control (ABC)
brightness gain
camera tube
charge-coupled device (CCD)

continuous fluoroscopy
conversion factor
electrostatic focusing lenses
fluoroscopy
flux gain
image intensification
input phosphor

magnification mode
minification gain
output phosphor
photocathode
pulsed fluoroscopy
spatial resolution

The previous chapters discussed radiographic imaging for producing static radiographs of anatomic tissues. Furthermore, imaging of the functioning or motion (dynamics) of anatomic structures is needed for evaluation and is accomplished by fluoroscopy. For example, in order to visualize the stomach emptying its contents into the small bowel, images must be created in a continuous form for accurate evaluation of the functioning. Most fluoroscopic procedures also require the use of contrast media to visualize internal structures and their functioning. This chapter discusses the components of fluoroscopic units, viewing and recording systems, and the digital fluoroscopy process in use today.

FLUOROSCOPY

Fluoroscopy allows imaging of the movement of internal structures. It differs from radiographic imaging by its use of a continuous beam of x-rays to create images of moving internal structures that can be viewed on a monitor. Internal structures, such as vascular or gastrointestinal systems, can be visualized in their normal state of motion with the aid of special liquid or gas substances (contrast media) that are either injected or instilled.

In image-intensified fluoroscopy, the milliamperage (mA) used during imaging is considerably lower (0.5 to 5 mA) than that in the radiographic mode, which is operated at a higher mA of 50 to 1200 mA. A low mA provides for the increased time the fluoroscope is operated. Because the time of exposure is lengthened, the control panel includes a timer that buzzes audibly when 5 min of x-ray fluoroscopic time has been used. Another important feature of a fluoroscopic unit is the deadman switch. The continuous x-ray beam is activated by either a hand switch on the unit or a foot pedal that must be continuously depressed for the x-rays to be produced. Releasing the pressure applied to the pedal or switch terminates the radiation exposure.

Image Intensification

Image intensification (Figure 10-1) is the process in which the exit radiation from the anatomic area of interest interacts with the **input phosphor** (a light-emitting material, such as cesium iodide) for conversion to visible light. The light intensities are equal to the intensities of the exit radiation and are converted to electrons by a **photocathode** (photoemission). The electrons are focused by **electrostatic focusing lenses** and accelerated toward an anode to strike the **output phosphor** (coated with light-emitting crystals, such as zinc cadmium sulfide) and create a brighter image.

IMPORTANT RELATIONSHIP

Image-Intensified Fluoroscopy

Dynamic imaging of internal anatomic structures can be accomplished with the use of an image intensifier. The exit radiation is absorbed by the input phosphor, converted to electrons, sent to the output phosphor, released as visible light, and converted to an electronic video signal for transmission to the television monitor.

The image light intensities from the output phosphor are converted to an electronic video signal and sent to a television monitor for viewing. Figure 10-2 is an example of a typical radiographic and image-intensified fluoroscopic unit. Additional filming devices, such as spot film or cine (movie film), can be attached to the fluoroscopic system to create permanent radiographic images of specific areas of interest.

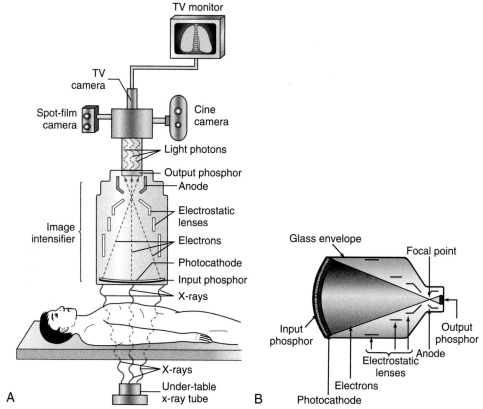

FIGURE 10-1 A, Fluoroscopic system used for dynamic imaging of internal structures. **B,** Major components of an image intensifier.

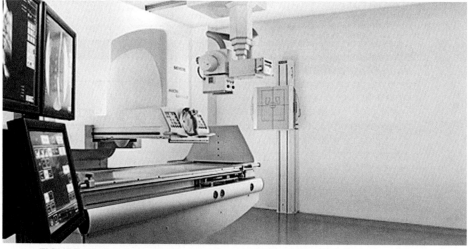

FIGURE 10-2 A typical radiographic and image-intensified fluoroscopic unit.

Brightness Gain

A brighter image is a result of high-energy electrons striking a small-output phosphor. Accelerating the electrons increases the light intensities at the output phosphor (**flux gain**). The reduction in the size of the output phosphor image compared with that of the input phosphor image also increases the light intensities (**minification gain**). **Brightness gain** is the product of both flux gain and minification gain and results in a brighter image on the output phosphor.

 IMPORTANT RELATIONSHIP

Brightness Gain

A brighter image is created on the output phosphor when accelerated electrons strike a smaller output phosphor.

Although the term *brightness gain* continues to be used, it is now a common practice to express this increase in brightness with the term *conversion factor*. **Conversion factor** is an expression of the luminance at the output phosphor divided by the input exposure rate, and its unit of measure is the candela per square meter per milliroentgen per second ($cd/m^2/mR/s$). The numeric conversion factor value is roughly equal to 1% of the brightness gain value. For example, a brightness gain of 20,000 would have a conversion factor of 200. The higher the conversion factor or brightness gain value, the greater the efficiency of the image intensifier. See Box 10-1 for brightness gain and conversion factor formulas.

Automatic Brightness Control

The radiographer must also be familiar with **automatic brightness control (ABC)**, a function of the fluoroscopic unit that maintains the overall appearance of the fluoroscopic image (contrast and density) by automatically adjusting the kilovoltage peak (kVp), mA, or both. ABC generally operates by monitoring the current through the image intensifier or the output phosphor intensity and adjusting the exposure factor if the monitored value falls below preset levels. The fluoroscopic unit allows the operator to select a desired brightness level, and this level is subsequently maintained by ABC. ABC is slightly slow in its response to changes in patient tissue thickness and tissue density as the fluoroscopy tower is moved about over the patient; this is visible to the radiographer as a lag in the image brightness on the monitor as the tower is moved.

BOX 10-1 Brightness Gain and Conversion Factor Formulas

$$\text{Brightness gain} = \text{Minification gain} \times \text{Flux gain}$$

$$\text{Flux gain} = \frac{\text{Number of output light photons}}{\text{Number of input x–ray photons}}$$

$$\text{Minification gain} = \left(\frac{d_i}{d_o}\right)^2$$

$$\text{Conversion factor} = \frac{\text{Output phosphor illumination (cd/m}^2)}{\text{Input exposure rate (mR/s)}}$$

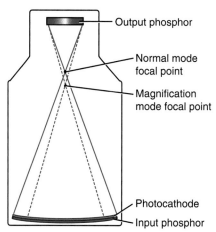

FIGURE 10-3 Magnification mode. When the image intensifier is operated in magnification mode, the voltage to the electrostatic focusing lenses is increased. This increase tightens the diameter of the electron stream, and the focal point is shifted farther from the output phosphor, resulting in a magnified image.

Magnification Mode

Another function of some image intensifiers is the multifield mode or magnification mode. Most image intensifiers in use today have this capability. When operated in **magnification mode**, the voltage to the electrostatic focusing lenses is increased. This increase tightens the diameter of the electron stream, and the focal point is shifted farther from the output phosphor (Figure 10-3). The effect is that only the electrons from the central area of the input phosphor interact with the output phosphor and contribute to the image, giving the appearance of magnification. For example, a 30/23/15 cm trifocus image intensifier can be operated in any of these three modes. When operated in the 23 cm mode, only the electrons from the central 23 cm of the input phosphor interact with the output phosphor; the electrons about the periphery miss and do not contribute to the image. The same is true for the 15 cm mode. Selecting the magnification mode automatically adjusts the x-ray beam collimation to match the displayed tissue image and avoids irradiating tissue that does not appear in the image. The degree of magnification (magnification factor [MF]) may be found by dividing the full-size input diameter by the selected input diameter. For example: MF = 30 ÷ 15 = 2× magnification.

This magnification improves the operator's ability to see small structures (spatial resolution, discussed shortly) but at the expense of increasing the patient dose. Remnant x-ray photons are converted to light and then to electrons and are focused on the output phosphor. If fewer electrons are incident on the output phosphor, the output intensity decreases. To compensate, more x-ray photons are needed at the beginning of the process to produce more light, resulting in more electrons at the input end of the image intensifier. ABC automatically increases x-ray exposure to achieve this. Again, with an increase in x-rays used comes an increase in patient dose.

⬥ IMPORTANT RELATIONSHIP
Magnification Mode and Patient Dose

Operating the image intensifier in one of the magnification modes increases the operator's ability to see small structures but at the price of increasing the radiation dose to the patient.

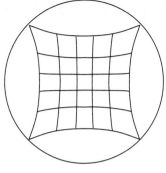

Image displaying
"pincushion" distortion

FIGURE 10-4 Pincushion distortion. Appearance of the pincushion effect. The circle represents the television monitor display, and the grid represents the effect on the image.

Magnification modes improve **spatial resolution**, which refers to the smallest structure that may be detected in an image. Spatial resolution is measured in line pairs per millimeter (Lp/mm), and typical fluoroscopic systems have spatial resolution capabilities of 4 to 6 Lp/mm but greatly depend on the rest of the imaging chain (i.e., the viewing and recording systems).

Distortion is also an issue with image-intensified fluoroscopy. In radiography, distortion is a misrepresentation of the true size or shape of an object. In the case of fluoroscopy, shape distortion can be a problem. In fluoroscopy, distortion is a result of inaccurate control or focusing of the electrons released at the periphery of the photocathode and the curved shape of the photocathode. The combined result is an unequal magnification (distortion) of the image, creating what is called a "pincushion appearance" (Figure 10-4). This problem also causes a loss of brightness around the periphery of the image, which is referred to as *vignetting*.

One last factor to consider with image intensifiers is noise. Image noise results when insufficient information is present to create the image. In the case of fluoroscopy, this lack of image-forming information ultimately goes back to an insufficient quantity of x-rays. If too few x-rays exit the patient and expose the input phosphor, not enough light will be produced, decreasing the number of electrons released by the photocathode to interact with the output phosphor. This results in a "grainy" or "noisy" image (Figure 10-5). Although other factors in the fluoroscopic chain may contribute to noise, the solution generally comes back to increasing the mA (quantity of radiation). See Box 10-2 for fluoroscopic equipment inspection checklist.

Viewing Systems

The original image intensifiers produced an image that was viewed using a mirror optics system—something akin to a sophisticated way of looking at the output phosphor with a "rearview mirror." Conventionally, the viewing system is now a closed-circuit television monitor system. To view the image from the output phosphor on a television monitor, it must first be converted to an electrical signal (often referred to as *video signal*) by the television camera. Two devices are commonly used today to accomplish this: a camera tube and a charge-coupled device (CCD). The camera tube and CCD differ in their size and readout process.

Television Cameras

Television cameras used in order to display the fluoroscopic image include the older camera tube (vidicon/Plumbicon) and the newer CCD. The **camera tube** has a vacuum tube approximately

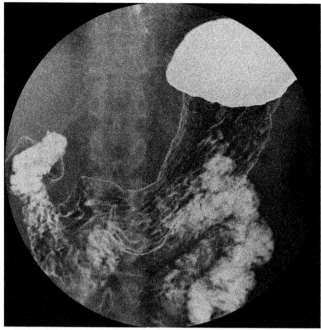

FIGURE 10-5 Quantum noise. If too few x-rays exit the patient and expose the input phosphor, not enough light will be produced, decreasing the number of electrons released by the photocathode to interact with the output phosphor. A "grainy" or "noisy" image results.

BOX 10-2 Fluoroscopic Equipment Inspection Checklist

Inspect:	Ensure that:
Bucky slot cover	When the Bucky is parked at the foot of the table, the metal cover should expand and cover the entire opening.
Protective curtain	The curtain should be in good condition and move freely into place when the tower is moved to the operating position.
Tower—locks, power assist, control panel	The electromagnetic locks are in good working order, the power assist moves the tower about easily in all directions, and all control panel indicator lights are operational.
Exposure switch (deadman switch)	The switch is not sticking and operates the x-ray tube only while in the depressed position (also test the switch with the tower in the park position; it should not activate the x-ray tube while parked).
Collimator shutters	In the fully open position, the shutters should restrict the beam to the size of the input phosphor and be accurate to within ±3%.
Fluoroscopic timer	The timer should buzz audibly after 5 min of fluoroscopic "beam-on" time.
Monitor brightness	While exposing a penetrometer through a fluoroscopic phantom, the monitor image is adjusted to display as many of the penetrometer steps as possible.
Table tilt motion	The table tilts smoothly to its limit in both directions, and the angulation indicator is operational.

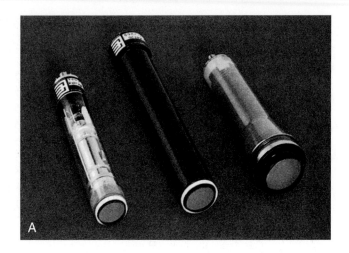

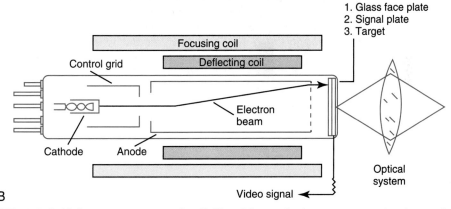

FIGURE 10-6 A, Vidicon-type camera tube. **B,** The vidicon tube has a vacuum tube that encloses an electron gun and a photoconductive target assembly. The electrical signal leaving the camera tube varies in strength proportionally based on the varying brightness of the image being scanned.

15 cm (6 in) in length that encloses an electron gun and a photoconductive target assembly (Figure 10-6). The diameter of the tube is the same size as that of the output phosphor. The light from the output phosphor arrives at the target assembly either by fiber optics or by a lens system. A steady stream of electrons from the electron gun scans the target assembly very quickly from left to right and top to bottom (raster pattern). As the stream of electrons bombards the target, anywhere there is light intensity from the output phosphor image there will be an electrical signal leaving the tube. Scanning a brighter or higher light intensity results in the electrical signal leaving the camera tube with a higher strength. The darker or lower the light intensities scanned, the lower the strength of the electrical signal. The electrical signal leaving the camera tube varies in strength in proportion to the varying brightness of the image being scanned. This electrical (video) signal goes to the television monitor to complete the display process.

The **charge-coupled device (CCD)** is a light-sensitive semiconducting device that generates an electrical charge when stimulated by light and stores this charge in a capacitor. The charge is proportional to the light intensity and is stored in rows of pixels. The CCD consists of a series of semiconductor capacitors, with each capacitor representing a pixel. Each pixel is

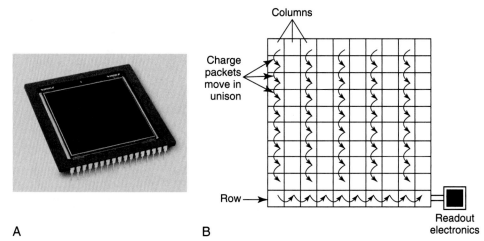

A   B

FIGURE 10-7 **A,** The charge-coupled device (CCD) is a light-sensitive semiconducting device that generates an electrical charge when stimulated by light and stores this charge in a capacitor. **B,** To digitize the charge from the CCD, the electrodes between each pixel, called *row gates*, are charged in sequence, moving the signal down the row where it is transferred into a capacitor. From the capacitors, the charge is sent as an electronic signal to the television monitor.

composed of photosensitive material that dislodges electrons when stimulated by light photons. To digitize the charge from this device, the electrodes between each pixel, called *row gates*, are charged in sequence, moving the signal down the row, where it is transferred into the capacitors. From the capacitors, the charge is sent as an electronic signal to the television monitor. In this way, each pixel is individually "read" and sent to the television monitor (Figure 10-7).

Compared with the vidicon-type camera tube, the CCD is read out by the charge in each pixel, whereas the vidicon is read out by an electronic beam. CCD TV cameras have some advantages over the camera tubes in that they are more sensitive to a wider range of light intensities and show no geometric distortion of the fluoroscopic display image. The CCD is smaller in size than the vidicon camera tube and works well in digital imaging.

Coupling of Devices

As mentioned earlier, the camera tube or CCD may be coupled to the output phosphor of the image intensifier by either a fiber-optic bundle or an optical lens system. The fiber-optic bundle is simply a bundle of very thin optical glass filaments. This system is very durable and simple in design but does not allow spot filming.

The optical lens system is a series of optical lenses that focus the image from the output phosphor on the television camera (camera tube or CCD). When spot filming is desired, a beam-splitting mirror (a partially silvered mirror that allows some light to pass through and reflects some in a new direction) is moved into the path of the output image and diverts some of the light to the desired spot-filming device (e.g., the photospot or cine camera) (Figure 10-1). This system, although allowing spot filming of this type, is more susceptible to rough handling, which may cause maladjustment of the mirror and lenses and result in a blurred image.

Television Monitor

The varying electrical (video) signals reach the television display monitor (cathode ray tube [CRT]) almost instantaneously. The CRT (Figure 10-8) includes an electron gun that scans the

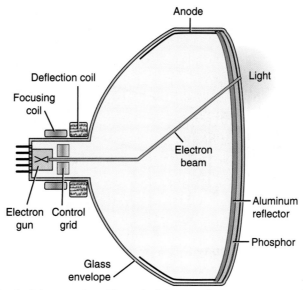

FIGURE 10-8 CRT television monitor. The television monitor reconstructs the image from the output phosphor as a visible image. The CRT includes an electron gun that scans the phosphor layer found on the inside of the glass front of the monitor in a raster pattern.

phosphor layer found on the inside of the glass front of the monitor, again in the raster pattern. As the video signal increases and decreases, so does the number of electrons emitted from the electron gun. The greater the number of electrons leaving the gun, the brighter the fluorescence of the phosphor, resulting in a bright spot on the display monitor. The lower the video signal, the fewer the electrons emitted from the gun and the lower the brightness of the displayed image.

In essence, the television monitor reconstructs the image from the output phosphor as a visible image. The image is created on the fluorescent screen one line at a time starting in the upper left-hand corner and moving to the right (active trace). It then blanks (turns off) and returns to the left side (horizontal retrace). This process continues to the bottom of the screen. It then returns to the top (vertical retrace) and begins again by placing a line between each of the previously drawn lines. This action creates a television frame. Typical television monitors are called *525-line systems* because the traces create a 525-line frame. High-resolution monitors have 1024 lines per frame. However, the monitor continues to be the weak link in terms of the resolution of the fluoroscopic chain. The image intensifier is capable of resolving approximately 5 Lp/mm, whereas the monitor can display only 1 to 2 Lp/mm.

IMPORTANT RELATIONSHIP

Coupling Systems and the Television Monitor

The camera tube and CCD are devices that couple the image intensifier to the television monitor to convert the image from the output phosphor to an electronic (video) signal that can be reconstructed on the television monitor.

Liquid Crystal Display (LCD) Monitors

LCD monitors are a modern display monitor option. LCD monitors offer superior resolution and brightness over television monitors. They work in a completely different way than television

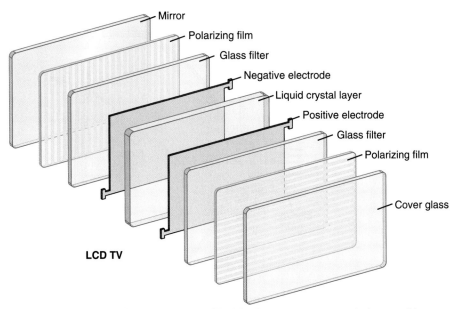

FIGURE 10-9 Liquid Crystal Display (LCD) Monitors are composed of several layers.

monitors. LCD monitors are made up of several layers (See Figure 10-9). The heart of the LCD is the liquid crystal layer sandwiched between polarizing layers. The liquid crystal layer contains nematic liquid crystals. These crystals are typically rod-shaped and are semi-liquid. They exist in an unorganized "twisted" state. When an electric current is applied, they organize or "untwist." In the untwisted state, they organize into configurations that block or allow light to pass through depending on the polarizing filters. The polarized layers on each side are oriented perpendicular to one other, meaning that light that may be able to pass through one would be at the wrong orientation to pass through the other. When electric current is applied to the liquid crystal layer, the "untwisting" changes the orientation of light passing through the back layer and allows it to pass through the front. A TFT panel is located behind the liquid crystal layer. The number of TFTs is equal to the number of pixels displayed. The TFTs control the current to each pixel and switch it on or off by causing the liquid crystals to twist or untwist. A monochromatic LCD monitor will display the light as shades of gray. A color LCD monitor has a color filter layer added to display shades of color. The intensity of light is controlled by the current to the crystals, which is controlled by the TFTs. This in turn determines the shade of gray if monochromatic or the shade of color if using a color monitor.

Plasma Monitors
Plasma monitors are another modern display option. Plasma monitors are very similar in construction to LCD monitors, but instead of a liquid crystal layer, they have a thin layer of pixels (see Figure 10-10). Each pixel contains three neon- and xenon-gas-filled cells (sub-pixels). Each of these cells is coated with a different phosphor layer formula that will produce red, green, or blue light when stimulated. On each side of this layer of pixels are dielectric layers. When electricity is passed between these dielectric layers through the pixels, the gas within is ionized. The liberated electrons release ultraviolet radiation in order to return to the shell of an atom. The ultraviolet radiation in turn stimulates the phosphor coating in the cell, producing visible light of a color corresponding to the phosphor formula. The current through the pixels (and sub-pixels) is modulated by the electrodes several thousand times per second, thereby controlling the intensity

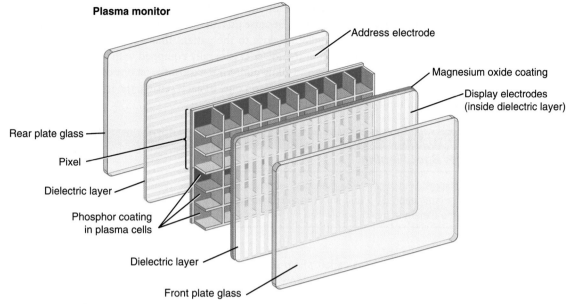

FIGURE 10-10 Plasma monitors are very similar in construction to LCD monitors, but instead of a liquid crystal layer, they have a thin layer of pixels.

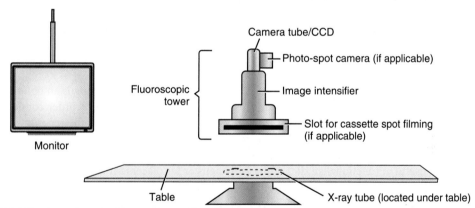

FIGURE 10-11 A typical image-intensified fluoroscopic unit showing two types of recording systems, cassette spot filming and a photo-spot camera.

of light produced. This control and modulation process makes it possible for plasma monitors to produce billions of different shades of color.

Recording Systems

Cassette spot filming has been a standard of image-intensified fluoroscopic imaging for many years (Figure 10-11). This is a static imaging process in which a standard radiographic cassette is used to obtain an image. With this system, the cassette is loaded into the lower part of the fluoroscopic tower and "parked" in a protective envelope in the back. When the spot-film exposure button is pressed, the cassette is moved into position between the patient and image intensifier, and the machine shifts from fluoroscopic to radiographic mode and exposes the film. In the shift to radiographic mode, the mA increases from one of the 0.5 to 5 mA fluoroscopic modes to one of the 50 to 1200 mA radiographic modes. Because this method of imaging uses the radiographic mode, it requires a much higher radiation dose to the patient than the other methods. As an alternative to exposing the entire film, the tower is generally equipped with a series of masking shutters that can "divide" the cassette and allow numerous exposures on one cassette, such as two exposures on one cassette, four on one, and six on one. In each setting, the image is smaller and organized as one of multiple images on one film.

> ### IMPORTANT RELATIONSHIP
> #### *Cassette Spot Filming*
>
> Cassette spot-film devices are a means of recording static images during an image-intensified fluoroscopic examination. The unit shifts to radiographic mode (using a higher mA), and the radiation dose to the patient is much higher than in the fluoroscopic mode.

Film cameras (sometimes called *photo-spot cameras*) have also been a mainstay of image-intensified fluoroscopy (refer back to Figure 10-11). 105 mm film or 70 mm roll film are the most commonly used varieties. The photo-spot camera is also a static imaging system that is used with an optical lens system incorporating a beam-splitting mirror. When the spot-film exposure switch is pressed, the beam-splitting mirror is moved into place, diverting some of the beam toward the photo camera and exposing the film. This device uses the visible light image from the output phosphor of the image intensifier and photographically exposes the 105 mm (or 70 mm) film, similar to a 35 mm film camera used in photography. This system allows very fast imaging of up to 12 frames per second, and because it "photographs" the image off of the output phosphor of the image intensifier, it requires approximately half the radiation dose of the cassette spot-filming system.

With image-intensified fluoroscopy, videotape or DVD recording is an option when dynamic imaging is desired. This process uses a VHS videotape or DVD recorder connected to the television monitor. From this point, it operates quite similar to a home recording system. During fluoroscopic examinations, the "record" button is pressed on the system, and it records the image from the monitor. Although not typically used in today's fluoroscopic systems, such imaging is useful in functional studies of the esophagus or for placement of catheters or medical devices.

As more departments transition to fully digital environments and eliminate film and chemical processing, a greater dependence is being placed on digital imaging and storage means. Without chemical processing and film, cassette spot filming and photo-spot imaging go away. If the fluoroscopic signal is in digital form, the size of the data files makes it impossible to record any length of dynamic images on a VHS tape.

MOBILE C-ARM UNITS

Mobile C-arm units have fluoroscopic capabilities that are typically used in the operating room when imaging is necessary during surgical procedures. Display monitors are also included, offering both static and dynamic imaging during the procedure. Because it is a fluoroscopic system, many of the features of a fixed fluoroscopic unit are also made available with a C-arm. A C-arm unit is designed with an x-ray tube and image intensifier attached in a C configuration (Figure 10-12). As a result, the unit can be positioned in a variety of planes, enabling viewing from different perspectives. Generally, three sets of locks are provided to move and hold the

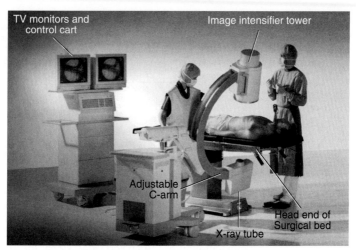

FIGURE 10-12 A mobile C-arm unit.

C-arm in place. One set moves the entire "c" toward or away from the base (the equivalent of moving a table side to side). Another set allows the "c" to pivot about its axis (the equivalent of angling a general radiographic tube head assembly). The last set allows the "c" to slide along its arc (the equivalent of moving the patient from anteroposterior or posteroanterior positions to oblique to lateral positions without having to move the patient).

As a general rule, the x-ray tube should be positioned under the patient and the image intensifier above the patient. Positioning the C-arm in this manner during the imaging procedure reduces the radiation exposure to the operator. Because the C-arm uses fluoroscopy, standard radiation exposure techniques and safety practices used during fluoroscopy in the radiology department must also be adhered to during operation of a C-arm unit. The radiographer should also pay particular attention to the distance between the patient and the x-ray tube as well as to total fluoroscopy time. Here, too, fluoroscopy is being used in an "uncontrolled" environment, and it is the radiographer's responsibility to monitor and apply radiation safety measures.

DIGITAL FLUOROSCOPY

Similar to image-intensified fluoroscopy, digital fluoroscopy has evolved over time. Early versions of digital fluoroscopy used an image-intensified fluoroscopic chain but added an analog-to-digital converter (ADC) and a computer between the TV camera and the monitor (Figure 10-13). An **analog-to-digital converter (ADC)** is a device that takes the video (analog) signal and divides it into a number of bits (1s and 0s) that the computer "understands." The number of bits into which the signal is divided determines the contrast resolution (number of shades of gray) of the system. The ADC is necessary for the computer to process and display the image. Once in digital form, the image can be postprocessed and stored in that format or printed onto film using a dry laser printer.

The incorporation of a CCD into this setup further improved digital fluoroscopy. The CCD eliminated some of the problems associated with the camera tube. The CCD is more light sensitive (higher detective quantum efficiency [DQE]) and exhibits less noise and no spatial distortion. It also has a higher spatial resolution and requires less radiation in the system, reducing patient dose.

A more recent advance in digital fluoroscopy is the introduction of a flat-panel detector in place of an image intensifier (Figure 10-14). Two forms of flat-panel detectors may be used for fluoroscopic applications: the cesium iodide amorphous silicon indirect-capture detector and the

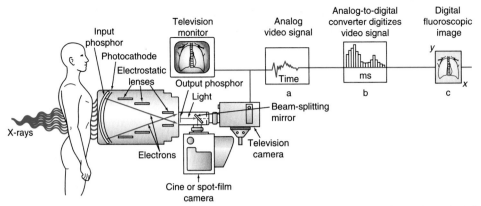

FIGURE 10-13 Analog and digital signals in fluoroscopy. The video signal from the television camera is analog, where the voltage signal continuously varies. This analog signal is sampled *(a)*, producing a stepped representation of the analog video signal *(b)*. The numerical values of each step are stored *(c)*, producing a matrix of digital image data. The binary representation of each pixel value in the matrix is stored and can be manipulated by a computer. The value of each pixel can be mapped to a brightness level for viewing on a display monitor or to an optical density for hard copy on film.

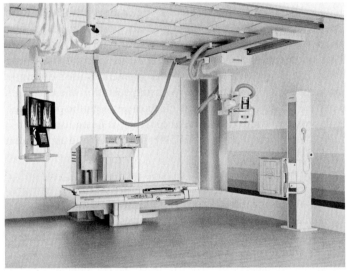

FIGURE 10-14 Digital fluoroscopy using flat-panel-detector technology.

amorphous selenium direct-capture detector. For use as a dynamic digital detector (i.e., in digital fluoroscopy applications), there are a few differences between the two. Generally, the digital detectors must respond in rapid sequences to create a dynamic image. Current dynamic digital detectors are capable of up to 60 frames per second. To accomplish this, rapid readout speeds (by which the active matrix processes the image data) are necessary.

Currently, the most commonly used flat-panel detector for fluoroscopic applications is the cesium iodide amorphous silicon indirect-capture detector. The scintillator of this system uses cesium iodide or gadolinium oxysulfide as the phosphor. The photodetector is amorphous silicon, which is a liquid that can be painted onto a substrate (foundation or underlying layer) and is the material that makes flat-panel detectors possible. The other component is a TFT array. TFTs are electronic components layered onto a glass substrate that includes a readout, charge collector, and light-sensitive elements. The panel is configured into a network of pixels (or detector elements [DELs]) covered by the scintillator plate with each pixel containing a photodetector and a TFT. With this system, x-ray energy is absorbed by the scintillator and converted to light energy. This light is then absorbed by the photodetectors and converted to electrical charges, which are in turn captured and transmitted by the TFT array to the monitor for display.

Flat-panel detectors are very popular in interventional and cardiology applications and are gaining ground in general fluoroscopy. They are much lighter and more compact, they produce a digital signal directly (no need for a camera tube or ADC), and because it is a digital system producing a digital signal (without the electronic components of the old image-intensified system), there is less electronic noise. Detector arrays are currently available in sizes of 25×25 cm to 40×40 cm.

Although the cesium iodide amorphous silicon indirect-capture detector is essentially the same as that for DR, there are a few differences for use as a dynamic digital detector in digital fluoroscopy applications. In general, dynamic versions of these detectors must respond in rapid sequences to create a dynamic image. Current dynamic versions are capable of up to 60 frames per second. To accomplish this, rapid readout speeds (how the active matrix processes the image data) are necessary. The design is a two-dimensional rectilinear array of pixels that can be electronically processed line by line in a fraction of a second. Furthermore, for fluoroscopic applications, very-low-noise flat-panel-detector systems are needed. Fluoroscopy generally operates at a low dose output; hence, any operational noise degrades the fluoroscopic image, making noise a greater factor in detectors used for this application.

The use of flat-panel detectors in place of an image intensifier offers several advantages. The first is a reduction in the size, bulk, and weight of the fluoroscopic tower. A flat-panel detector greatly reduces all three, allowing easier manipulation of the tower, greater flexibility of movement, and greater access to the patient during the examination. A flat-panel detector with a 12" × 16" active area occupies less than 25% of the volume of a 12" image intensifier tube and less than 15% of the volume of a 16" image intensifier tube. The flat-panel detectors also replace the spot filming and other recording devices. They are capable of operating in radiographic mode, so that in many cases, additional radiographic images are not needed. The images, both dynamic and static, are recorded by the system and can be readily archived with the patient record in a Picture Archiving and Communication System (PACS). It should be noted that the images produced are very large data files, as spot images can be 8 MB or larger and dynamic images as large as 240 MB per second. Furthermore, flat-panel detectors do not degrade with age; are more durable; present a rectangular field providing more information; and have better contrast resolution, higher DQE, wider dynamic range, and all the postprocessing options common to digital images. The spatial resolution of flat-panel detectors is the same for all field of view options provided binning (the process of grouping and averaging adjacent DELS) is not used and is higher than that of an image-intensified system (2.5–3.2 Lp/mm versus 1–2 Lp/mm). Finally, flat-panel detectors do not exhibit most image artifacts seen with image intensifiers. Flat-panel detectors have a 60 times larger operational dynamic range than image intensifier systems and, because of this, do not exhibit veiling glare. Because the DELs of a flat-panel detector are arranged in a grid pattern (uniform columns and rows), they do not exhibit the pincushion and S distortion artifacts. Vignetting (unequal brightness) and defocusing artifacts are also eliminated with flat-panel detectors. They do all of this with as much as a 50% lower radiation dose to the patient.

IMPORTANT RELATIONSHIP

Digital Fluoroscopic Systems

The use of flat-panel detectors in place of an image intensifier offers several advantages, such as a reduction in the size, bulk, and weight of the fluoroscopic tower, allowing for easier manipulation of the tower and greater access to the patient during the examination. The flat-panel detectors also replace the spot filming and other recording devices, and, because they are capable of operating in radiographic mode, in many cases, additional radiographic images are not needed. The images, both dynamic and static, can also be readily archived with the patient record in a PACS.

The mA used to operate a digital fluoroscopic unit is similar to the mA used in the radiographic mode, in the hundreds, as opposed to image intensified fluoroscopy in the low mA range. In addition, the x-ray beam is not continuously operated, but is rather automatically pulsed to reduce the heat loading on the tube. Similar to image-intensified fluoroscopy, the average exposure to the image receptor or detector signal needs to be maintained in order to produce a diagnostic-quality digital fluoroscopic image. Generator controls, such as automatic dose rate and automatic exposure rate, are similar to the concept of automatic brightness control (ABC) previously discussed. These controls change the kVp, mA, or both in combination to adjust the exposure factors to maintain the brightness and contrast needed for the fluoroscopic image. Maintaining the average exposure or signal to the image receptor will also vary the radiation dose to the patient and therefore the operator needs to monitor any available dose measurements displayed.

CONTINUOUS VERSUS PULSED FLUROSCOPY

With modern image-intensified fluoroscopic units, the operator has the option of selecting a continuous or pulsed x-ray beam during the fluoroscopic procedure (Figure 10-15). When operated in the **continuous fluoroscopy** mode, the x-ray exposure continues without interruption while the exposure pedal/button is activated. This results in 30 frames of fluoroscopic images each second. When a fluoroscope is operated in the continuous mode, the patient receives a high amount of radiation exposure due to the increased number of fluoroscopic images. In addition, because there are many more images per second, patient motion may be visible.

 IMPORTANT RELATIONSHIP

Continuous Fluoroscopy

Operating the fluoroscope in a continuous mode will produce 30 frames of images each second, increase patient dose, and may increase the visibility of patient motion.

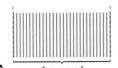

FIGURE 10-15 Continuous versus Pulsed Fluoroscopy. **A,** Continuous fluoroscopy produces 30 images (frames) during a period of 1 s. **B,** Pulsed fluoroscopy can vary the number of images (frames) per second. This example has 7 frames per second.

Operating in a **pulsed fluoroscopy** mode means the x-ray exposure is not continuous and has gaps of no exposure between each image frame. These units may have several options in the pulsed mode, such as selecting the number of images (frames) per second or pulse rate (for example between 2–15 frames per second). The operator selects the pulse rate and the x-ray exposure pulses automatically occur while the fluoro pedal/button is depressed. When pulsed fluoroscopy is used, exposure parameters (kV and mA) are increased to maintain a satisfactory signal-to-noise ratio (SNR) for a quality image. However, because there are fewer image frames per second when compared to continuous fluoroscopy, the patient dose can be reduced. In addition, using the pulsed fluoroscopic mode will decrease the visibility of patient motion. It is recommended to use the lowest pulsed fluoroscopic mode required for the specific procedure.

A related feature of modern fluoroscopic units is the dose rate feature, low to high. Using a low fluoroscopic dose rate will reduce the dose to the patient but at the cost of increased noise in the images. Using a higher dose rate will reduce image noise but increase the dose to the patient. The operator needs to understand these features and how they affect patient dose. For example, if the lowest pulsed mode is used along with a high dose rate, patient dose is higher, when compared to a lower pulse mode and low dose rate.

 IMPORTANT RELATIONSHIP

Pulsed Fluoroscopy

> Operating the fluoroscope in a pulsed mode will reduce the number of images each second, decrease patient dose, and reduce the visibility of patient motion.

RADIATION SAFETY

Radiation safety is just as important during fluoroscopic imaging as it is with radiographic imaging. It is the fluoroscopic operator's responsibility to be knowledgeable about the equipment and methods to reduce patient radiation dose. A few methods of minimizing radiation dose to the patient during fluoroscopic procedures include omission of the grid during fluoroscopy, minimal use of the magnification feature, and the use of the last image hold where the x-ray exposure is not activated while the operator reviews the image.

Because older image-intensified fluoroscopic units use a continuous stream of x-rays, the exposure should be intermittently pulsed by the operator. Applying pressure to the exposure switch or pedal intermittently significantly reduces the exposure of both patients and personnel and reduces the heat load on the x-ray tube. Modern image-intensified and digital fluoroscopy use a controlled pulsed x-ray exposure, and the operator is not required to intermittently release the pressure. Operating the fluoroscope in the lowest pulsed mode along with a lower dose rate will minimize patient radiation dose.

Time, distance, and shielding are the standard radiation safety practices used during fluoroscopic imaging. Reducing the x-ray exposure time reduces the exposure to the patient and any personnel remaining in the room. The control panel timer produces an audible noise when 5 min of x-ray fluoroscopic time have been used. It is the operator's responsibility to minimize the x-ray fluoroscopy, and the radiographer should document the total amount of x-ray fluoroscopic time used during the procedure. Modern fluoroscopic units provide dose monitoring in addition to the cumulative fluorotimer. The dose area product (DAP) and cumulative air kerma (kinetic energy released in a mass) provides radiation exposure data and need to be recorded in the patient's medical record. If these dose-monitoring systems are not available, then the cumulative exposure time and number

TABLE 10-1   Methods of Reducing Patient and Personnel Exposure During Fluoroscopy

- Operating the fluoroscope in the lowest pulsed mode along with a lower dose rate and the use of last image hold will minimize patient radiation dose.
- Reducing the amount of x-ray fluoroscopic time reduces patient and personnel exposure.
- Increase collimation, remove the grid, and minimize the use of magnification.
- Monitor and document the amount of total x-ray fluoroscopic time displayed in 5 min increments on the control panel in addition to the number of acquired radiographic images. If provided, cumulative radiation dose data should be recorded.
- The intensity of x-ray exposure at the tabletop should not exceed 10 R/min for units equipped with ABC and 5 R/min for units without ABC.
- The SSD should be not less than 38 cm (15 in) for stationary fluoroscopic units and not less than 30 cm (12 in) on mobile C-arm fluoroscopic units.
- Personnel in the fluoroscopic room during procedures should increase their distance from the patient to reduce exposure to scatter radiation.
- Personnel should wear appropriate lead shielding during fluoroscopic procedures.
- The Bucky slot cover must contain at least 0.25 mm of lead-equivalent shielding and cover the opened space on the side of the table.
- A protective curtain placed between the patient and operator must have at least 0.25 mm of lead equivalent.

of acquired images need to be documented. In addition, the intensity of the x-ray exposure at the tabletop should not exceed 10 R per minute for units equipped with ABC and 5 R per minute for units without ABC. Whenever the patient's exposure is reduced, personnel exposure also is reduced.

The source-to-skin distance (SSD) should be no less than 38 cm (15 in) for stationary fluoroscopic units and no less than 30 cm (12 inches) on a mobile C-arm fluoroscopic unit. Increasing the SSD and decreasing the distance between the patient and the image receptor (OID) will decrease patient exposure. Increasing collimation and decreasing the number of acquired (radiographic) images will reduce patient exposure. If the fluoroscopic unit has features such as virtual collimation (x-ray field size can be adjusted without irradiating the patient) and the ability to save a sequence of fluoroscopic images without acquiring radiographic images, patient exposure will be further decreased. In addition, personnel other than the operator should increase their distance from the patient to reduce exposure to scatter radiation from the patient.

In addition to all personnel in the room wearing lead aprons (recommended 0.5 mm of lead equivalent), two additional types of shielding are required during fluoroscopy. Because the Bucky tray is positioned at the end of the table for operation of the under-table x-ray tube, a Bucky slot cover with at least 0.25 mm of lead equivalent should automatically cover the opened space at the side of the table. In addition, a protective lead curtain with at least 0.25 mm of lead equivalent must be placed between the patient and the operator to reduce exposure to the operator. Table 10-1 lists methods of reducing patient and personnel exposure during fluoroscopy.

QUALITY CONTROL

Quality control programs are vitally important for all ionizing-radiation-producing equipment to monitor equipment performance and minimize patient dose. Fluoroscopic equipment is used extensively in health care and contributes significantly to the radiation dose received by the general population. Quality control is a team effort among the radiographer, radiologist, and medical physicist. Although some equipment monitoring and data may be collected by a radiographer, performance tests and their interpretation are typically performed by a medical physicist. However,

BOX 10-3   Quality Control (QC) Specific to Fluoroscopic Equipment

QC Test	Description
Fluoroscopic system resolution	Tests the system's ability to display details of small objects (high-contrast resolution) and larger objects (low-contrast resolution).
Fluoroscopic automatic brightness control (ABC) performance	Evaluates image quality for changes in exposure parameters such as high dose rate, pulsed modes, and field of view (FOV)
Fluoroscopic phantom image quality	Evaluates the quality of the displayed fluoroscopic image, including image distortion or lag.
Fluoroscopic exposure rates	Measures the intensity of the x-ray beam. Fluoroscopic exposure rate should not exceed 10 R/min for units with ABC systems and 5 R/min for those without ABC systems.
Fluoroscopic alignment test	Ensures the radiation beam aligns with the center of the image intensifier within 2% of the SID.
Patient dose monitoring system calibration, if present	Evaluates proper function of patient dose monitoring systems such as DAP meters.
Digital monitor performance	Evaluates the display characteristics of the monitor (described in Chapter 4)

the radiographer should be familiar with the monitoring and testing necessary to ensure that the fluoroscopic unit is operating correctly.

The radiographer, in particular, a quality control radiographer, may be responsible for the operational inspection of the equipment. This inspection should be conducted using a checklist of the items found in Box 10-2 at least every 6 months. The radiographer may also be responsible for an inspection of the imaging suite itself to examine the general physical condition of the room, unit, supporting electrical cables, and control booth, noting any wear or deterioration. This inspection of the physical condition should be placed on the same schedule and conducted along with the operational inspection.

The other important part of the quality program is the performance inspection and equipment testing (Box 10-3 lists a few common fluoroscopic quality control tests). Although a quality control radiographer may perform some of these tests, an appropriately trained and licensed medical physicist should conduct and interpret this portion of the program and oversee the entire quality control monitoring program.

CHAPTER SUMMARY

- Fluoroscopy allows imaging of the movement of internal structures by its use of a continuous beam of x-rays.
- Image intensification provides a brighter image for viewing. The exit radiation is absorbed by the input phosphor, converted to electrons, sent to the output phosphor, released as visible light, and converted to an electronic video signal for transmission to the television monitor.
- Brightness gain is the product of flux gain and minification gain and results in a brighter image on the output phosphor.
- Automatic brightness control (ABC) maintains the overall appearance of the image by monitoring the current through the image intensifier or the output phosphor intensity and adjusting exposure factors if the monitored values fall below preset levels.

- Image intensifiers provide a multifield mode that magnifies the image. When operating the unit in the magnification mode, spatial resolution improves but patient exposure increases.
- To view the fluoroscopic image on a television monitor, it must be converted to an electrical signal by a camera tube or charge-coupled device (CCD).
- Cassette spot film, photo-spot cameras, cine film, and videotape/DVD are all methods of recording static or dynamic images during image-intensified fluoroscopy.
- Cassette spot filming shifts to the radiographic mode using a higher mA and increases patient exposure.
- A C-arm unit is designed with an x-ray tube and image intensifier attached in a C configuration. As a result, the unit can be positioned in a variety of planes, enabling viewing from different perspectives.
- Digital fluoroscopy can be accomplished by attaching an analog-to-digital converter (ADC) between the camera tube or CCD and the television monitor.
- The use of flat-panel detectors in place of an image intensifier offers several advantages, such as reductions in the size, bulk, and weight of the fluoroscopic tower, allowing easier manipulation of the tower and greater access to the patient during the examination.
- Flat-panel detectors also replace spot filming and other recording devices, and, because they are capable of operating in radiographic mode, in many cases, additional radiographic images are not needed. The images, both dynamic and static, can also be readily archived with the patient record in a PACS.
- Image-intensified fluoroscopy uses a lower mA (0.5–5 mA), whereas digital fluoroscopy uses a higher mA (100–1200 mA). Digital fluoroscopy uses a pulsed x-ray beam, whereas older image intensifiers operate as a continuous x-ray beam exposure unless the operator produces intermittent x-ray exposures.
- Radiation safety practices include reducing the amount of fluoroscopic time and shielding the operator with the Bucky slot cover and a protective curtain placed between the patient and the operator. The source-to-skin distance (SSD) should be not less than 38 cm (15 in) for stationary fluoroscopic units and not less than 30 cm (12 in) on a mobile fluoroscopic unit, and the intensity of the x-ray exposure at the tabletop should not exceed 10 R/min.
- Quality control procedures are important for monitoring the performance of the fluoroscopic unit.

REVIEW QUESTIONS

1. In image-intensified fluoroscopy, the milliamperage range is typically _____.
   - **A.** 0.5 to 5 mA
   - **B.** 20 to 50 mA
   - **C.** 100 to 300 mA
   - **D.** 400 to 600 mA
2. During fluoroscopy, releasing the pressure applied to the pedal or switch terminates the radiation exposure and is known as the _____.
   - **A.** fluoroscopic timer
   - **B.** intensification switch
   - **C.** activation switch
   - **D.** deadman switch
3. What component of the image intensifier converts the exit or remnant radiation into visible light?
   - **A.** Output phosphor
   - **B.** Photocathode

    C. Input phosphor

    D. Electrostatic focusing lenses

4. What component of the image intensifier converts the visible light into electrons?

    A. Output phosphor

    B. Photocathode

    C. Input phosphor

    D. Electrostatic focusing lenses

5. In image intensified fluoroscopy, in order to view the images on a television monitor, the light intensities are converted by a _____.

    A. camera tube

    B. electrostatic lens

    C. charge-coupled device

    D. A or C

6. Brightness gain is a product of _____.

    A. minification gain and automatic brightness control

    B. flux gain and automatic brightness control

    C. minification gain and flux gain

    D. automatic brightness control and milliamperage

7. The numeric conversion factor value is equal to _____ of the brightness gain value.

    A. 0.001

    B. 0.01

    C. 0.1

    D. 1.0

8. A brightness gain of 40,000 would have a conversion factor of _____.

    A. 40

    B. 400

    C. 4000

    D. 40,000

9. A disadvantage of using the magnification mode during fluoroscopy is _____.

    A. decreased spatial resolution

    B. increased patient exposure

    C. decreased brightness

    D. decreased contrast

10. When spot filming during image-intensified fluoroscopy, the radiation dose to the patient is decreased.

    A. True

    B. False

11. In digital fluoroscopy, the x-ray beam is operated in a continuous mode similar to conventional fluoroscopy.

    A. True

    B. False

12. When operating a stationary fluoroscopic unit, the source-to-skin distance (SSD) should not be less than _____.

    A. 25 cm (10 in)

    B. 30 cm (12 in)

    C. 38 cm (15 in)

    D. 45 cm (18 in)

13. For fluoroscopic units with automatic brightness control (ABC), the x-ray exposure at the tabletop should not exceed _____.
    A. 0.01 R/min
    B. 0.1 R/min
    C. 1.0 R/min
    D. 10 R/min

14. The Bucky slot cover must have a lead equivalent thickness of _____.
    A. 0.10 mm
    B. 0.25 mm
    C. 0.50 mm
    D. 2.5 mm

15. Which of the following combinations will reduce patient radiation exposure during fluoroscopy?
    A. Highest pulse mode and highest dose rate
    B. Highest pulse mode and lowest pulse rate
    C. Lowest pulse mode and highest dose rate
    D. Lowest pulse mode and lowest dose rate

Summary of Important Relationships

CHAPTER 1: RADIATION AND ITS DISCOVERY

The Dual Nature of X-ray Energy

X-rays act like both waves and particles. (See p. 6)

Wavelength and Frequency

Wavelength and frequency are inversely related. Higher-energy x-rays have decreased wavelength and increased frequency. Lower-energy x-rays have increased wavelength and decreased frequency. (See p. 6)

CHAPTER 2: THE X-RAY BEAM

Filament

The filament is the source of electrons during x-ray production. (See p. 16)

Target

The target is the part of the anode that is struck by the focused stream of electrons coming from the cathode. The target stops the electrons and creates the opportunity for the production of x-rays. (See p. 17)

Tungsten

Because tungsten has a high atomic number (74) and a high melting point (3400° C [6152° F]), it efficiently produces x-rays. (See p. 18)

Dissipating Heat

The heat produced when the x-ray exposure is activated is transferred to the insulating oil that surrounds the x-ray tube. (See p. 18)

Rotating Anodes

Rotating anodes can withstand higher heat loads than stationary anodes because the rotation causes a greater physical area, or focal track, to be exposed to electrons. (See p. 19)

Production of X-rays

As electrons strike the target, their kinetic energy is transferred to the tungsten atoms in the anode to produce x-rays. (See p. 20)

Interactions that Produce X-ray Photons

Bremsstrahlung interactions and characteristic interactions both produce x-ray photons. (See p. 20)

Bremsstrahlung Interactions

Most x-ray interactions in the diagnostic energy range are bremsstrahlung. (See p. 21)

Characteristic Interactions

Characteristic x-rays can be produced in a tungsten target only when the kVp is set at 70 or greater because the binding energy of the K-shell electron is 69.5 keV. (See p. 22)

Thermionic Emission

When the tungsten filament gains enough heat (therm), the outer-shell electrons (ions) of the filament atoms are boiled off, or emitted, from the filament. (See p. 23)

Tube Current

Electrons flow only in one direction in the x-ray tube—from cathode to anode. This flow of electrons is called the *tube current* and is measured in milliamperes (mA). (See p. 24)

Energy Conversion in the X-ray Tube

As electrons strike the anode target, greater than 99% of their kinetic energy is converted to heat, whereas less than 1% of their energy is converted to x-rays. (See p. 25)

Kilovoltage and the Speed of Electrons

The speed of the electrons traveling from the cathode to the anode increases as the kilovoltage applied across the x-ray tube increases. (See p. 26)

Speed of Electrons and Quality of X-rays

The speed of the electrons in the tube current determines the quality or energy of the x-rays that are produced. The quality or energy of the x-rays in turn determines the penetrability of the primary beam. (See p. 27)

kVp and Beam Penetrability

As kVp increases, beam penetrability increases; as kVp decreases, beam penetrability decreases. (See p. 27)

Milliamperage, Tube Current, and X-ray Quantity

The quantity of electrons in the tube current and quantity of x-rays produced are directly proportional to the milliamperage. (See p. 30)

Exposure Time, Tube Current, and X-ray Quantity

The quantity of electrons flowing from the cathode to the anode and the quantity of x-rays produced are directly proportional to the exposure time. (See p. 30)

Quantity of Electrons, X-rays, and mAs

The quantity of electrons flowing from the cathode to the anode and the quantity of x-rays produced are directly proportional to mAs. (See p. 31)

Line-Focus Principle

The line-focus principle describes the relationship between the actual focal spot, where the electrons in the tube current bombard the target, and the effective focal spot, which is the same area as seen from directly below the tube. (See p. 32)

Anode Angle and Effective Focal Spot Size

Based on the line-focus principle, the smaller the anode target angle, the smaller the effective focal spot size. (See p. 33)

Anode Heel Effect

X-rays are more intense on the cathode side of the tube; their intensity decreases toward the anode side. (See p. 33)

Low-Energy Photons, Patient Dose, and Image Formation

Low-energy photons serve only to increase patient dose and do not contribute to image formation. (See p. 34)

CHAPTER 3: IMAGE FORMATION AND RADIOGRAPHIC QUALITY

Differential Absorption and Image Formation

A radiographic image is created when an x-ray beam passes through a patient and then interacts with an image receptor, such as a digital-imaging system. The variations in the absorption and transmission of the exiting x-ray beam structurally represent the anatomic area of interest. (See p. 43)

X-ray Photon Absorption

During attenuation of the x-ray beam, the photoelectric effect is responsible for total absorption of the incoming x-ray photon. (See p. 44)

X-ray Beam Scattering

During attenuation of the x-ray beam, the incoming x-ray photon may lose energy and change direction as a result of the Compton effect. (See p. 45)

Factors Affecting Beam Attenuation

Increasing tissue thickness, atomic number, and tissue density increases x-ray beam attenuation because more x-rays are absorbed by the tissue. Increasing the quality of the x-ray beam decreases beam attenuation because the higher-energy x-rays penetrate the tissue. (See p. 49)

X-ray Interaction with Matter

When the diagnostic primary x-ray beam interacts with anatomic tissues, three processes occur: absorption, scattering, and transmission. (See p. 50)

Image Brightness

The range of image brightness levels visible after processing is a result of the variation in x-ray absorption and transmission as the x-ray beam passes through anatomic tissues. (See p. 52)

Creating the Latent Image

The process of differential absorption for image formation is the same for digital and film-screen imaging. The varying x-ray intensities exiting the anatomic area of interest form the latent image. (See p. 52)

Brightness and Radiographic Quality

A radiographic image must have sufficient brightness to visualize the anatomic structures of interest. (See p. 53)

Differentiating Among Anatomic Tissues

The ability to distinguish among types of tissues is determined by the differences in brightness levels in the image or contrast. Anatomic tissues that attenuate the beam similarly have low subject contrast. Anatomic tissues that attenuate the beam very differently have high subject contrast. (See p. 54)

Sharpness of Anatomic Detail

The accuracy of the anatomic structural lines recorded in the radiographic image is determined by its spatial resolution. (See p. 57)

Size Distortion

Radiographic images of objects are always magnified in terms of the true object size. The SID and OID play important roles in minimizing the amount of size distortion or magnification created. (See p. 59)

Shape Distortion

Shape distortion can occur from inaccurate central ray (CR) alignment of the tube, the part being radiographed, or the image receptor. Elongation refers to images of objects that appear longer than the true objects. Foreshortening refers to images that appear shorter than the true objects. (See p. 60)

Number of Photons and Quantum Noise

Decreasing the number of photons reaching the image receptor may increase the amount of quantum noise within the radiographic image; increasing the number of photons reaching the image receptor may decrease the amount of quantum noise within the radiographic image. (See p. 61)

Dynamic Range and Film-Screen Imaging

The range of exposure intensities that film can accurately detect is limited (limited dynamic range). This renders film more susceptible to overexposure and underexposure and restricts its ability to display tissues that vary greatly in x-ray attenuation. (See p. 63)

CHAPTER 4: DIGITAL IMAGING

Pixel Size, FOV, and Matrix Size

The pixel size is directly related to FOV and inversely related to matrix size. Increasing the FOV for the same matrix size will increase the size of the pixel and decrease spatial resolution, whereas increasing the matrix size for the same FOV will decrease the pixel size and increase spatial resolution. (See p. 70)

Pixel Bit Depth and Contrast Resolution

The greater the pixel bit depth (i.e., 16 bit), the more precise the digitization of the analog signal, and the greater the number of shades of gray available for image display. Increasing the number of shades of gray available to display on a digital image improves its contrast resolution. (See p. 71)

Pixel Density and Pitch and Spatial Resolution

Increasing the pixel density and decreasing the pixel pitch increases spatial resolution. Decreasing pixel density and increasing pixel pitch decreases spatial resolution. (See p. 72)

Spatial Frequency and Spatial Resolution

The unit of measure for spatial frequency is line pairs per millimeter (lp/mm). Increasing the number of line pairs per millimeter resolved in the imaging system (higher spatial frequency) results in improved spatial resolution. (See p. 74)

Modulation Transfer Function (MTF) and Anatomic Detail

MTF is a measure of the imaging system's ability to accurately display small anatomic objects having high spatial frequency. An imaging system that has a high MTF can display anatomic detail with improved visibility. (See p. 75)

Computed Radiography Digital Image Receptors

The CR latent image is acquired in the PSP layer of the IP. Most energy from the exit radiation intensities is stored in the PSP for extraction in the reader unit. (See p. 76)

Sampling Frequency and Spatial Resolution

Increasing the sampling frequency results in a smaller sampling and pixel pitch, which improves the spatial resolution of the digital image. Decreasing the sampling frequency results in a larger sampling and pixel pitch and decreased spatial resolution. (See p. 79)

Imaging Plate Size and Matrix Size

For a fixed matrix size CR system, using a smaller IP for a given field of view (FOV) results in improved spatial resolution of the digital image. Increasing the size of the IP for a given FOV results in decreased spatial resolution. (See p. 79)

Digital Detectors and Dynamic Range

Digital IRs have a wide dynamic range; that is, they can accurately capture a wide range of x-ray intensities exiting the patient. The computer then processes the raw pixel data to compensate for exposure errors and create a radiographic image. However, lower- or higher-than-necessary exposure techniques do not guarantee a quality digital image with reasonable radiation exposure to the patient. (See p. 84)

Detective Quantum Efficiency (DQE) and X-ray Exposure

An image receptor with a higher DQE requires less x-ray exposure to produce a quality radiographic image when compared to an image receptor with a lower DQE value. (See p. 85)

Signal-to-Noise Ratio and Image Quality

Increasing the SNR increases the visibility of anatomic details, whereas decreasing the SNR decreases the visibility. (See p. 86)

Contrast-to-Noise Ratio and Image Quality

Increasing the CNR increases the visibility of anatomic details, whereas decreasing the CNR decreases the visibility. (See p. 86)

Histogram Analysis

With digital systems, the computer creates a histogram of the data set. The histogram is a graph of the exposure received to the pixel elements and the prevalence of the exposures within the image. This created histogram is compared with a stored histogram model for that anatomic part; VOIs are identified, and the image is displayed. (See p. 88)

Exposure Indicators

The radiographer should strive to select techniques that result in exposure indicator values falling within the indicated optimum range for the corresponding digital imaging system. However, the radiographer also needs to recognize the limitations of exposure indicators for providing accurate information. (See p. 90)

Lookup Tables

Lookup tables provide the means to alter the original pixel values to improve the brightness and contrast of the image. (See p. 92)

Window Level and Image Brightness

A direct relationship exists between window level and image brightness on the display monitor. Increasing the window level increases the image brightness; decreasing the window level decreases the image brightness. (See p. 99)

Window Width and Image Contrast

A narrow (decreased) window width displays higher radiographic contrast, whereas a wider (increased) window width displays lower radiographic contrast. (See p. 100)

CHAPTER 5: FILM-SCREEN IMAGING

Dynamic Range and Film-Screen Imaging

The range of exposure intensities that film can accurately detect is limited (limited dynamic range). This renders film more susceptible to overexposure and underexposure and restricts its ability to display tissues that vary greatly in x-ray attenuation. (See p. 112)

Sensitivity Specks and Latent Image Centers

Sensitivity specks serve as the focal points for the development of latent image centers. After exposure, these specks trap the free electrons and then attract and neutralize the positive silver ions. After enough silver is neutralized, the specks become a latent image center and are converted into metallic silver after chemical processing. (See p. 114)

Silver Halide and Film Sensitivity

As the number and/or size of silver halide crystals increase, film sensitivity or speed increases. A faster film speed requires less radiation exposure to produce a specific density. (See p. 114)

Screen Speed and Recorded Detail

As screen speed increases, recorded detail decreases; as screen speed decreases, recorded detail increases. (See p. 116)

Screen Speed, Light Emission, and Patient Dose

The faster an intensifying screen, the more light is emitted for the same intensity of x-ray exposure. As screen speed increases, less radiation is necessary, and radiation dose to the patient is decreased; as screen speed decreases, more radiation is necessary, and the radiation dose to the patient is increased. (See p. 117)

Film-Screen System Speed and mAs

Increasing the film-screen speed requires a decrease in the mAs to maintain density. Decreasing the film-screen speed requires an increase in the mAs to maintain density. (See p. 118)

Developing or Reducing Agents

The developing agents are responsible for reducing the exposed silver halide crystals to metallic silver, visualized as radiographic densities. Phenidone is responsible for creating the lower densities, and hydroquinone is responsible for creating the higher densities. Their combined effect results in a range of visible densities on the radiograph. (See p. 120)

Clearing the Unexposed Crystals

The fixing agent, ammonium thiosulfate, is responsible for removing the unexposed crystals from the emulsion. (See p. 121)

Archival Quality of Radiographs

Maintaining the archival (long-term) quality of radiographs requires most of the fixing agent to be removed (washed) from the film. Staining or fading of the permanent image results when too much thiosulfate remains on the film. (See p. 121)

Archival Quality of Radiographs

Permanent radiographs must retain a moisture content of 10%–15% to maintain archival quality. Excessive drying can cause the emulsion layers to crack. (See p. 122)

Replenishment and Solution Performance

The replenishment system provides fresh chemicals for the developing and fixing solutions to maintain their chemical activity and volume when they become depleted during processing. (See p. 123)

Developer Temperature and Radiographic Quality

Variations in developer temperature can adversely affect the quality of the radiographic image. Increasing developer temperature increases the density, and decreasing it decreases the density. Further, radiographic contrast may be adversely affected by changes in the developer temperature. (See p. 124)

Silver Recovery

Silver is a natural resource, is a heavy metal that can be toxic to the environment, and it must be removed from the used fixer. (See p. 128)

CHAPTER 6: EXPOSURE TECHNIQUE FACTORS

mAs and Quantity of Radiation

As mAs increases, the quantity of radiation reaching the IR increases. As mAs decreases, the amount of radiation reaching the IR decreases. (See p. 149)

Milliamperage and Exposure Time

Milliamperage and exposure time have an inversely proportional relationship when maintaining the same mAs. (See p. 150)

mAs and Digital Image Brightness

The level of mAs does not directly affect image brightness when using digital IRs. During computer processing, image brightness is maintained when the mAs is too low or too high. A lower-than-needed mAs produces an image with increased quantum noise, and a higher-than-needed mAs exposes a patient to unnecessary radiation. (See p. 150)

Exposure Indicator Value

A numerical value or exposure indicator is displayed on the processed digital image to indicate the level of x-ray exposure received (incident exposure) on the IR. If the exposure indicator value falls outside the manufacturer's suggested range, image quality, patient exposure, or both could be compromised. (See p. 151)

mAs and Film-Screen Density

The amount of mAs has a direct effect on the amount of radiographic density produced when using a film-screen IR. The minimum change needed to correct a density error is determined by multiplying or dividing the mAs by 2. (See p. 152)

kVp and the Radiographic Image

Increasing or decreasing the kVp changes the amount of radiation exposure to the IR and the contrast produced within the image. (See p. 152)

Exposure Errors in Digital Imaging

kVp and mAs exposure errors should be reflected in the exposure indicator value; however, image brightness can be maintained during computer processing. (See p. 153)

Exposure Errors and Film-Screen Imaging

kVp directly affects the density produced on a film-screen image; however, its effect is not equal throughout the range of kVp (low, middle, and high). (See p. 153)

kVp and the 15% Rule

A 15% increase in kVp has the same effect on exposure to the IR as doubling the mAs. A 15% decrease in kVp has the same effect on exposure to the IR as halving the mAs. (See p. 154)

kVp and Radiographic Contrast

A high kVp results in less absorption and more transmission in the anatomic tissues, which results in less variation in the x-ray intensities exiting the patient (lower subject contrast), producing a low-contrast image. A low kVp results in more absorption and less x-ray transmission but with more variation in the x-ray intensities exiting the patient (higher subject contrast), producing a high-contrast image. (See p. 155)

Kilovoltage and Digital Image Quality

Assuming that the body part has been adequately penetrated, changing the kVp affects the radiation exposure to the digital IR in a way similar to changing mAs; but unlike mAs, kVp also affects image contrast. However, image brightness and contrast are primarily controlled during computer processing. (See p. 157)

Kilovoltage, Scatter Radiation, and Radiographic Contrast

At higher kVp, more x-rays are transmitted with fewer overall interactions; however, a greater proportion of the interactions are from Compton scattering than x-ray absorption (photoelectric effect), which decreases the radiographic contrast. Decreasing the kVp will increase x-ray absorption and increase the number of interactions, but the proportion of Compton scattering will decrease compared to photoelectric interactions, increasing radiographic contrast. (See p. 157)

Focal Spot Size and Spatial Resolution

As focal spot size increases, unsharpness increases and spatial resolution decreases; as focal spot size decreases, unsharpness decreases and spatial resolution increases. (See p. 158)

SID and X-ray Beam Intensity

As SID increases, the x-ray beam intensity becomes spread over a larger area. This decreases the overall intensity of the x-ray beam reaching the IR. (See p. 159)

SID and mAs

Increasing the SID requires the mAs to be increased to maintain exposure to the IR, and decreasing the SID requires a decrease in the mAs to maintain exposure to the IR. (See p. 160)

SID, Size Distortion, and Spatial Resolution

As SID increases, size distortion (magnification) decreases and spatial resolution increases; as SID decreases, size distortion (magnification) increases and spatial resolution decreases. (See p. 161)

OID, Size Distortion, and Spatial Resolution

Increasing the OID increases magnification and decreases the spatial resolution, whereas decreasing the OID decreases magnification and increases the spatial resolution. (See p. 163)

Grids, Scatter, and Contrast

Placing a grid between the anatomic area of interest and the IR absorbs scatter radiation exiting the patient and increases radiographic contrast. (See p. 167)

Grids and Image Receptor Exposure

Adding, removing, or changing a grid requires an adjustment in mAs to maintain radiation exposure to the IR. (See p. 167)

Beam Restriction and Image Receptor Exposure

Changes in beam restriction alter the amount of tissue irradiated and therefore affect the amount of exposure to the IR. The effect of collimation is greater when imaging large anatomic areas, performing examinations without a grid, and using a high kVp. (See p. 169)

Tube Filtration, Radiation Quantity and Energy

Increasing tube filtration will decrease radiation quantity and increase the average energy of the x-ray beam. Decreasing tube filtration will increase radiation quantity and decrease the average energy of the x-ray beam. (See p. 170)

CHAPTER 7: SCATTER CONTROL

kVp and Scatter

The amount and energy of scatter radiation exiting the patient depends, in part, on the kVp selected. Examinations using higher kVp produce a greater proportion of higher-energy scattered x-rays compared with examinations using low kVp. (See p. 179)

X-ray-Beam Field Size, Thickness of the Part, and Scatter

The larger the x-ray-beam field size, the greater the amount of scatter radiation produced. The thicker the part being imaged, the greater the amount of scatter radiation produced. (See p. 180)

Volume of Tissue Irradiated and Scatter

The volume of tissue irradiated is affected by both the part thickness and the x-ray-beam field size. Therefore, the greater the volume of tissue irradiated, because of either or both factors, the greater the amount of scatter radiation produced. (See p. 180)

Beam Restriction and Patient Dose

As beam restriction or collimation increases, the field size decreases, and patient dose decreases. As beam restriction or collimation decreases, the field size and patient dose increases. (See p. 180)

Collimation and Scatter Radiation

As collimation increases, the field size and quantity of scatter radiation decreases; as collimation decreases, the field size and quantity of scatter radiation increases. (See p. 181)

Collimation and Radiographic Contrast

As collimation increases, the quantity of scatter radiation decreases, and radiographic contrast increases; as collimation decreases, the quantity of scatter radiation increases and radiographic contrast decreases. (See p. 181)

Collimation and Exposure to the Image Receptor

As collimation increases, exposure to the IR decreases; as collimation decreases, exposure to the IR increases. (See p. 182)

Scatter Radiation and Image Quality

Scatter radiation adds unwanted exposure to the IR and decreases image quality. (See p. 188)

Grid Ratio and Radiographic Contrast

As the grid ratio increases for the same grid frequency, scatter cleanup improves and radiographic contrast increases; as grid ratio decreases for the same grid frequency, scatter cleanup becomes less effective and radiographic contrast decreases. (See p. 189)

Focused versus Parallel Grids

Focused grids have lead lines that are angled to approximately match the divergence of the primary beam. Thus, focused grids allow more transmitted photons to reach the IR than parallel grids. (See p. 192)

Grid Ratio and Exposure to Image Receptor

As the grid ratio increases, exposure to the IR decreases; as the grid ratio decreases, exposure to the IR increases. (See p. 194)

Grid Ratio and Patient Dose

As the grid ratio increases, patient dose increases; as the grid ratio decreases, patient dose decreases. (See p. 196)

Upside-Down Focused Grids and Grid Cutoff

Placing a focused grid upside-down on the IR causes the lateral edges of the IR to be highly underexposed. (See p. 197)

Off-Level Error and Grid Cutoff

Angling the x-ray tube across the grid lines or angling the grid itself during exposure produces an overall decrease in exposure to the image receptor. (See p. 197)

Off-Center Error and Grid Cutoff

If the center of the x-ray beam is not aligned from side to side with the center of a focused grid, grid cutoff occurs. (See p. 198)

Off-Focus Error and Grid Cutoff

Using an SID outside the focal range creates a loss of exposure at the periphery of the radiograph. (See p. 198)

Air Gap Technique and Scatter Control

The air gap technique is an alternative to using a grid to control the scatter reaching the IR. By moving the IR away from the patient, more scatter radiation will miss the IR. The greater the gap, the lesser the scatter reaches the IR. (See p. 203)

CHAPTER 8: EXPOSURE TECHNIQUE SELECTION

Principle of Automatic Exposure Control Operation

Once a predetermined amount of radiation is transmitted through a patient, the x-ray exposure is terminated. This determines the exposure time and therefore the total amount of radiation exposure to the IR. (See p. 209)

Radiation-Measuring Devices

Detectors are the AEC devices that measure the amount of radiation transmitted. The radiographer selects the combination of the three detectors to use. (See p. 210)

Function of the Ionization Chamber

The ionization chamber interacts with exit radiation before it reaches the IR. Air in the chamber is ionized, and an electrical charge proportional to the amount of radiation is created. (See p. 212)

Automatic Exposure Control and mAs Readout

If the radiographic unit has an mAs readout display, the radiographer should take note of the reading after an exposure is made. This information can be invaluable. (See p. 212)

kVp and Automatic Exposure Control Response

The radiographer must set the kVp as needed to ensure adequate penetration while producing the appropriate level of contrast. The kVp selected determines the length of exposure time when using AEC. A low kVp requires more exposure time to reach the predetermined amount of exposure. A high kVp decreases the exposure time to reach the predetermined amount of exposure and reduces the overall radiation exposure to the patient. (See p. 212)

mA and Automatic Exposure Control Response

If the radiographer can set the mA when using AEC, it will affect the time of exposure for a given procedure. Increasing the mA decreases the exposure time to reach the predetermined amount of exposure. Decreasing the mA increases the exposure time to reach the predetermined amount of exposure. (See p. 213)

Function of Backup Time

Backup time, the maximum exposure time allowed during an AEC examination, serves as a safety mechanism when AEC is not used properly or is not functioning properly. (See p. 214)

Setting Backup Time

Backup time should be set to 150%–200% of the expected exposure time. This allows the properly used AEC system to appropriately terminate the exposure but protects the patient and tube from excessive exposure if a problem occurs. (See p. 214)

Detector Selection

The combination of detectors affects the amount of exposure reaching the IR. If the area of radiographic interest is not directly over the selected detectors, that area will likely be overexposed or underexposed.

When performing a radiographic study where the IR is located outside the Bucky, the AEC system should be deactivated and a manual technique should be used. (See p. 215)

Patient Centering

Accurate centering of the area of interest over the detectors is critical to ensure proper exposure to the IR. If the area of interest is not properly centered to the detectors, overexposure or underexposure may occur. (See p. 216)

Collimation and Automatic Exposure Control Response

Excessive or insufficient collimation may affect the amount of exposure reaching the IR. Insufficient collimation may result in excessive scatter reaching the detectors, causing the exposure time to terminate too quickly. Excessive collimation may result in an extremely long exposure time. (See p. 219)

Type of Image Receptor and Automatic Exposure Control Response

The AEC system is calibrated based on the type of IR used. If an IR of a different type is used, the detectors will not sense the difference and the exposure time will terminate at the preset value, which may jeopardize image quality. (See p. 219)

Digital Image Receptors and the Automatic Exposure Control Response

Because the visual cues of increased or decreased radiographic density when using film-screen IRs are lacking in digital imaging, the radiographer must be very conscientious about excessive radiation exposure to the patient. (See p. 220)

Exposure Technique Charts and Radiographic Quality

Exposure technique charts are just as important for digital imaging because digital systems have a wide dynamic range and can compensate for exposure technique errors. Technique charts should be developed and used with all types of radiographic imaging systems to maintain patient radiation exposure as low as reasonably achievable (ALARA). (See p. 224)

Variable kVp/Fixed mAs Technique Chart

The variable kVp chart adjusts the kVp for changes in part thickness while maintaining a fixed mAs. (See p. 226)

Fixed kVp/Variable mAs Technique Charts

Fixed kVp/variable mAs technique charts identify optimal kVp values and alter the mAs for variations in part thickness. (See p. 227)

CHAPTER 10: DYNAMIC IMAGING: FLUOROSCOPY

Image-Intensified Fluoroscopy

Dynamic imaging of internal anatomic structures can be accomplished with the use of an image intensifier. The exit radiation is absorbed by the input phosphor, converted to electrons, sent to the output phosphor, released as visible light, and converted to an electronic video signal for transmission to the television monitor. (See p. 263)

Brightness Gain

A brighter image is created on the output phosphor when accelerated electrons strike a smaller output phosphor. (See p. 265)

Magnification Mode and Patient Dose

Operating the image intensifier in one of the magnification modes increases the operator's ability to see small structures but at the price of increasing the radiation dose to the patient. (See p. 266)

Coupling Systems and the Television Monitor

The camera tube and CCD are devices that couple the image intensifier to the television monitor to convert the image from the output phosphor to an electronic (video) signal that can be reconstructed on the television monitor. (See p. 271)

Cassette Spot Filming

Cassette spot-film devices are a means of recording static images during an image-intensified fluoroscopic examination. The unit shifts to radiographic mode (using a higher mA), and the radiation dose to the patient is much higher than in the fluoroscopic mode. (See p. 274)

Digital Fluoroscopic Systems

The use of flat-panel detectors in place of an image intensifier offers several advantages, such as a reduction in the size, bulk, and weight of the fluoroscopic tower, allowing for easier manipulation of the tower and greater access to the patient during the examination. The flat-panel detectors also replace the spot filming and other recording devices, and, because they are capable of operating in radiographic mode, in many cases, additional radiographic images are not needed. The images, both dynamic and static, can also be readily archived with the patient record in a PACS. (See p. 278)

Continuous Fluoroscopy

Operating the fluoroscope in a continuous mode will produce 30 frames of images each second, increases patient dose, and may increase the visibility of patient motion. (See p. 278)

Pulsed Fluoroscopy

Operating the fluoroscope in a pulsed mode will reduce the number of images each second, decrease patient dose, and reduce the visibility of patient motion. (See p. 279)

Summary of Mathematical Applications

CHAPTER 2: THE X-RAY BEAM

Calculating mAs

$$mAs = mA \times seconds$$

Examples:

$$200 \, mA \times 0.25 \, s = 50 \, mAs$$

$$500 \, mA \times 2/5 \, s = 200 \, mAs$$

$$800 \, mA \times 100 \, ms \text{ (milliseconds or 0.1 s)} = 80 \, mAs$$

(See p. 31)

Calculating Heat Units

An exposure is made with a three-phase x-ray unit at 600 mA and 75 kVp over 0.05 s. How many heat units are produced from this exposure?

$$HU = mA \times time \times kVp \times generator \, factor$$

$$HU = 600 \times 0.05 \times 75 \times 1.35$$

$$= 3037.5 \, HU$$

(See p. 37)

CHAPTER 4: DIGITAL IMAGING

Pixel Size and FOV

FOV = 17 in (431.8 mm) and matrix size = 1024

$$\frac{431.8}{1024} = 0.42 \, mm \, pixel \, size$$

If the FOV was decreased to 12 in (304.8 mm) for the same matrix size of 1024

$$\frac{304.8}{1024} = 0.30 \, mm \, pixel \, size$$

Decreasing the FOV for a given matrix size will decrease the size of the pixels and increase spatial resolution.
(See p. 70)

Pixel Size and Matrix Size

FOV = 17 in (431.8 mm) and matrix size = 1024:

$$\frac{431.8}{1024} = 0.42 \, mm \, pixel \, size$$

If the matrix size was increased to 2048 for the same FOV:

$$\frac{431.8}{2048} = 0.21 \, mm \, pixel \, size$$

Increasing the matrix size for a given FOV will decrease the size of the pixels and increase spatial resolution.
(See p. 70)

CHAPTER 5: FILM-SCREEN IMAGING

Adjusting mAs for Changes in Film-Screen System Speed

A quality radiograph is obtained using 10 mAs at 65 kVp and 100-speed film-screen system. What new mAs is used to maintain radiographic density when changing to a 400-speed film-screen system?

$$\frac{10 \text{ mAs}}{X} = \frac{400 \text{ speed}}{100 \text{ speed}}$$

$$10 \text{ mAs} \times 100; \; 1000 = 400 \text{ X}; \; \frac{1000}{400} = 2.5 \text{ mAs} = X$$

(See p. 118)

CHAPTER 6: EXPOSURE TECHNIQUE FACTORS

Adjusting Milliamperage or Exposure Time

$$200 \text{ mA} \times 0.1 \text{ s} = 20 \text{ mAs}$$

To increase the mAs to 40, one could use the following formulas:

$$400 \text{ mA} \times 0.1 \text{ s} = 40 \text{ mAs}$$

$$200 \text{ mA} \times 0.2 \text{ s} = 40 \text{ mAs}$$

(See p. 149)

Adjusting Milliamperage and Exposure Time to Maintain mAs

$$200 \text{ mA} \times 100 \text{ ms} \; (0.1 \text{ s}) = 20 \text{ mAs}$$

To maintain the mAs, use the following formulas:

$$400 \text{ mA} \times 50 \text{ ms} \; (0.05 \text{ s}) = 20 \text{ mAs}$$

$$100 \text{ mA} \times 200 \text{ ms} \; (0.2 \text{ s}) = 20 \text{ mAs}$$

(See p. 150)

Using the 15% Rule

To increase exposure to the IR, multiply the kVp by 1.15 (original kVp + 15%):

$$75 \text{ kVp} \times 1.15 = 86 \text{ kVp}.$$

To decrease exposure to the IR, multiply the kVp by 0.85 (original kVp − 15%):

$$75 \text{ kVp} \times 0.85 = 64 \text{ kVp}.$$

To maintain exposure to the IR, when increasing the kVp by 15% (kVp × 1.15), divide the original mAs by 2:

$$75 \text{ kVp} \times 1.15 = 86 \text{ kVp and mAs/2}.$$

When decreasing the kVp by 15% (kVp × 0.85), multiply the mAs by 2:

$$75 \text{ kVp} \times 0.85 = 64 \text{ and mAs} \times 2.$$

(See p. 155)

Inverse Square Law Formula

$$\frac{I_1}{I_2} = \frac{(D_2)^2}{(D_1)^2}$$

If the intensity of radiation at an SID of 40 in is equal to 400 mR, what is the intensity of radiation when the distance is increased to 72 in?

$$\frac{400 \text{ mR}}{X} = \frac{(72)^2}{(40)^2} \; 400 \text{ mR} \times 1600 = 640,000$$

$$= 5184 \text{ X};$$

$$\frac{640,000}{5184} = X; \; 123.5 \text{ mR} = X$$

(See p. 159)

mAs-Distance Compensation Formula

$$\frac{\text{mAs}_1}{\text{mAs}_2} \; \frac{(\text{SID}_1)^2}{(\text{SID}_2)^2}$$

Optimal exposure to the IR is achieved at an SID of 40 in using 25 mAs. The SID must be increased to 72 in. What adjustment of mAs is needed to maintain exposure to the IR?

$$\frac{25}{X} = \frac{(40)^2}{(72)^2}; \; 1600X = 129,600;$$

$$\frac{129,600}{1600}; \; X = 81 \text{ mAs}_2$$

(See p. 160)

Magnification Factor

An anteroposterior projection (AP) of the knee is produced with a SID of 40 in and an OID of 3 in (SOD is equal to 37 in). What is the MF?

$$SOD = SID - OID, \; MF = \frac{40}{37}; \; MF = 1.081,$$

$$37 = 40 - 3$$

(See p. 164)

Determining Object Size

On an AP image of a knee taken with an SID of 40 in and an OID of 3 in (SOD = 37 in), the size of a lesion measures 0.5 in in diameter on the radiograph. The MF has been determined to be 1.081. What is the object size of this lesion?

$$\frac{40}{37} = 1.081 \text{ MF}; \quad \text{Object size} = \frac{0.5 \text{ in}}{1.081}$$

The object size is 0.463 in.
(See p. 165)

Determining Object % of Magnification

A lesion on the radiographic image measures 1.16 cm and the lesion's (object's) true size measures 1.06 cm. What is the object % of magnification?

$$\text{Object \% of magnification} = \frac{1.16 - 1.06}{1.06 \text{ cm}} \times 100$$

$$\frac{0.10}{1.06} = 0.09434 \times 100 =$$

$$9.43 \text{ \% object magnification}$$

(See p. 165)

Adjusting mAs for Changes in the Grid

A quality radiograph is obtained using 5 mAs at 70 kVp without using a grid. What new mAs is needed when adding a 12:1 grid to maintain the same exposure to the IR?

$$\frac{5 \text{ mAs}}{X} = \frac{1}{5}; \quad 1X = 25; X = 25 \text{ mAs}$$

The new mAs produces an exposure comparable with the IR.
(See p. 168)

CHAPTER 7: SCATTER CONTROL

Calculating Grid Ratio

What is the grid ratio when the lead strips are 2.4 mm high and separated by 0.2 mm?

$$\text{Grid ratio} = h/D$$

$$\text{Grid ratio} = \frac{2.4}{0.2} = 12 \text{ or } 12:1$$

(See p. 189)

Adding a Grid

If a radiographer produced a shoulder radiograph with nongrid exposure using 3 mAs and then wanted to use a 12:1 ratio grid, what value of mAs should be used to produce the same exposure to the IR?

Nongrid exposure = 3 mAs
GCF (for 12:1 grid) = 5 (from Table 7-2)

$$\text{GCF} = \frac{\text{mAs with the grid}}{\text{mAs without the grid}}$$

$$5 = \frac{\text{mAs with the grid}}{3}$$

$$15 = \text{mAs with the grid}$$

When adding a 12:1 ratio grid, mAs must be increased by a factor of 5 (in this case to 15 mAs).
(See p. 194)

Removing a Grid

If a radiographer produced a knee radiograph using an 8:1 ratio grid and 10 mAs and on the next exposure wanted to use nongrid exposure, what mAs should be used to produce the same exposure to the IR?

Grid exposure = 10 mAs
GCF (for 8:1 grid) = 4 (from Table 7-2)

$$\text{GCF} = \frac{\text{mAs with the grid}}{\text{mAs without the grid}}$$

$$4 = \frac{10 \text{ mAs}}{\text{mAs without the grid}}$$

$$2.5 = \text{mAs without the grid}$$

When removing an 8:1 ratio grid, mAs must be decreased by a factor of 4 (in this case to 2.5 mAs).
(See p. 195)

Decreasing the Grid Ratio

If a radiographer used 40 mAs with a 12:1 ratio grid, what mAs should be used with a 6:1 ratio grid to produce the same exposure to the IR?

Exposure 1: 40 mAs, 12:1 grid, GCF = 5
Exposure 2: _____ mAs, 6:1 grid, GCF = 3

$$\frac{mAs_1}{mAs_2} = \frac{GCF_1}{GCF_2}$$

$$\frac{40}{mAs_2} = \frac{5}{3}$$

$$mAs_2 = 24$$

Decreasing the grid ratio requires less mAs.
(See p. 195)

Increasing the Grid Ratio

If a radiographer performed a routine portable pelvic examination using 40 mAs with an 8:1 ratio grid, what mAs should be used if a 12:1 ratio grid is substituted?

Exposure 1: 40 mAs, 8:1 grid, GCF = 4
Exposure 2: _____ mAs, 12:1 grid, GCF = 5

$$\frac{mAs_1}{mAs_2} = \frac{GCF_1}{GCF_2}$$

$$\frac{40}{mAs_2} = \frac{4}{5}$$

$$mAs_2 = 50$$

Increasing the grid ratio requires additional mAs.
(See p. 196)

Summary of Radiation Protection Alerts

CHAPTER 1: RADIATION AND ITS DISCOVERY

ALARA Principle

It is the radiographer's responsibility to minimize the radiation dose to the patient, to themselves, and to others in accordance with the **As Low As Reasonably Achievable** (ALARA) Principle. (See p. 9)

Cardinal Principles for Minimizing Radiation dose

Time- Limit the amount of time exposed to ionizing radiation.
Distance- Maintain a safe distance from source of ionizing radiation exposure.
Shielding- Maximize the use of shielding from ionizing radiation exposure.
(See p. 10)

Beam Restriction

Limiting the size of x-ray exposure field reduces the volume of tissue irradiated and limits the radiation dose to the patient. (See p. 11)

Primary Exposure Factors

The combination of kVp and mAs is selected based on a number of considerations, including the anatomic part being examined, patient age, condition, and pathology, and should be ideally suited to the circumstance to minimize radiation dose while producing a quality image. (See p. 11)

Avoid Duplicate Exams

The radiographer must recognize and accept his/her role as a patient advocate and do what is necessary to avoid duplication of exams. (See p. 11)

Screening for Pregnancy

Screening for pregnancy is another important task for minimizing unnecessary exposure to a developing fetus. When it is necessary to perform a radiographic exam on a pregnant patient, shielding materials and precise collimation should be used to minimize the radiation dose administered to the fetus. (See p. 12)

CHAPTER 2: THE X-RAY BEAM

Beam Filtration

Low-energy photons, created during x-ray production, are unable to penetrate the patient. Patients are protected from unnecessary exposure to this low-energy radiation by the placement of inherent and added filtration in the path of the x-ray beam. (See p. 36)

CHAPTER 4: DIGITAL IMAGING

Digital Detectors and Dynamic Range

Because digital image receptors have a wide dynamic range, a quality image can be produced when using more radiation exposure than necessary. Radiographers must take extra precautions to not unnecessarily overexpose patients. (See p. 85)

CHAPTER 6: EXPOSURE TECHNIQUE FACTORS

Excessive Radiation Exposure and Digital Imaging

Although the computer can adjust image brightness for technique exposure errors, routinely using more radiation than required for the procedure in digital radiography unnecessarily increases patient exposure. Even though the digital system can adjust for overexposure, it is an unethical practice to knowingly overexpose a patient. (See p. 153)

kVp/mAs

Whenever possible, a higher kilovoltage and lower mAs should be used to reduce patient exposure. Increasing kilovoltage requires a lower mAs to maintain the desired exposure to the IR and decreases the radiation dose to the patient. For example, changing kVp from 75 to 86 when imaging a pelvis is a 15% increase and would require half the mAs needed for the original 75 kVp. Higher kVp increases the beam penetration, and therefore, less radiation is needed to achieve a desired exposure to the IR. (See p. 155)

Grid Selection

Decisions regarding the use of a grid and grid ratio should be made by balancing image quality and patient protection. To keep patient exposure as low as possible, grids should be used only when appropriate, and the grid ratio should be the lowest that would provide sufficient contrast improvement. (See p. 168)

Beam Restriction

In performing a radiographic examination, the radiographer should be aware of the anatomic area of interest and limit the x-ray field size to just beyond this area. Collimating to the appropriate field size is a basic method for protecting patients from unnecessary exposure. (See p. 169)

CHAPTER 7: SCATTER CONTROL

Appropriate Beam Restriction

In performing a radiographic examination, the radiographer should be aware of the anatomic area of interest and limit the x-ray field size to just beyond this area. Collimating to the appropriate field size is a basic method for protecting patients from unnecessary exposure. (See p. 180)

Limit Field Size to Image Receptor Size

Whether or not automatic collimation is being used, the radiographer should always be sure that the size of the x-ray field is the same as or less than the size of

the IR except for digital flat-panel detectors. When using a digital flat-panel detector, the x-ray field size should be restricted to the anatomic area of interest. These digital IRs are typically of a similar size, and, in many instances, larger than the anatomic area of interest. Therefore, it is even more crucial for the radiographer to appropriately collimate for the imaging procedure so that the patient is not unnecessarily exposed to radiation. (See p. 187)

Grid Selection

Decisions regarding the use of a grid and grid ratio should be made by balancing image quality and patient protection. In order to keep patient exposure as low as possible, grids should be used only when appropriate and the grid ratio selected should be the lowest capable of providing sufficient contrast improvement. (See p. 196)

Grid Errors

A radiographic image with suboptimal exposure can be the result of many factors, one of which is grid cutoff. Before assuming that an underexposed image is due to technique factors and then re-exposing the patient, the radiographer should evaluate grid alignment. If misalignment is the cause of the underexposure, the patient can be protected from re-exposure with a technique factor adjustment. (See p. 199)

CHAPTER 8: EXPOSURE TECHNIQUE SELECTION

Kilovoltage Selection

Using a higher kVp with AEC decreases the exposure time and the overall mAs needed to produce a diagnostic image, significantly reducing patient exposure. The kVp selected for an examination should produce the desired image contrast for the part examined while being as high as possible to minimize the patient's radiation exposure. (See p. 213)

Monitoring Backup Time

To minimize patient exposure, the backup time should be neither too long nor too short. Backup time that is too short results in the exposure being stopped prematurely, and the image may need to be repeated because of poor image quality. Backup time that is too long results in the patient receiving unnecessary radiation if a problem occurs and the exposure does not end until the backup time is reached. In addition, the image may have to be repeated because of poor image quality. (See p. 214)

Patient Variability

Factors related to the patient affect the time of exposure reaching the IR and ultimately the image quality; such factors include pathology, contrast media, foreign objects, and pockets of gas. Increases or decreases in patient thickness result in changes in the time of exposure if the AEC system is functioning properly. (See p. 218)

Anatomically Programmed Technique and Patient Exposure

When using a preprogrammed set of exposure factors, the radiographer must evaluate the appropriateness of the selected exposure technique factors.

Adjustment of the preprogrammed exposure factors may be necessary for that patient or procedure. (See p. 220)

Exposure Technique Charts and Digital Imaging

Exposure technique charts are just as important, if not more so, when using digital IRs. Underexposure or overexposure of a film-screen IR can result in a radiograph with decreased or increased density. Because image brightness is controlled by computer processing, the visual cues for overexposure or underexposure are missing. Exposure technique charts are an effective tool in selecting appropriate exposure techniques for a quality digital image. (See p. 223)

Answer Key for Chapter 9: Image Evaluation

ACTIVITY 1

Image Quality
Digital

An optimal digital image of the hip was produced using the following exposure technique:

200 mA	12:1 grid ratio
50 ms	CR image receptor
70 kVp	8×12 in collimation
40-inch SID	Patient thickness 10 cm
0.6 mm small focal spot	Minimal OID

Without compensation, the proposed changes are made one by one. On the following chart, indicate the effect, if any, that each change has on the exposure to IR, contrast, and spatial resolution of the radiographic image.

1. If the exposure to the IR, contrast, or spatial resolution of the image is increased, mark a + in the space provided.
2. If the exposure to the IR, contrast, or spatial resolution of the image is decreased, mark a − in the space provided.
3. If the exposure to the IR, contrast, or spatial resolution of the image is unchanged, mark a 0 in the space provided.

Proposed Individual Change	Exposure to IR	Contrast	Spatial Resolution
85 kVp	+	-	0
1.25 mm focal spot size	0	0	-
45″ SID	-	0	+
50 mA @ 0.20 s	0	0	0
Patient thickness 6 cm	+	+	+
Remove grid	+	-	0
Increase OID 4″	-	+	-
14 × 17 collimation	+	-	0

❓ ACTIVITY 2

Image Quality

Film

An optimal film radiograph of the pelvis was produced using the following exposure technique:

100 mA	12:1 grid ratio
0.5 s	400 speed F/S
70 kVp	14×17 in collimation
40-inch SID	Patient thickness 14 cm
1.25-mm large focal spot	Minimal OID
92° F development temperature	
90-s processing time	

Without compensation, the proposed changes are made one by one. On the following chart, indicate the effect, if any, that each change has on the density, contrast, and recorded detail of the radiographic image.

1. If the radiographic density, contrast, or recorded detail of the image is increased, mark a + in the space provided.
2. If the radiographic density, contrast, or recorded detail of the image is decreased, mark a – in the space provided.
3. If the radiographic density, contrast, or recorded detail of the image is unchanged, mark a 0 in the space provided.

Proposed Change	Density	Contrast	Recorded Detail
Increase SID to 48″	-	0	+
Use 200 mAs	+	-*	0
Increase kVp to 80	+	-	0
Film-screen speed 200	-	0	+
Increase patient thickness to 18 cm	-	-	-
10 × 12 in collimation	-	+	0
Development temperature decreased	-	-	0
Patient moves during exposure	0	0	-
Angle tube 20°	-	0	-
Change to 8:1 grid ratio	+	-	0
Use 0.6 mm focal spot size	0	0	+
Increase OID 3″	-	+	-

*excessive density will decrease contrast.

ACTIVITY 3

Image Quality Calculations

Solve for the missing variable or calculate the new exposure factor to maintain exposure to the IR as in the initial exposure technique. Show all calculations.

mAs

mA = 100	mA = **500**	mA = 50
time = 0.25 s	time = 100 ms	time = **0.3 s**
mAs = **25**	mAs = 50	mAs = 15
$100 \times 0.25 = 25$ mAs	$50 \div 0.100 = 500$ mA	$15 \div 50 = 0.3$ s

15% rule

Initial kVp = 70
Initial mAs = 10
New kVp = 70 + 15% = **80.5**
New mAs = **5**
$70 \times 1.15 = 80.5$ kVp
$10 \div 2 = 5$ mAs

Initial kVp = 80
Initial mAs = 100
New kVp = 80 − 15% = **68**
New mAs = **200**
$80 \times 0.85 = 68$ kVp
$100 \times 2 = 200$ mAs

Initial kVp = 75
Initial mAs = 35
New kVp = 75 + 2(15%) = 99.19
New mAs = **8.75**
$75 \times 1.15 = 86.25 \times 1.15 = 99.19$ kVp
$35 \div 2 = 17.5 \div 2 = 8.75$ mAs

mAs-Distance Conversions

Initial mAs = 100
Initial SID = 40 in
New SID = 72 in
New mAs = **324**
$$\frac{100}{X} = \frac{40^2}{72^2}$$
$1600\,X = 518{,}400$
$X = 324$ mAs

Initial time = 0.5 s
Initial SID = 60 in
New SID = 25 in
New time = **0.0868**
$$\frac{0.5}{X} = \frac{60^2}{25^2}$$
$3600X = 312.5$
$X = 0.0868$ s

Initial mAs = 125
Initial SID = 56 in
New SID = 40 in
New mAs = **63.78**
$$\frac{125}{X} = \frac{56^2}{40^2}$$
$3136\,X = 200{,}000$
$X = 63.78$ mAs

Grid Conversions

No grid, initial mAs = 10
Add 8:1 grid, new mAs = **40**
$$\frac{10}{X} = \frac{1}{4}$$
$X = 40$ mAs

12:1 grid, initial mAs = 50
6:1 grid, new mAs = **30**
$$\frac{50}{X} = \frac{5}{3}$$
$5X = 150$
$X = 30$ mAs

5:1 grid, initial time = 0.05 s
12:1 grid, new time = **0.125 s**
$$\frac{0.05}{X} = \frac{2}{5}$$
$2X = 0.25$
$X = 0.125$ S

Film-Screen Speed (F/s Spd.)

Initial mAs = 25	Initial mAs = 10	Initial time = 0.25
Initial F/s Spd. = 200	Initial F/s Spd. = 600	Initial F/s Spd. = 100
New F/s Spd. = 400	New F/s Spd. = 300	New F/s Spd. = 50
New mAs = **12.5**	New mAs = **20**	New time = **0.5s**

$\dfrac{25}{X} = \dfrac{400}{200}$; $400X = 5000$ $\dfrac{10}{X} = \dfrac{300}{600}$; $300X = 6000$ $\dfrac{0.25}{X} = \dfrac{50}{100}$; $50X = 25$

$X = 12.5$ mAs $X = 20$ mAs $X = 0.5$ s

WORD PROBLEMS

1. A digital image of the hip was created using 75 kVp @ 5 mAs, a 12:1 grid, a 40-inch SID and a small focal spot size. The exposure indicator value denotes insufficient exposure to the IR and the image displays excessive noise. What adjustments to the exposure technique would improve the quality of the image if repeated?

   A general rule of thumb for insufficient exposure to the IR is to double the mAs. Because exposure indicators vary by manufacturer, it is important for the radiographer to assess how far the exposure indicator is below its desired value and then adjust the mAs appropriately.

2. During a fluoroscopic procedure, the radiation exposure is 50 mR at a distance of 100 cm from the radiation source. Calculate the radiation exposure at a distance of 150 cm.

   Using the Inverse Square Law:

   $$\frac{50 \; mR}{X} = \frac{(150)^2}{(100)^2}; \; 10{,}000 \times 50 = 22{,}500X; \; \frac{500{,}000}{22{,}500} = 22.22 \; mR \; at \; a \; distance \; of \; 150 \; cm$$

3. A good-quality AP pelvis image was created in the radiology department using 80 kVp @ 15 mAs, a 40-in SID, and a 12:1 grid ratio. A request to image a similar-sized patient's pelvis with the mobile x-ray unit requires the SID to be increased to 48 in and the use of an 8:1 grid ratio. What adjustments in the exposure technique would provide a similar quality image?

   Assuming that the mobile unit has a comparable radiation output to the stationary x-ray unit, calculate the new mAs for changes in SID and grid ratio:

   a. $\dfrac{15 \; mAs}{X} = \dfrac{(40)^2}{(48)^2}; 2304 \times 15 = 1600X; \dfrac{34{,}560}{1{,}600} = X; X = 21.6 \; mAs$

   b. $\dfrac{21.6 \; mAs}{X} = \dfrac{5}{4}; \; 21.6 \times 4 = 5X; \dfrac{86.4}{5} = X; X = 17.28 \; mAs$

4. A good-quality KUB image was created on a patient measuring 10 cm using 80 kVp @ 20 mAs, a 40-in SID, a 12:1 grid, and a large focal spot size. What adjustment in exposure technique would be done if the next patient requiring a KUB measured 15 cm?

   A general rule of thumb for patient variations is to adjust the mAs by a factor of 2 for every 4-5 cm change in thickness:

   80 kVp @ 40 mAs (20 mAs × 2), 40" SID, 12:1 grid, and a large focal spot size

⚡ ACTIVITY 4

Image Quality Exposure Conversions

Calculate the new exposure factor to maintain a similar exposure to the IR as in the initial exposure technique. Show all calculations.

Initial Digital Exposure Technique		**New Digital Exposure Technique**
100 mAs		**40.82** mAs
80 kVp	TO	58 kVp
12:1 grid		No grid
56-in SID		40-in SID

Calculations

1. *The kVp is decreased by 15% twice and requires a factor of 2 increase of the mAs for each decrease.*

$$100 \times 2 = 200 \text{ mAs}$$
$$200 \times 2 = 400 \text{ mAs}$$

2. *The grid is removed and requires a decrease in mAs.*

$$\frac{400}{X} = \frac{5}{1}$$
$$5X = 400$$
$$X = 80 \text{ mAs}$$

3. *The SID is decreased and requires a decrease in mAs.*

$$\frac{80}{X} = \frac{56^2}{40^2}$$
$$3,136X = 128,000$$
$$X = 40.82 \text{ mAs}$$

❓ ACTIVITY 5

Image Quality Exposure Conversions

Calculate the new exposure factor for maintaining a similar exposure to the IR as in the initial exposure technique. Show all calculations.

Initial Film-Screen Exposure Technique

200 mA

0.05 s

65 kVp   TO

6:1 grid

40-in SID

400 F/S speed

New Film-Screen Exposure Technique

261.4 mA

⅕ s

75 kVp

8:1 grid

56-in SID

100 F/S speed

Calculations

1. *The kVp is increased by 15% and requires a decrease in mAs by a factor of 2:*

$$\frac{10}{2} = 5\ mAs$$

2. *The grid ratio is increased and requires an increase in mAs:*

$$\frac{5}{X} = \frac{3}{4}$$
$$3X = 20$$
$$X = 6.67\ mAs$$

3. *The SID is increased and requires an increase in mAs:*

$$\frac{6.67}{X} = \frac{40^2}{56^2}$$
$$1{,}600X = 20{,}917.12$$
$$X = 13.07\ mAs$$

4. *The film-screen speed is decreased and requires an increase in mAs:*

$$\frac{13.07}{X} = \frac{100}{400}$$
$$100X = 5{,}228$$
$$X = 52.28\ mA$$

5. *The new mA needs to be calculated:*

$$\frac{52.28}{0.2} = 261.4\ mA$$

IMAGE EVALUATION

The ability to recognize exposure technique errors and their resultant effects on the radiographic image is an important problem-solving skill. The following exercises provide you with an opportunity to apply the knowledge gained from previous chapters in identifying causes of poor-quality images for both digital and film-screen IRs.

💡 ACTIVITY 6

Image Evaluation
Matching

One of the four computed radiography (CR) images is of good quality, whereas the others are the results of errors. Match each image with its corresponding statement:

1. Good-quality lateral   <u>D</u>   A.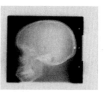
   skull image

2. Imaging plate placed   <u>A</u>   B.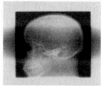
   upside down

3. Grid placed upside-down   <u>B</u>   C.
   on an imaging plate

4. Grid removed with   <u>C</u>   D.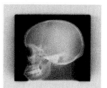
   the mAs adjustment

ACTIVITY 7

Image Evaluation
Multiple Choice

Select the most likely exposure technique error responsible for the poor-quality image, and write your answer in the middle column:

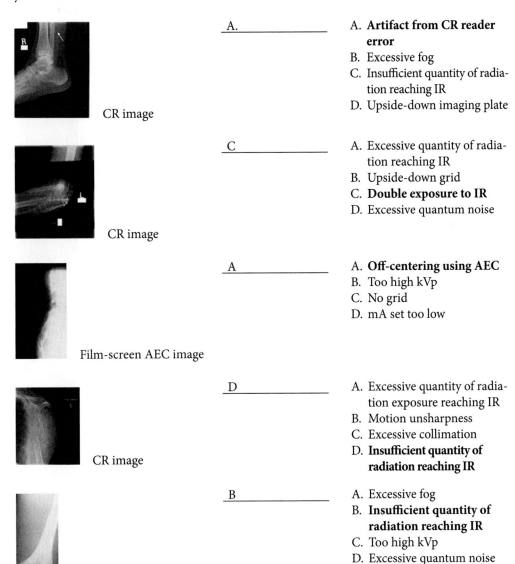

A. _____

A. **Artifact from CR reader error**
B. Excessive fog
C. Insufficient quantity of radiation reaching IR
D. Upside-down imaging plate

CR image

C _____

A. Excessive quantity of radiation reaching IR
B. Upside-down grid
C. **Double exposure to IR**
D. Excessive quantum noise

CR image

A _____

A. **Off-centering using AEC**
B. Too high kVp
C. No grid
D. mA set too low

Film-screen AEC image

D _____

A. Excessive quantity of radiation exposure reaching IR
B. Motion unsharpness
C. Excessive collimation
D. **Insufficient quantity of radiation reaching IR**

CR image

B _____

A. Excessive fog
B. **Insufficient quantity of radiation reaching IR**
C. Too high kVp
D. Excessive quantum noise

Film-screen image

IMAGE ANALYSIS

The ability to evaluate image quality and problem solve for improvement involves several skills. Knowledge of how exposure factors affect image quality individually and in combination is the first step toward successful problem solving. In addition, the ability to accurately calculate exposure factor changes is necessary for improving image quality.

The following image quality exercises are opportunities to develop problem-solving skills by applying the knowledge learned in previous chapters.

❓ ACTIVITY 8

Image Analysis
Film Image Evaluation: Image Quality Analysis
Radiograph 1
kVp = 70
F/S speed = 400
mAs = 4
Grid ratio = 12:1
SID = 40 in
Focal spot = small
Optical density = 1.04

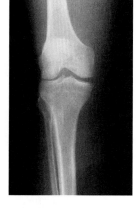

Radiograph 2
kVp = 60
F/S speed = 100
mAs = 6.3
Grid ratio = 6:1
SID = 34 in
Focal spot = large
Optical density = 0.30

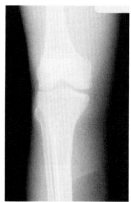

Evaluation:
- *Visually compare Radiograph 1 and Radiograph 2, and comment on the quality of the density, contrast, and sharpness of Radiograph 2. State whether Radiograph 2 needs to be repeated and explain why.*
- *Evaluate each change in exposure factor, and discuss its appropriateness and how it affects the density, contrast, or sharpness (even if not apparent) of the image and patient exposure.*
- *Calculate the appropriate mAs value for each of the cumulative changes to determine why Radiograph 2 displays its level of density, contrast, and sharpness.*
- *Identify the correct mAs value that should have been used for each of the exposure factor changes to maintain density as in Radiograph 1. Last, compare the actual mAs used in Radiograph 2 with the calculated mAs value that was needed to maintain density and contrast. In addition, make other exposure factor recommendations to improve the quality of the image.*

Calculate and Respond

➤ The kVp decreased by 15% in image 2 and requires an increase in mAs by a factor of 2:

$$4 \ mAs \times 2 = 8 \ mAs$$

➤ The SID was decreased from 40 in to 34 in, and the mAs would need to decrease:

$$\frac{8}{X} = \frac{(40)^2}{(34)^2}$$
$$1,600X = 9,248$$
$$X = 5.78 \ mAs$$

➤ The film-screen speed was decreased from 400 to 100 and requires an increase in mAs:

$$\frac{5.78}{X} = \frac{100}{400}$$
$$100X = 2,312$$
$$X = 23.12 \ mAs$$

➤ The grid ratio was changed from 12:1 to 6:1, and the mAs would need to decrease:

$$\frac{23.12}{X} = \frac{5}{3}$$
$$5X = 69.36$$
$$X = 13.87 \ mAs$$

➤ In comparing Radiograph 2 with Radiograph 1, there is decreased density in Radiograph 2. In the area of interest, Radiograph 2 had an OD of 0.30, which is below the diagnostic range. This image would be considered unacceptable and needs to be repeated because the visibility of the area of interest is too low for diagnostic interpretation.

➤ Radiograph 2 has a decrease in kVp of 15% (70 to 60), which would decrease the density and increase the contrast; an increase in mAs by a factor of 2 would be needed to compensate. The mAs would need to be 8 instead of 4. A kVp of 60 for the knee is lower than needed, and requires a higher mAs resulting in increased patient exposure.

➤ The SID was decreased from 40 in to 34 in, which would increase the radiation intensity reaching the body part and increase the density. The mAs would need to be decreased from 8 to 5.78. Decreasing the SID would also increase the magnification and decrease recorded detail in the image.

➤ The film-screen speed was decreased from 400 to 100, which would require an increase in mAs from 5.78 to 23.12. Decreasing the film-screen speed would not only increase the recorded detail in the image but also increase patient exposure.

➤ The grid was changed to a lower grid ratio from 12:1 to 6:1, which would decrease contrast because more scatter radiation reached the film and density was increased. Radiographic contrast was decreased because of the excessive scatter reaching the film. The mAs needs to be decreased to compensate and should have been 13.87 instead of 23.12. Using a lower grid ratio for the knee would decrease patient exposure.

➤ Finally, a large focal spot was used instead of a small focal spot, and this would have decreased the recorded detail in the image.

➤ After all the changes in exposure factors, Radiograph 2 is too light because 6.3 mAs was used instead of 13.87 mAs. The SID should be 40 inches to improve the sharpness in addition to using a smaller focal spot. The film-screen speed should be faster to reduce patient exposure.

ACTIVITY 9

Image Analysis
Computed Radiography Image Evaluation (Recommended S Number Between 100 and 300)

Radiograph 1
kVp = 81
mAs = 5
Focal spot = small
Grid ratio = 12:1
SID = 40 in
Central ray perpendicular
S number = 156

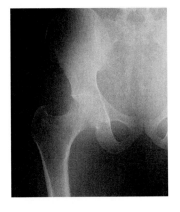

Radiograph 2
kVp = 59
mAs = 1.1
Focal spot = large
Tabletop = no grid
SID = 30 in
Central ray angled 20° caudad
S number = 620

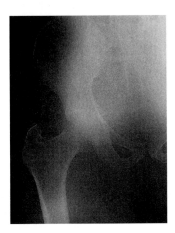

Evaluation

- *Visually compare Radiograph 1 and Radiograph 2, and comment on the quality of the contrast and spatial resolution of Radiograph 2. State whether Radiograph 2 should be repeated and explain why.*
- *Evaluate each change in exposure factor, and discuss its appropriateness and how it affected the exposure to the IR, contrast, and/or spatial resolution (even if not apparent) of the image and patient exposure.*
- *Calculate the appropriate mAs value for each of the cumulative changes to determine why Radiograph 2 displays its level of contrast, spatial resolution, and S number.*
- *Identify the correct mAs value that should have been used for each of the exposure factor changes to maintain the quality as in Radiograph 1. Last, compare the actual mAs used in Radiograph 2 with the calculated mAs value that was needed to maintain sufficient exposure to the IR. In addition, make other exposure factor recommendations to improve the quality of the image.*

Calculate and Respond

➤ The kVp decreased by 15% twice in image 2 and would require an increase in mAs by a factor of 4:

$$5 \ mAs \times 4 = 20 \ mAs$$

➤ The SID was decreased from 40 in to 30 in, and the mAs would need to decrease:

$$\frac{20}{X} = \frac{(40)^2}{(30)^2}$$
$$1{,}600X = 18{,}000$$
$$X = 11.25 \ mAs$$

➤ The grid ratio was removed, and the mAs would need to decrease:

$$\frac{11.25}{X} = \frac{5}{1}$$
$$5X = 11.25$$
$$X = 2.25 \ mAs$$

➤ In comparing Radiograph 2 with Radiograph 1, the brightness levels are similar; however, the contrast is decreased, and there is an increase in quantum noise visible. This image would be considered unacceptable and needs to be repeated because the visibility of the area of interest is too low for diagnostic interpretation.

➤ Radiograph 2 has a decrease in kVp of 15% twice (81 to 59), which would decrease the exposure to the IR and increase contrast; an increase in mAs by a factor of 4 would be needed to compensate. The mAs would need to be 20 instead of 5. A kVp of 59 for the hip is lower than needed, which requires more mAs and results in increased patient exposure.

➤ The SID was decreased from 40 inches to 30 inches, which would increase the radiation intensity reaching the anatomic part and IR. The mAs would need to be decreased from 20 to 11.25. Decreasing the SID would also increase magnification and decrease spatial resolution in the image.

➤ The grid was removed, which would decrease contrast because more scatter radiation reached the IR, thereby reducing radiographic contrast by adding fog to the image. The mAs would need to be decreased to compensate and should be 2.25 instead of 11.25. A grid should be used with the hip because of the amount of scatter radiation reaching the IR. However, removing the grid requires a decrease in mAs, and this would reduce patient exposure.

➤ A large focal spot was used instead of a small focal spot, and this would decrease the spatial resolution in the image.

➤ The central ray was angled 20° caudad, which caused increased shape distortion and decreased the spatial resolution in the image.

➤ In comparing the S number between the two images, the S number is increased from 156 in Radiograph 1 to 620 in Radiograph 2. This indicates a low exposure to the IR and is outside of the recommended range for the hip.

➤ After all the changes in the exposure factors, the mAs should have been 2.25 mAs instead of the 1.1 mAs actually used in Radiograph 2. The insufficient exposure to the IR is indicated by the high S number. The brightness was maintained in Radiograph 2 as a result of automatic rescaling during computer processing. The SID should be 40 in to improve the spatial resolution in addition to using a smaller focal spot and remove the 20°- central ray angulation.

Chapter Review Questions Answer Key

CHAPTER 1: RADIATION AND ITS DISCOVERY

1. B	4. A	7. B	10. C
2. C	5. D	8. D	11. C
3. D	6. C	9. A	12. D

CHAPTER 2: THE X-RAY BEAM

1. B	4. A	7. D	10. D	13. D
2. D	5. C	8. A	11. C	14. D
3. B	6. A	9. C	12. B	15. A

CHAPTER 3: IMAGE FORMATION AND RADIOGRAPHIC QUALITY

1. D	4. B	7. A	10. C	13. B
2. D	5. D	8. A	11. B	14. D
3. C	6. B	9. C	12. D	

CHAPTER 4: DIGITAL IMAGING

1. D	5. D	9. B	13. C	17. D
2. C	6. C	10. C	14. D	18. A
3. A	7. D	11. C	15. B	19. D
4. D	8. A	12. A	16. A	20. B

CHAPTER 5: FILM-SCREEN IMAGING

1. D	5. B	9. D	13. C
2. B	6. A	10. C	14. A
3. A	7. A	11. B	15. D
4. D	8. D	12. C	16. A

CHAPTER 6: EXPOSURE TECHNIQUE FACTORS

1. D	4. B	7. C	10. D
2. C	5. D	8. D	11. B
3. A	6. C	9. A	12. B

CHAPTER 7: SCATTER CONTROL

1. C	5. B	9. B	13. C	17. C
2. B	6. A	10. A	14. D	18. D
3. D	7. D	11. D	15. A	
4. B	8. D	12. A	16. B	

CHAPTER 8: EXPOSURE TECHNIQUE SELECTION

1. B	5. B	9. C	13. B
2. C	6. D	10. B	14. C
3. D	7. B	11. D	15. A
4. D	8. A	12. C	16. C

CHAPTER 9: IMAGE EVALUATION

1. C	3. A	5. C	7. A	9. A
2. D	4. B	6. B	8. C	10. D

CHAPTER 10: DYNAMIC IMAGING: FLUOROSCOPY

1. A	4. B	7. B	10. B	13. D
2. D	5. D	8. B	11. B	14. B
3. C	6. C	9. B	12. C	15. D

Illustration Credits

Chapter 1

Figures 1-1 and 1-3, From *Glasser O: Wilhelm Conrad Roentgen and the early history of the roentgen rays, 1933.*

Figure 1-7, A, Courtesy *Royal Philips.* **B,** From *Bontrager K, Lampignano J: Textbook of Radiographic Positioning and Related Anatomy, 7e, St. Louis, 2010, Mosby.*

Chapter 2

Figures 2-9, 2-12, 2-14, 2-15, and 2-20, From *Johnston JN, Fauber TL: Essentials of Radiographic Physics and Imaging, 2e, St. Louis, 2016, Mosby.*

Figure 2-23, Courtesy *Varian Medical Systems, North Charleston, South Carolina.*

Chapter 3

Figures 3-1, 3-2, 3-3, 3-4, 3-5, 3-6, 3-7, 3-8, 3-9, 3-10, 3-11, and 3-26, From *Johnston JN, Fauber TL: Essentials of Radiographic Physics and Imaging, ed 2, St. Louis, 2016, Mosby.*

Figures 3-13 and 3-22, From *Mosby's Instructional Radiographic Series: Radiographic Imaging, St. Louis, 1998, Mosby.*

Figure 3-23, Modified from *Sprawls P: Physical Principles of Medical Imaging Online, 2e,* http://www.sprawls.org/ppmi2/.

Figure 3-27, From *Long B, Rollins J, Smith B: Merrill's Atlas of Radiographic Positioning and Procedures, 13e, St. Louis, 2016, Mosby.*

Chapter 4

Figures 4-4, 4-10, and 4-17, From *Johnston JN, Fauber TL: Essentials of Radiographic Physics and Imaging, ed 2, St. Louis, 2016, Mosby.*

Figure 4-5, Courtesy *Fluke Biomedical.*

Figures 4-6 and 4-21, From *Bushong SC: Radiologic Science for Technologists, 10e, St. Louis, 2013, Mosby.*

Figures 4-7, 4-22, 4-24, 4-30, 4-31, 4-43, and 4-44, Courtesy of *Andrew Woodward.*

Figures 4-11 and 4-12, Courtesy *Fujifilm Medical Systems, USA, Inc., Stamford, Connecticut.*

Figures 4-19 and 4-20, Modified from *Bushong SC: Radiologic Science for Technologists, 10e, St. Louis, 2013, Mosby.*

Figure 4-21, From *Bushong SC: Radiologic Science for Technologists, 10e, St. Louis, 2013, Mosby.*

Figure 4-23, A, *From Cesar LJ: Computed radiography: its impact on radiographers, J ASRT 68(3):225-232, 1997.* **B,** *Modified from Sprawls P: Physical Principles of Medical Imaging Online, 2e,* http://www.sprawls.org/ppmi2/.

Figures 4-25, 4-26, 4-27, 4-28, 4-29, 4-37, and 4-38, Modified from *Sprawls P: Physical Principles of Medical Imaging Online, 2e,* http://www.sprawls.org/ppmi2/.

Figure 4-32, ©*Barco.*

Figure 4-34, From *Bushberg J: The Essential Physics of Medical Imaging, 2e, Philadelphia, 2001, Lippincott Williams & Wilkins.*

Figures 4-35 and 4-36, From *Kuni C: Introduction to Computers and Digital Processing in Medical Imaging, Chicago, 1988, Year Book Medical Publishers.*

Chapter 5

Figure 5-3, From *Johnston JN, Fauber TL: Essentials of Radiographic Physics and Imaging, ed 2, St. Louis, 2016, Mosby.*

Figures 5-8 and 5-9, Courtesy *Nuclear Associates.*

Chapter 6

Figures 6-2, 6-14, 6-16, and 6-17, From *Johnston JN, Fauber TL: Essentials of Radiographic Physics and Imaging, ed 2, St. Louis, 2016, Mosby.*

Chapter 7

Figures 7-6 and 7-8, From *Mosby's Radiographic Instructional Series: Radiographic Imaging, St. Louis, 1998, Mosby.*
Figure 7-20, From *Johnston JN, Fauber TL: Essentials of Radiographic Physics and Imaging, ed 2, St. Louis, 2016, Mosby.*
Figure 7-26, Courtesy *Andrew Woodward.*
Figure 7-28, From *Bontrager KL, Lampignano JP: Textbook of radiographic positioning and related anatomy, ed 7, St Louis, 2010, Mosby.*

Chapter 8

Figures 8-1 and 8-7, From *Johnston JN, Fauber TL: Essentials of Radiographic Physics and Imaging, ed 2, St. Louis, 2016, Mosby.*
Figure 8-6, Courtesy *Philips Healthcare, Andover, Massachusetts.*
Figure 8-8, From *Long B, Rollins, J, Smith B: Merrill's Atlas of Radiographic Positioning and Procedures, 13e, St. Louis, 2016, Mosby.*

Chapter 9

Figure 9-10, Courtesy *Andrew Woodward.*
Activity 7, Figure 1 and Figure 2, Courtesy *Andrew Woodward.*

Activity 7, Figure 4, From *Bontrager KL, Lampignano JP: Textbook of radiographic positioning and related anatomy, ed 7, St Louis, 2010, Mosby.*

Chapter 10

Figure 10-1, A, From *Fauber TL: Radiographic Imaging and Exposure, ed 4, St. Louis, 2013, Mosby.* **B,** From *Bushong SC: Radiologic Science for Technologists, 10e, St. Louis, 2013, Mosby.*
Figure 10-2 and 10-14, Courtesy *Siemens Healthcare, Malvern, Pennsylvania.*
Figures 10-3, 10-4, 10-8, 10-9, 10-10, 10-11, and 10-12, From *Johnston JN, Fauber TL: Essentials of Radiographic Physics and Imaging, ed 2, St. Louis, 2016, Mosby.*
Figure 10-5, From *Bontrager K, Lampignano J: Textbook of Radiographic Positioning and Related Anatomy, 7e, St. Louis, 2010, Mosby.*
Figure 10-6, A, Courtesy *Royal Philips.* **B,** From *Curry T, Dowdey J, Murry R: Christensen's Physics of Diagnostic Radiology, 4e, Philadelphia, 1990, Lippincott Williams & Wilkins.*
Figure 10-7, A, From *Bushong SC: Radiologic Science for Technologists, 10e, St. Louis, 2013, Mosby.* **B,** From *Bushberg J: The Essential Physics of Medical Imaging, 2e, Philadelphia, 2001, Lippincott Williams & Wilkins.*
Figure 10-10, From *Johnston JN, Fauber TL: Essentials of Radiographic Physics and Imaging, ed 2, St. Louis, 2016, Mosby.*

GLOSSARY

15% rule Rule stating that changing the kilovoltage peak by 15% has the same effect on image receptor exposure as doubling or halving the mAs.

absorbed dose The transfer of radiation energy into matter (e.g., tissue).

absorption As the energy of the primary x-ray beam is deposited within the atoms comprising the tissue, some x-ray photons are completely absorbed. Complete absorption of the incoming x-ray photon occurs when it has enough energy to remove (eject) an inner-shell electron.

active layer The radiation-sensitive and light-sensitive layer of the film.

actual focal spot size The size of the area on the anode target that is exposed to electrons from the tube current. Actual focal spot size depends on the size of the filament producing the electron stream.

added filtration The filtration that is added to the port of the x-ray tube.

air gap technique Based on the simple concept that much of the scatter will miss the image receptor if there is an increased distance between the patient and the image receptor (increased OID).

air kerma The amount of energy deposited in a unit mass of air.

ambient lighting The level of light in the room while viewing images.

ALARA As Low As Reasonably Achievable.

anatomically programmed techniques A radiographic system that allows the radiographer to select a particular button on the control panel that represents an anatomic area; a preprogrammed set of exposure factors is displayed and selected for use.

anode A positively charged electrode within the x-ray tube composed of molybdenum, copper, tungsten, and graphite. It consists of a target and, in rotating anode tubes, a stator and rotor.

anode heel effect The x-ray beam has greater intensity (number of x-rays) on the cathode side of the tube, with the intensity diminishing toward the anode side. The heel effect occurs because of the angle of the target.

aperture diaphragm A flat piece of lead (diaphragm) containing a hole (aperture) for beam restriction.

artifact Any unwanted image on a radiograph.

attenuation Reduction in the energy or number of the primary x-ray beam as it passes through anatomic tissue.

automatic brightness control (ABC) A function of the fluoroscopic unit that maintains the overall appearance of the fluoroscopic image (contrast and density) by automatically adjusting the kilovoltage peak (kVp) or milliamperage (mA) or both.

automatic collimator/positive beam-limiting device Automatically limits the size and shape of the primary beam to the size and shape of the image receptor.

automatic exposure control (AEC) A system used to consistently control the amount of radiation reaching the image receptor by terminating the length of exposure.

automatic film processor A device that encompasses chemical tanks, a roller transport system, and a dryer system for the processing of radiographic film.

automatic rescaling Occurs during histogram analysis and is employed to maintain consistent image brightness despite overexposure or underexposure of the digital image receptor.

average gradient The slope of the straight-line region of a film's sensitometric curve.

backup time The maximum length of time for which the x-ray exposure continues when using an AEC system.

base plus fog (B + F) The lowest amount of density on the radiographic film due to the tint added to its base and any slight amount of fog added during processing.

beam-restricting device Changes the shape and size of the primary beam, located just below the x-ray tube housing.

beam restriction/collimation Interchangeably used terms that refer to a decrease in the size of the projected radiation field.

bit 0 or 1 that refers to the computer's basic unit of information.

bit depth Number of bits.

body habitus Refers to the general form or build of the body, including size. The four types of body habitus are *sthenic, hyposthenic, hypersthenic,* and *asthenic.*

bremsstrahlung interactions Occur when a projectile electron completely avoids the orbital electrons of the tungsten atom and travels very close to its nucleus. The very strong electrostatic force of the nucleus causes the electron suddenly to "slow down." As the electron loses energy, it suddenly changes its direction and the energy loss reappears as an x-ray photon.

brightness The amount of luminance (light emission) of a display monitor.

brightness gain The product of both flux gain and minification gain; this results in a brighter image on the output phosphor.

Bucky Located directly below the radiographic tabletop, the grid is found just above the tray that holds the image receptor. More accurately called the *Potter-Bucky diaphragm.*

Bucky factor/grid conversion factor Used to determine the adjustment in mAs needed when changing from using a grid to nongrid (or vice versa) or when changing to grids with different grid ratios.

byte 8 bits combined.

caliper A device that measures part thickness.

camera tube A device used to convert the light emitted from the output phosphor to an electrical signal sent to the television monitor.

cassette Container for both the intensifying screens and the film.

cathode A negatively charged electrode (within the x-ray tube). It comprises a filament and a focusing cup.

characteristic interactions Produced when a projectile electron interacts with an electron from the inner (K) shell of the tungsten atom and ejects it. An outer-shell electron drops into vacancy and the energy difference is emitted as an x-ray photon.

charge-coupled device (CCD) A light-sensitive semiconducting device that generates an electrical charge when stimulated by light and stores this charge in a capacitor.

coherent scattering An interaction that occurs with low-energy x-rays, typically below the diagnostic range. The incoming photon interacts with the atom, causing it to become excited. The x-ray does not lose energy but changes direction.

collimator Two sets of adjustable lead shutters located 3–7 in below the tube that consist of longitudinal and lateral leaves or blades, each with its own control; this makes the collimator adjustable in terms of its ability to produce projected fields of varying sizes.

comparative anatomy Concept stating that different parts of the same size can be radiographed using the same exposure factors, provided the minimum kVp value needed to penetrate the part is used in each case.

compensating filter Special filters added to the primary beam to alter its intensity. These types of filters are used to image anatomic areas that are nonuniform in makeup and assist in producing more consistent exposure to the image receptor.

Compton effect The loss of energy of the incoming photon when it ejects an outer-shell electron from the atom. The remaining lower-energy x-ray photon changes direction and may leave the anatomic part.

Compton electron/secondary electron The ejected electron resulting from the Compton effect interaction.

cone An aperture diaphragm that has an extended flange attached to it. The flange can vary in length and is shaped as a cone. The flange can also be made to telescope, increasing its total length.

continuous fluoroscopy The x-ray exposure continues without interruption while the exposure pedal/button is activated.

contrast medium A substance instilled into the body by injection or ingestion that is used when imaging anatomic tissues that have low subject contrast. Also called *contrast agent*.

contrast resolution The ability of the image receptor to distinguish between objects having similar subject contrast.

contrast-to-noise ratio A method of describing the contrast resolution with the amount of noise apparent in a digital image.

convergent line If points were connected along the length of the grid, they would form an imaginary line.

convergent point If imaginary lines were drawn from each of the lead lines in a linear focused grid, these lines would meet to form an imaginary point.

conversion factor An expression of the luminance at the output phosphor divided by the input exposure rate; its unit of measurement is candela per square meter per milliroentgen per second.

crossed/cross-hatched grid A grid containing lead lines that are perpendicular to one another. Crossed grids remove more scattered photons than linear grids because they contain more lead strips, oriented in two directions.

cylinder An aperture diaphragm that has an extended flange attached to it. The flange can vary in length and is shaped as a cylinder.

densitometer A device used to numerically determine the amount of blackness on the radiograph.

density The amount of overall blackness of the processed image.

density controls Controls that allow the radiographer to adjust the amount of preset radiation detection values. Each control changes the exposure time by a certain predetermined amount or increment.

detective quantum efficiency (DQE) A measurement of the efficiency of an image receptor in converting the x-ray exposure it receives to a quality radiographic image.

detectors The sensors, cells, or chambers within an AEC device that sense how much radiation has reached the imaging plate in order to terminate the exposure.

developing or reducing agents Agents that reduce exposed

silver halide to metallic silver and add electrons to exposed silver halide during film processing.

deviation index (DI) A value that reflects the difference between the desired or target exposure to the image receptor and the actual exposure to the image receptor.

diagnostic densities The appropriate range of optical densities.

differential absorption A process whereby some of the x-ray beam is absorbed in the tissue and some passes through (transmits) the anatomic part.

digital imaging Constructing an image from numeric data.

digital imaging and communications in medicine (DICOM) A communication standard for information sharing between PACS and imaging modalities.

distortion Results from the radiographic misrepresentation of either the size (magnification) or the shape of the anatomic part.

D_{max} The point on the sensitometric curve where maximum density has been produced.

D_{min} The point on the sensitometric curve where the minimum amount of radiation exposure produced the minimum amount of optical density.

dose equivalent Units of radiation exposure used in measuring occupational exposure.

dosimeter A device that measures x-ray exposure.

double-emulsion film Has an emulsion coating on both sides of the base.

dynamic range Refers to the range of exposure intensities an image receptor can accurately detect.

effective focal spot size Focal spot size as measured directly under the anode target.

electromagnetic radiation Radiation that has both electrical and magnetic properties. All radiations that are electromagnetic make up a spectrum.

electronic masking Also known as *shuttering*. A postprocessing function that can remove regions of the digital image.

electrostatic focusing lenses Focuses and accelerates the electrons through the image intensifier toward the anode.

elongation Refers to images of objects that appear longer than the true objects.

emulsion layer The radiation- and light-sensitive layers of the film.

exit radiation When the attenuated x-ray beam leaves the patient, the remaining x-ray beam is composed of both transmitted and scattered radiation.

exposure The amount of ionizations or electrical charge in a specified amount of air expressed by Roentgen (R).

exposure indicator A numeric value that is displayed on the processed image to indicate the level of x-ray exposure received on the digital image receptor.

exposure intensity The amount and energy of the x-rays reaching an area of the image receptor.

exposure latitude The range of exposures that produce optical densities within the straight-line region of the sensitometric curve.

exposure technique charts Pre-established guidelines used by the radiographer to select standardized manual or AEC exposure factors for each type of radiographic examination.

exposure time Determines the length of time that the x-ray tube produces x-rays.

extrapolated Mathematically estimated; the mathematical process used to create technique charts.

feed tray A flat metal surface with an edge on either side that permits the film to enter the processor easily and correctly aligned.

filament A coiled tungsten wire that is the source of electrons during x-ray production.

filament current Heats the tungsten filament. This heating of the filament causes thermionic emission.

fill factor The percentage of the x-rays reaching the sensitive area of the detector element (DEL).

film contrast Controlled by the design and manufacturing of the film components and the effect of processing.

film speed The degree to which the emulsion is sensitive to x-rays or light. The greater the speed of a film, the more sensitive it is.

fixed kVp/variable mAs technique chart A type of exposure technique chart that is based on the concept of selecting an optimal kVp value that is required for the radiographic examination and adjusting the mAs for variations in part thickness.

fixing agent Clears undeveloped silver halide from the film during processing.

flat-panel detectors (FPD) Solid-state image receptors using a large-area active matrix array of electronic components ranging in sizes from 43 × 35 cm to 43 × 43 cm.

fluorescence The ability of phosphors to emit visible light only while exposed to x-rays (with little or no afterglow).

fluoroscopy Allows imaging of the movement of internal structures. It differs from film-screen imaging in that it uses a continuous beam of x-rays to create images of moving internal structures that can be viewed on a television monitor.

flux gain The increase in light intensities at the output phosphor by accelerating the electrons.

focal distance The distance between the grid and the convergent line or point, sometimes referred to as *grid radius*.

focal range The recommended range of SIDs that can be used with a focused grid. The convergent line or point always falls within the focal range.

focused grid Grid that has lead lines that are angled, or canted, to approximately match the angle of divergence of the primary beam.

focusing cup Made of nickel and nearly surrounds the filament. It is open at one end to allow electrons to flow freely across the tube from cathode to anode. It has a negative charge, which keeps the cloud of electrons emitted from the filament from spreading apart. Its purpose is to focus the stream of electrons.

fog Scatter radiation (Compton interactions) that reach the image receptor and creates unwanted exposure on the radiographic image.

foreshortening Refers to images that appear shorter than the true objects.

frequency The number of waves passing a given point per given unit of time. Frequency is represented by a lowercase *f* or by the Greek letter *nu (ν)*, and values are given in Hertz (Hz).

gradient point The slope along any portion of the sensitometric curve.

gray scale The number of different shades of gray that can be stored and displayed by a computer system.

grid A device that has very thin lead strips with radiolucent interspaces, intended to absorb scatter radiation emitted from the patient.

grid cap Contains a permanently mounted grid and allows the image receptor to slide in behind it.

grid cassette An image receptor that has a grid permanently mounted to its front surface.

grid cutoff A decrease in the number of transmitted photons that reach the image receptor because of some misalignment of the grid.

grid focus The orientation of the lead lines to one another.

grid frequency Expresses the number of lead lines per unit length, in inches or centimeters or both. Grid frequencies can range from 25 to 45 lines/cm (60 to 110 lines/in).

grid pattern The linear pattern of the lead lines of a grid. The two types of grid pattern are linear and crossed or crosshatched.

grid ratio The ratio of the height of the lead strips to the distance between them.

half-value layer (HVL) The amount of filtration that reduces the intensity of the x-ray beam to one-half of its original value is considered the best method for describing x-ray quality. The HVL also can be used as an indirect measure of the total filtration in the path of the x-ray beam. It is expressed in millimeters of aluminum (mm-Al).

health level seven standard (HL7) A communication standard for medical information.

heat unit (HU) The amount of heat produced from any given exposure.

high contrast A radiograph with few densities but great differences among them.

histogram analysis Graphic display of the distribution of pixel values. Each image has its own histogram, and it is evaluated to determine the adequacy of the image receptor exposure to x-rays.

illuminator Device that provides light illumination so that the anatomy, displayed as various shades of optical densities, can be visualized. It is also known as a *viewbox*.

image intensification The process whereby the exit radiation from the anatomic area of interest interacts with a light-emitting material (input phosphor) for conversion to visible light to create a brighter image.

image receptor (IR) A device that receives the radiation leaving the patient.

imaging plate (IP) Located in the CR image receptor, where the photon intensities are absorbed by the phosphor.

immersion heater A heating coil that is immersed in the bottom of the developer and fixer tank. It is thermostatically controlled to heat the developer solution to its proper temperature and maintain that temperature as long as the processor is turned on.

inherent filtration The filtration that is permanently in the path of the x-ray beam. Three components contribute to inherent filtration: (1) the glass envelope of the tube, (2) the oil that surrounds the tube, and (3) the window in the tube housing.

input/output phosphor Phosphors within the image intensifier. The input phosphor converts incoming radiation into visible light energy, and the output phosphor converts the electrons into a brighter image.

intensifying screen A device in radiographic cassettes that contains phosphors that convert x-ray energy into light, which exposes the radiographic film.

intensity of radiation exposure The amount and energy of the x-rays reaching an area of the image receptor.

interspace material Radiolucent strips between the lead lines of a grid; generally made of aluminum.

inverse square law The relationship between distance and x-ray beam intensity, which states that the intensity of the x-ray beam is inversely proportional to the square of the distance from the source.

invisible image The latent image not visible within the image receptor.

ionization The ability to remove (eject) electrons; a property of x-rays.

ionization/ion chamber A hollow cell that contains air and is connected to the AEC timer circuit via an electrical wire.

kilovoltage (kVp) Potential difference applied across the x-ray tube at the time the exposure is initiated, kVp determines the speed at which the electrons in the tube current move.

latent image The invisible image within the image receptor.

latent image centers Several sensitivity specks with many silver ions attracted to them.

latent image formation The Gurney–Mott theory used to explain what happens to silver halide crystals when exposed to x-rays and light.

leakage radiation Any x-rays, other than the primary beam, that escape the tube housing.

line focus principle Describes the relationship between the actual and the effective focal spots in the x-ray tube. A smaller target angle produces a smaller effective focal spot.

linear grid Contains lead lines that run in only one direction.

long-dimension linear grid Contains lead strips that run parallel to the long axis of the grid.

long-scale/low contrast A radiograph with a large number of densities but little differences among them.

lookup tables (LUT) Provides a method of altering the image to change the display of the digital image in a variety of ways.

luminescence The emission of light from the screen when stimulated by radiation.

magnification An increase in the image size of the object compared with its true or actual size. Also known as *size distortion*.

magnification factor (MF) Indicates how much size distortion or magnification is shown on a radiograph. MF = SID divided by SOD.

magnification mode Image intensifiers have a multifold function to increase the size of the area of interest displayed on the television monitor. Changing the voltage of the electrostatic focusing lenses tightens the diameter of the electron stream, giving the appearance of magnification.

manifest/visible image The visible image after processing.

mAs/distance compensation formula A formula that provides a mathematical calculation for adjusting mAs when changing the SID.

mAs readout The actual mAs used for the image is displayed immediately after the AEC exposure, sometimes for only a few seconds.

matrix A digital image is displayed as a combination of rows and columns (array) of small, usually square, "picture elements" called *pixels*.

maximum contrast The greatest difference in optical densities.

milliamperage (mA) The unit used to measure the tube current.

minification gain Increased light intensities as a result of the reduction in size of the output phosphor image compared with that of the input phosphor image.

minimum response time Refers to the shortest exposure time that the AEC system can produce.

modulation transfer function (MTF) A measure of the imaging systems ability to display contrast of anatomic objects varying in size.

Moiré effect An artifact that can occur when a stationary grid is used during computed radiography (CR) imaging if the grid frequency is similar to the scanning frequency. Also known as the *Zebra pattern*.

object-to-image-receptor distance (OID) Distance created between the object radiographed and the image receptor.

off-focus radiation Occurs when projectile electrons are reflected and x-rays are produced outside the focal spot.

optical density (OD) A numeric calculation that compares the intensity of light transmitted through an area on the film (I_t) to the amount of light originally striking (incident) the area (I_0).

optimal density Densities that lie within the straight-line region of the sensitometric curve.

optimal kVp The kVp value that is high enough to ensure penetration of the part but not too high to diminish radiographic contrast.

parallel/nonfocused grid A grid with lead lines that run parallel to one another.

penetrometer A device comprising uniform absorbers of increasing thicknesses.

phosphor layer Active layer that is the most important screen component because it contains the material that absorbs the transmitted x-rays and converts them to visible light.

photocathode Converts the visible light in the image intensifier into electrons.

photoelectric effect Complete absorption of the incoming x-ray photon occurs when it has enough energy to remove (eject) an inner-shell electron. The ionized atom has a vacancy, or electron hole, in its inner shell, and an electron from an outer shell drops down to fill the vacancy.

photoelectron The ejected electron resulting from ionization during the photoelectric effect.

photomultiplier (PM) tube An electronic device that converts visible light energy into electrical energy.

photon A small, discrete bundle of energy.

photostimulable luminescence (PSL) The emission of visible light from the photostimulable phosphor when stimulated by a high-intensity laser beam.

photostimulable phosphor (PSP) The phosphor layer of the imaging plate (IP) composed of barium fluorohalide crystals doped with europium.

phototimer Uses a fluorescent (light-producing) screen and a device that converts light to electricity in an AEC device.

picture archival and communication system (PACS) A computer system designed for digital imaging that can receive, store, distribute, and display digital images.

pixel The smallest component of the matrix. Also known as *picture elements*.

pixel density The number of pixels per unit area.

pixel pitch The pixel spacing or distance measured from the center of a pixel to an adjacent pixel.

pulsed fluoroscopy The x-ray exposure has gaps of exposure between each image frame.

quantum A small, discrete bundle of energy.

quantum noise Visible as brightness or density fluctuations on the image as a result of too few photons reaching the image receptor to form the image. *Quantum mottle* is the term typically used when referring to noise on a film image.

radioactivity Unstable atoms spontaneously emitting particles and energy from the nucleus in an effort to attain stability.

rare earth elements Chemical compounds of elements that are relatively difficult and expensive to extract from the earth and range in atomic number from 57 to 71 on the periodic table of elements.

recirculation system Acts to circulate solution in a film processing tank by pumping the solution out of one portion of the tank and returning it to a different location within the same tank from which it was removed.

reducing agents Developing agents that reduce exposed silver halide to metallic silver and add electrons to the exposed silver halide during film processing.

relative speed Results by comparing film-screen systems on the basis of the amount of light produced for a given exposure.

remnant radiation When the attenuated x-ray beam leaves the patient, the remaining x-ray beam is composed of both transmitted and scattered radiation. Also known as *exit radiation*.

replenishment The replacement of fresh chemicals after the loss of chemicals during film processing, specifically, developer solution and fixer solution.

rotor A device in the x-ray tube that causes the target to rapidly rotate during x-ray production.

sampling frequency How often the analog signal is reproduced in its discrete digitized form.

sampling pitch The distance between the sampling points.

scale of contrast The range of densities visible in a film image.

scattering Some incoming photons are not absorbed but instead lose energy during interactions with atoms comprising tissue.

scintillator A phosphor material that converts the exit radiation into visible light.

screen film Radiographic film sensitive to light emitted by the intensifying screen.

screen speed The capability of an intensifying screen to produce visible light. The greater the speed, the more sensitive it is.

secondary electron The ejected electron resulting from the Compton effect interaction. Also known as a *Compton electron*.

sensitometer A device designed to produce consistent step-wedge densities.

sensitometric curve A graph of step-wedge optical densities that visually demonstrates the relationship between the intensity of radiation exposure (x-axis) and the resultant optical densities (y-axis).

sensitometric strip A density step-wedge image.

sensitometry The study of the relationship between the intensity of radiation exposure to a film and the amount of blackness produced after processing (density).

shape distortion Images of objects that appear longer or shorter than the true objects.

short-dimension linear grid Contains lead strips running perpendicular to the long axis of the grid.

short-scale contrast A film radiograph with few densities but great differences among them is said to have *high contrast*.

shoulder region A point on the sensitometric curve where changes in exposure intensity no longer affect the optical density.

signal-to-noise ratio (SNR) A method of describing the strength of the radiation exposure compared with the amount of noise apparent in a digital image.

silver halide A material sensitive to radiation and light.

silver recovery Refers to the removal of silver from used fixer solution.

size distortion/magnification Refers to an increase in the image size of an object compared with its true, or actual, size.

slope Steepness of the sensitometric curve indicated by the ratio of the change in y (optical density) for a unit change in x (log relative exposure).

source-to-image-receptor distance (SID) The distance between the source of the radiation and the image receptor.

source-to-object distance (SOD) Refers to the distance from the x-ray source (focal spot) to the object being radiographed.

space charge The electrons liberated from the filament during thermionic emission that form a cloud around the filament.

space charge effect The tendency of the space charge not to allow more electrons to be boiled off the filament.

spatial frequency Variation in anatomic details imaged as white to black brightness levels that can be defined by the unit of line pairs per millimeter (lp/mm).

spatial resolution The smallest detail that can be detected in an image; the term typically used in digital imaging.

spectral emission The color of light produced by a particular intensifying screen.

spectral matching Correctly matching the color sensitivity of the film to the color emission of the intensifying screen.

spectral sensitivity The color of light to which a particular film is most sensitive.

speed A film's sensitivity to radiation exposure.

speed exposure point The area on the x axis (log of exposure) that produced the optical density of 1.0 plus B + F.

speed point The point on a sensitometric curve that corresponds to the optical density of 1.0 plus B + F.

standby control An electric circuit that shuts off power to the roller assemblies when the film processor is not being used.

stator An electric motor that turns the rotor at very high speed during x-ray production.

step-wedge densities A radiograph of uniform densities resembling a step wedge.

straight-line region The area on the sensitometric curve where the diagnostic or most useful range of densities is produced.

subject contrast A result of the absorption characteristics of the anatomic tissue radiographed along with the quality of the x-ray beam.

target A metal that abruptly decelerates and stops electrons in the tube current, allowing the production of x-rays.

thermionic emission The boiling off of electrons from the cathode filament.

tissue density Matter per unit volume or the compactness of the anatomic particles comprising the anatomic part.

toe region The area of low density on the sensitometric curve.

total filtration The sum of the x-ray tube's added and inherent filtration.

transmission The incoming x-ray photon passes through the anatomic part without any interaction with the atomic structures.

trough filter A double-wedge compensating filter added to the primary beam to produce more consistent exposure to the image receptor.

tube current The flow of electrons from cathode to anode, measured in milliamperage (mA).

values of interest (VOI) Determines the range of the histogram data set included in the displayed image.

variable kVp/fixed mAs technique chart A type of exposure technique chart based on the concept that kVp can be increased as the anatomic part size increases. The baseline kVp is increased by 2 for every 1 cm increase in part thickness, and the mAs is maintained.

voltage ripple The amount of consistency in voltage waveforms during x-ray production.

wafer grid A type of stationary grid placed on top of the image receptor.

wavelength The distance between two successive crests or troughs.

wedge filter The most common type of compensating filter. The thicker part of the wedge filter is lined up with the thinner portion of the anatomic part that is being imaged, allowing fewer x-ray photons to reach that end of the part.

window level Sets the midpoint (center) of the range of brightness visible in the digital image.

window width The range or number of shades of gray visible on the digital image.

x-ray emission spectrum The range and intensity of emitted x-rays.

INDEX

A

ABC. *see* Automatic brightness control (ABC)
Abdomen, image contrast in, 54, 56f
Absorbed dose, 7–8
Absorption, 44
  differential. *see* Differential absorption
Absorption efficiency, and screen speed, 117
Accuracy, of structural lines, 237–238
Active layer, of film, 111
Actual focal spot size, 32, 32f
ADC. *see* Analog-to-digital converter (ADC)
Added filtration, 35, 35f
AEC. *see* Automatic exposure control (AEC)
Air gap, object-to-image-receptor distance (OID) and, 162, 162f
Air gap technique, 203, 203f, 203b
Air kerma, 7
ALARA principle. *see* As low as reasonably achievable (ALARA) principle
Alignment considerations, in automatic exposure control, 215–218
Ambient light, 95–96
Ammonium thiosulfate, as fixing agent, 121, 121b
Amorphous selenium direct-capture detector, for digital fluoroscopy, 275–276
Analog-to-digital converter (ADC)
  in computed radiography, 77, 78f
  in digital fluoroscopy, 275, 276f
Anatomic detail, modulation transfer function and, 75b
Anatomically programmed technique, 220, 220b, 223f
Anode, 17–18
  heat dissipation in, 18, 18b
  rotating, 17, 17f–18f, 19b
    focal track and focal spot of, 18, 19f
    heat loads of, 18
    rotor of, 17, 18f
    stator of, 17, 18f
    tungsten of, 17, 17f–18f, 18b
  stationary, 17, 17f, 19f
  target of, 17, 17b
Anode angle, and effective focal spot size, 33f, 33b

Anode heel effect, 33–34, 33b, 34f
Aperture diaphragms, for beam restriction, 183, 183f–184f
Archival quality, of radiographs, 121b–122b
Artifacts
  due to foreign bodies, 62
  film, 125, 126f–127f
  image, 62–63
    digital, 93, 94f
    in image evaluation, 243–244, 244f
    minus-density, 243
    plus-density, 243
As low as reasonably achievable (ALARA) principle, 9b
Automatic brightness control (ABC), in fluoroscopy, 265
Automatic collimators, 187–188, 187b
Automatic exposure control (AEC), 209–220
  alignment and positioning considerations in, 215–218
    detector selection as, 215, 215b, 216f
    detector size as, 217–218
    patient centering as, 215–217, 216b, 217f
  backup time in, 213–214
    function of, 214b
    monitoring, 214b
    setting, 214, 214b
  compensating issues in, 218–220
    calibration as, 219–220, 219b–220b
    collimation as, 218, 219b
    image receptor variations as, 219, 219b
    patient considerations as, 218, 218b
  defined, 209
  density adjustment in, 214
  with digital imaging, 221t
  with film-screen radiography, 222t
  kVp and mA selections in, 212–213, 212b–213b
  mAs readout, 212, 212b
  minimum response time in, 213
  principle of, 209, 209b
  radiation detectors in, 209–212, 210f, 210b
    ionization chamber systems as, 210–212, 211f, 212b
    phototimers as, 210, 211f

Page numbers followed by *b*, *t*, and *f* indicate boxes, tables, and figures, respectively.

Automatic film processing, 119–124
  automatic film processor for, 119, 120f
  stages of, 119, 120t
    developing as, 119–121, 120t
    drying as, 120t, 122
    fixing as, 121
    washing as, 120t, 121–122
  systems for, 122–124, 123f
    feed tray in, 122, 123f
    immersion heater in, 124
    inadequate processing in, 124, 124t
    recirculation system in, 123
    replenishment in, 122, 123b
    solution performance in, 123b
    standby control in, 122
    temperature control in, 123
Automatic film processor, 119, 120f
Automatic rescaling, 88, 89f
Average gradient, 137–138, 138f

B

Back screen, of intensifying screen, 116
Backup time, in automatic exposure control, 213–214
    defined, 213
    function of, 214b
    monitoring, 214b
    setting, 214, 214b
Bariatric patients, in exposure technique, 229
Barium platinocyanide, 2
Base, of intensifying screen, 115b
Beam alignment, quality control check for, 187b
Beam attenuation, 43–46
    defined, 43
    factors affecting, 47–49, 49b, 50t
    and photoelectric effect, 44, 45f
    and photon absorption, 44, 44b
    and scattering, 44–46, 45b
    and tissue density, 48–49, 50t
    and tissue thickness, 47, 47f–48f, 50t
    and tissue type, 47–49, 48f, 50t
    and x-ray beam quality, 49, 49f, 50t
Beam filtration, 34–35
    added, 35, 35f
    compensating filters with, 36, 37f
    inherent, 35, 35f
    low-energy photons and, 34, 34b
    quality-control check for, 36b
    radiation protection and, 36b
    total, 35
    and x-ray quality and quantity, 36f
Beam penetrability, kilovoltage and, 27, 27b
Beam restriction, 10, 11b, 180
    appropriate, 180b
    compensation for, 182
    and contrast, 181, 181b

Beam restriction *(Continued)*
  defined, 180
  devices for, 182–188
    aperture diaphragms as, 183, 183f–184f
    collimators as, 184–186, 186f–187f
      automatic, 187–188, 187b
      quality-control check for, 187b
    cones and cylinders as, 183–184, 184f–186f
    positive beam-limiting, 187–188, 187b
  and exposure, to image receptor, 182, 182b
  as exposure technique factors, 169, 169b
  in image receptors
    digital, 245t
    film-screen, 246t
  and patient dose, 180b
  purposes of, 180
  result of, 182t
  and scatter radiation, 180–182, 181b, 182f
  unrestricted primary beam and, 180, 181f
Binary digits, 72b
Binary number system, 72b
Bit, 72b
Bit depth. *see* Pixel bit depth
Black/white reversal, postprocessing, 102, 103f
Blue-sensitive film, 114–115
Body habitus, 170, 171f
Bremsstrahlung interactions, 20, 21f, 21b
Bremsstrahlung x-rays, 23f
Brightness. *see* Image brightness
Brightness gain, in fluoroscopy, 265, 265b
Bucky, 193
Bucky, Gustave, 188
Bucky factor, 194, 195t
Bucky slot cover, in fluoroscopic equipment inspection, 268b
Byte, 72b

C

Calibration, in automatic exposure control, 219–220, 219b–220b
Calipers, 224–225, 225f
Camera tube, in viewing systems, of fluoroscopy, 267–269, 269f
Cassette
    for computed tomography, 75, 75f
    for film-screen imaging, 111, 118–119
Cassette spot filming, in fluoroscopy, 273–274, 273f
Casts, in exposure technique, 230
Cathode, 16, 16f, 18f
Cathode ray tube (CRT) monitor, 94
    in fluoroscopy, 270–271, 271f
CCD. *see* Charge-coupled device (CCD)
Central ray
    angulation of, 60
    in image receptors

Central ray (Continued)
  digital, 245t
  film-screen, 246t
  misalignment of, 59
Characteristic interactions, 21–22, 22f, 22b
Characteristic x-rays, 21, 22f–23f
Charge-coupled device (CCD)
  in digital fluoroscopy, 275
  in viewing systems, of fluoroscopy, 269–270, 270f
Cine camera, in fluoroscopy, 264f, 270
Coherent scattering, 46
Collimation, in automatic exposure control, 218, 219b
Collimator shutters, in fluoroscopic equipment
    inspection, 268b
Collimators, 184–186
  automatic, 187–188, 187b
  lead shutters of, 184–186, 186f
  quality-control check for, 187b
  x-ray field measurement guide on, 184–186, 187f
Comparative anatomy, in exposure technique chart
    development, 228
Compensating filters, 36, 37f, 170
Compton effect, 44–45, 46f
  and photoelectric effect, 47b
Compton electron, 44–45
Computed radiography (CR), 68, 75–81, 78f
  digital image receptors, 76f, 76b
    analog-to-digital converter of, 77, 78f
    helium-neon laser beam or solid state laser diode
        in, 77, 78f
    imaging plate of, 75, 75f–77f
    matrix size in, 79b, 80f
    photomultiplier tube of, 77, 78f
    photostimulable phosphor, 75, 76f
    pixel pitch of, 77–79, 79f
    reader unit of, 77, 77f
    sampling frequency of, 77–79, 79f
    sampling pitch of, 77–79
    trapped electrons in, 77
  exposure indicator for, 242, 242b
  in image analysis, activity on, 257–258, 257f–258f
  vendor-specific exposure indicators, 89t
Cones, for beam restriction, 183–184, 184f–186f
Continuous fluoroscopy, 278–279, 278f, 278b
Contrast
  beam restriction and, 181, 181b
  in image evaluation, 238–239
    high (short-scale), 239, 239f–240f
    low (long-scale), 239, 239f–240f
Contrast enhancement, postprocessing, 101, 102f
Contrast media, in exposure technique, 232, 233f
Contrast resolution, 55, 71b, 73f
  of digital image, 96
  processing, 99

Contrast-to-noise ratio, of digital imaging system, 86,
    86b, 87f
Convergent line, 192–193, 192f
Convergent point, 192–193, 192f
Conversion efficiency, and screen speed, 117
Conversion factor, in fluoroscopy, 265, 265b
Coupling of devices, in viewing systems, of
    fluoroscopy, 270
Coupling systems, television monitor and, 271b
CR. see Computed radiography (CR)
Crookes tube, 1–2, 3f
Crossed grid, 190, 190f
Cross-hatched grid, 190, 190f
CRT monitor. see Cathode ray tube (CRT) monitor
Cylinders, for beam restriction, 183–184, 184f–186f

D
Darkroom, quality control in, 125, 128b
Deadman switches, 23
Degree of quantization, in computed radiography,
    79–81
Densitometer, 129, 130f–131f
Density
  image, 52
    and image contrast, 53–54, 55f
    milliamperage and, 151, 152f, 152b
    and quantity of radiation, 53
  in image evaluation, 238, 238f
  optical, 131
    diagnostic range of, 131
    formula for, 132b
    and transmittance, 131
  optimal, 140–141, 140f
  tissue
    and beam attenuation, 48–49, 50t
    and image brightness, 51–53, 51f, 52b, 53f–54f
Density adjustment, in automatic exposure control, 214
Density controls, in automatic exposure control, 214
Destructive diseases, exposure techniques with, 231t
Detail screens, 117–118
Detective quantum efficiency (DQE), of digital imaging
    system, 85, 85b
Detector(s)
  flat-panel
    for digital fluoroscopy, 275–277, 276f
    in direct radiography, 81–82, 81f–82f
      direct conversion, 83, 84f
      indirect conversion, 82–83
  radiation, in automatic exposure control, 209–212,
      210f, 210b
    ionization chamber systems as, 210–212, 211f, 212b
    phototimers as, 210, 211f
  selection of, 215, 215b, 216f
  size of, 217–218

Detector elements (DEL), in direct digital radiography, 81

Developing, of film, 119–121, 120t

Developing agents, 119, 120b

Differential absorption, 43–51, 44f
  beam attenuation in, 43–46
    defined, 43
    factors affecting, 47–49, 49b, 50t
    and photoelectric effect, 44, 45f
    and photon absorption, 44, 44b
    and scattering, 44–46, 45b
    and tissue density, 48–49, 50t
    and tissue thickness, 47, 47f–48f, 50t
    and tissue type, 47–49, 48f, 50t
    and x-ray beam quality, 49, 49f, 50t
  defined, 43
  and image brightness, 51–53, 51f, 52b, 53f–54f
  and image formation, 43b

Diffusion, in washing process, 121

Digital communication networks, 104–105, 105f

Digital fluoroscopy, 275–278, 276f, 278b

Digital image display, 93–104
  display monitors in, 94–103
    cathode ray tube (CRT), 94, 95f
    contrast resolution of, 96
    landscape, 94
    liquid crystal display, 94, 96f
    luminance of, 96
    performance criteria for, 96
    portrait, 94, 95f
    primary, 96
    types of, 94–95, 95f
    viewing conditions for, 95–96
  laser printers for, 104
  postprocessing in, 98–103
    black/white reversal in, 102, 103f
    brightness, 98–99, 99f
      window level, 99f, 99b
    contrast enhancement in, 101, 102f
    contrast resolution in, 99
    edge enhancement in, 102, 102f
    electronic masking, 98
    smoothing in, 102
    subtraction in, 101, 101f
  soft copy viewing for, 93–94, 94f

Digital image processing, 86–92
  automatic rescaling in, 88, 89f
  exposure indicator in, 88–90, 90b
  histogram analysis in, 87–90, 87f–88f, 88b
  lookup tables in, 90–92, 91f, 92b, 93f
    with change in pixel values, 91f
    with no change in pixel values, 91f

Digital image quality, activity on, 246–247, 247f, 247t

Digital image receptors
  computed radiography, 76f, 76b
    analog-to-digital converter of, 77, 78f
    helium-neon laser beam or solid state laser diode in, 77, 78f
    imaging plate of, 75, 75f–77f
    matrix size in, 79b, 80f
    photomultiplier tube of, 77, 78f
    photostimulable phosphor, 75, 76f
    pixel depth, 79–81
    pixel pitch of, 77–79, 79f
    quality control checks for, 97b–98b
    reader unit of, 77, 77f
    sampling frequency of, 77–79, 79f
    sampling pitch of, 77–79
    trapped electrons in, 77
  detective quantum efficiency with, 85, 85b
  direct radiography, 81–83
    flat-panel detectors as, 81–82, 81f–82f
      direct conversion, 83, 84f
      indirect conversion, 82–83, 83f
    dynamic range, 83–84, 85f, 85b
    exposure technique factors and, 245t
    signal-to-noise ratio with, 85–86, 86b

Digital imaging, 67–109
  artifacts, 93, 94f
  automatic exposure control with, 221t
  contrast resolution in, 71b, 73f
  dynamic range in, 83–84, 84b–85b
  excessive radiation exposure and, 153b
  exposure errors in, 152, 153b
  exposure technique charts with, 223b
  field of view in, 68, 69f, 70b
  image contrast in, 55
  kilovoltage peak and, 157, 157b
  matrix and pixels in, 68, 69f, 70b
  pixel bit depth in, 70b–71b, 79–81
  pixel density and pixel pitch in, 72, 72f, 72b
  pixel values, 71f, 87f
  receptors, 75–86
  scatter control and, 204
  terminology for, 70b
  vs. film-screen imaging, 63–64

Digital Imaging and Communications in Medicine (DICOM), 105
  Grayscale Standard Display Function (GSDF), 96

Direct conversion detectors, for direct digital radiography, 83, 84f

Direct radiography (DR), 75
  exposure indicator for, 243
  image receptors in, 81–83
    flat-panel detectors as, 81–82, 81f–82f
      direct conversion, 83, 84f
      indirect conversion, 82–83, 83f

Display monitors, 94–103
    cathode ray tube (CRT), 94, 95f
    contrast resolution of, 96, 99
    landscape, 94
    liquid crystal display, 94, 96f
    luminance of, 96
    performance criteria for, 96
    portrait, 94, 95f
    primary, 96
    types of, 94–95, 95f
    viewing conditions for, 95–96
Distance, radiation protection and, 10
Distortion, 58–60
    in fluoroscopy, 267, 267f
    in image evaluation, 240–241, 241f
    shape, 59–60, 60f, 60b, 165–167, 166f
    size, 58–59, 59b
        object-to-image-receptor distance (OID) and, 162,
            163f, 163b
        source-to-image-receptor distance and, 161, 161f,
            161b
Dose equivalent, 8
Dosimeter, 36b
Drying, of film, 120t, 122
Dual-focus tubes, 16
Duration (s), of x-ray beams, 11
Dynamic imaging. see Fluoroscopy
Dynamic range, 83–84, 84b–85b, 111, 112b
    of digital image receptors, 83–84, 85f

E
Edge enhancement, postprocessing, 102, 102f
Effective focal spot size, 32, 32f
    anode angle and, 33f, 33b
Electrolytic method, silver recovery by, 126
Electromagnetic radiation, 1, 5
Electromagnetic spectrum, 5, 5f
Electron speed, kilovoltage and, 26b
Electrostatic focusing lenses, in fluoroscopy, 263,
    264f
Elongation, 59, 60f
Emulsion, of film, 111–113
Energy
    defined, 5
    x-rays as, 5–8, 5f–7f
Energy conversion, in x-ray tube, 24, 25b
Envelope, of x-ray tube, 19, 19f
Erythema, due to x-ray exposure, 5
Exam, duplication of, x-rays and, 11, 11b
Exit-beam intensities, kilovoltage peak and, 155, 156f
Exit radiation, 49–51, 51f
Exposure, 7
    reproducibility of, 31b
Exposure button, 23

Exposure control
    automatic, 209–220
        alignment and positioning considerations in,
            215–218
            detector selection as, 215, 215b, 216f
            detector size as, 217–218
            patient centering as, 215–217, 216b, 217f
        backup time in, 213–214
            function of, 214b
            monitoring, 214b
            setting, 214, 214b
        compensating issues in, 218–220
            calibration as, 219–220, 219b–220b
            collimation as, 218, 219b
            image receptor variations as, 219, 219b
            patient considerations as, 218, 218b
        density adjustment in, 214
        with digital imaging, 221t
        with film-screen radiography, 222t
        kVp and mA selections in, 212–213, 212b–213b
        mAs readout, 212, 212b
        minimum response time in, 213
        principle of, 209, 209b
        radiation detectors in, 209–212, 210f, 210b
            ionization chamber systems as, 210–212, 211f,
                212b
            phototimers as, 210, 211f
    exposure technique charts for, 223–228
        conditions for, 224–225
        defined, 223
        development of, 228, 228b
        and digital imaging, 223b
        measurement with, 224, 225f
        and radiographic quality, 224b
        types of, 225–228
            fixed kVp/variable mAs, 227–228, 227t, 227b
            variable kVp/fixed mAs, 225–226, 226t, 226b
Exposure errors
    in digital imaging, 152, 153b
    in film-screen imaging, 153, 153f, 153b
Exposure index (EI) numbers, on exposure indicator, 89
Exposure indicator, 150–151, 151b
    in digital image processing, 88–90, 90b
    in image evaluation, 242–243, 242b
Exposure intensity, defined, 128–129
Exposure latitude, 138–140, 139f
Exposure switch, in fluoroscopic equipment inspection,
    268b
Exposure technique, 62
    selection of, 208–236
        special considerations in, 229–232
Exposure technique charts, 223–228
    conditions for, 224–225
    defined, 223

Exposure technique charts *(Continued)*
    development of, 228, 228b
    and digital imaging, 223b
    measurement with, 224, 225f
    and radiographic quality, 224b
    types of, 225–228
        fixed kVp/variable mAs, 227–228, 227t, 227b
        variable kVp/fixed mAs, 225–226, 226t, 226b
Exposure technique factors, 147–177
    beam restriction as, 169, 169b
    calculating magnification as, 163–165
        determining object size in, 164, 165b
        magnification factor in, 163, 164b
        object % of magnification in, 165, 165b
        source-to-object distance in, 163, 164f
    central ray alignment as, 165–167, 166f
    compensating filters as, 170
    effect on x-ray beams, 173t–174t
    focal spot size as, 158, 158b, 159f
    generator output as, 169
    grids as, 167–168
        adjusting mAs for, 168, 168b
        grid conversion chart for, 168, 169t
        and image receptor exposure, 167, 167b
        and radiographic contrast, 167, 167b, 168f
        and scatter absorption, 167, 167f, 167b
        selection of, 168b
    in image evaluation, 244–246
        with digital image receptors, 245t
        with film-screen image receptors, 246t
    and image quality, 174t–175t
    kilovoltage peak as, 152–158
        and 15% rule, 154, 154b–155b
        and density, 153, 154f
        and digital image quality, 157, 157b
        and exit-beam intensities, 155, 156f
        and exposure to image receptor, 152–155, 152b
            in digital imaging, 152, 153b
            in film-screen imaging, 153, 153f, 153b
        and radiographic contrast, 155–158, 155b, 157b
        and scatter radiation, 157, 157b
    mathematical calculations in, 173t
    milliamperage as
        and density, 151, 152f, 152b
        and digital image brightness, 150, 150b
        and exposure time, 150b
            adjustment of, 149, 149b
            exposure indicator for, 150–151, 151b
            maintaining mAs with, 149, 150b
        and quantum noise, 150, 151f
        and x-ray quality, 148–149, 149f, 149b
    object-to-image-receptor distance (OID) as,
        162–163
        and air gap, 162, 162f

Exposure technique factors *(Continued)*
    defined, 163
        and size distortion, 162, 163f, 163b
        and spatial resolution, 162, 163b
    patient, 170–172
        body habitus as, 170, 171f
        part thickness as, 172
    primary, 148–158
    secondary, 158–170
    source-to-image-receptor distance as, 158–161
        inverse-square law for, 158–159, 159b
        mAs-distance compensation formula for, 160,
            160b
        and size distortion, 161, 161f, 161b
        and x-ray beam intensity, 159, 159b, 160f
    tube filtration as, 169–170, 170b
Exposure time, 30
    milliamperage and, 30–31, 150b
        adjustment of, 149, 149b
        exposure indicator for, 150–151, 151b
        linearity of, 31b
        maintaining mAs with, 149, 150b
        and x-ray quality, 148–149, 149f, 149b
    quality-control check for, 30b
    and x-ray quantity, 30b
Extrapolation, in exposure technique chart
    development, 228
Extremity screens, 117–118

F
Feed tray, of processor system, 122, 123f
Field of view (FOV), 68, 69f, 70b
Field size
    result of increasing, 182t
    and scatter radiation, 179, 180b
15% rule, kilovoltage peak and, 154, 154b–155b
Filament, of x-ray tube, 16, 16f, 16b, 18f
    large and small, 16, 16f
    during x-ray exposure, 25f
Filament current, 23, 25f
Film, 112–115
    characteristics of, 135–140
    composition of, 112–113, 112b
    contrast of, 114, 137–138, 138f
        and average gradient, 137–138, 138f
        and determining slope of line, 137b
        and gradient point, 137
        maximum, 141, 141f–142f
    exposure latitude in, 138–140, 139f
    latent image formation on, 113–114, 113f
    latitude of, 114
    limitations of, 112b
    processing of, 119–128
    screen, 113

Film *(Continued)*
  sensitivity specks on, 113–114
  sensitometry of, 128–129
    equipment for, 129
      densitometer as, 129, 130f–131f
      penetrometer as, 129, 129f–130f
      sensitometer as, 129
  size of, 112–113
  spectral sensitivity of, 114–115
  speed of, 114, 135
    and speed exposure point, 135, 136f–137f
    and speed point, 135, 136f
  storage of, 125
Film artifacts, 125, 126f–127f
Film cameras, in fluoroscopy, 273f, 274
Film contrast, 114, 137–138, 138f
  and average gradient, 137–138, 138f
  and determining slope of line, 137b
  and gradient point, 137
  maximum, 141, 141f–142f
Film image evaluation, in image analysis, activity on,
    254–257, 254f, 256f
Film latitude, 114
Film processing, 119–128
  automatic, 119–124
    automatic film processor for, 119, 120f
    recirculation system in, 123
    stages of, 119, 120t
      developing as, 119–121, 120t
      drying as, 120t, 122
      fixing as, 121
      washing as, 120t, 121–122
    systems for, 122–124, 123f
      feed tray in, 122, 123f
      immersion heater in, 124
      inadequate processing in, 124t
      replenishment in, 122, 123b
      solution performance in, 123b
      standby control in, 122
      temperature control in, 123
  inadequate, 124
  quality control for, 125, 126f–127f, 128b
  silver recovery in, 125–128, 128b
Film sensitivity, and silver halide, 114b
Film speed, 114, 135
  and speed exposure point, 135, 136f–137f
  and speed point, 135, 136f
Film-screen image quality, activity on, 247–248, 247t, 248f
Film-screen image receptors
  exposure technique factors and, 246t
  intensifying screens in, 115–119, 115f
    absorption efficiency of, 117
    composition of, 115–116, 115b
    conversion efficiency of, 117

Film-screen image receptors *(Continued)*
    fluorescence of, 116
    luminescence, 116
    quality-control check for, 119b
    speed of, 116–119
      for detail or extremity, 117–118
      factors affecting, 117, 117t
      and light emission, 117b
      and milliamperage, 118, 118b
      and patient dose, 117b
      and recorded detail, 116, 116b, 117t
      relative, 117–118
  radiographic film in, 112–115
    composition of, 112–113, 112b
    contrast of, 114, 137–138, 138f
      and average gradient, 137–138, 138f
      and determining slope of line, 137b
      and gradient point, 137
      maximum, 141, 141f–142f
    double-emulsion, 113
    exposure latitude of, 138–140, 139f
    latent image formation on, 113–114, 113f
    latitude of, 114
    limitations of, 112b
    screen film as, 113
    size of, 112–113
    spectral sensitivity in, 114–115
    speed of, 114, 135
Film-screen imaging, 110–146
  active layer or emulsion in, 111
  automatic exposure control with, 217
  cassette of, 118–119
  clinical considerations for, 140–143
    image display in, 142–143
      illuminators for, 142–143
    maximum film contrast in, 141, 141f–142f
    optimal density in, 140–141, 140f
  and dynamic range, 63b
  image contrast in, 55
  intensifying screens in, 115–119, 115f
    absorption efficiency of, 117
    composition of, 115–116, 115b
    conversion efficiency of, 117
    fluorescence of, 116
    luminescence, 116
    quality-control check for, 119b
    speed of, 116–119
      for detail or extremity, 117–118
      factors affecting, 117, 117t
      and light emission, 117b
      and milliamperage, 118, 118b
      and patient dose, 117b
      and recorded detail, 116, 116b, 117t
      relative, 117–118

Film-screen imaging (Continued)
  and optical density, 131
    diagnostic range of, 131
    formula for, 132b
    and transmittance, 131
  practical tips for, 142b
  radiographic film in, 112–115
    composition of, 112–113, 112b
    contrast of, 114, 137–138, 138f
      and average gradient, 137–138, 138f
      and determining slope of line, 137b
      and gradient point, 137
      maximum, 141, 141f–142f
    double-emulsion, 113
    exposure latitude of, 138–140, 139f
    latent image formation on, 113–114, 113f
    latitude of, 114
    limitations of, 112b
    screen film as, 113
    size of, 112–113
    spectral sensitivity in, 114–115
    speed of, 114, 135
      and speed exposure point, 135, 136f–137f
      and speed point, 135, 136f
  sensitometric curve in, 132–135, 133f
    log of relative exposure and, 133, 134f
    other terms for, 133b
    regions of, 133–135, 134f
      shoulder, 135
      straight-line, 135
      toe, 135
  sensitometry, 128–129
    equipment for, 129
      densitometer as, 129, 130f–131f
      penetrometer as, 129, 129f–130f
      sensitometer as, 129
  vs. digital imaging, 63–64
Film-screen speed
  in image quality calculations, 250, 250t
  in image receptors
    digital, 245t
    film-screen, 246t
525-line systems, in fluoroscopy, 271
Fixed kVp/variable mAs technique chart, 227–228,
    227t, 227b
Fixing, in film processing, 121
Fixing agent, 121, 121b
Flat-panel detectors (FPD)
  for digital fluoroscopy, 275–277, 276f
  for direct radiography, 81–82, 81f–82f
    direct conversion, 83, 84f
    indirect conversion, 82–83, 83f
Fluorescence, 2
  of intensifying screens, 116

Fluoroscopic timer, in fluoroscopic equipment
    inspection, 268b
Fluoroscopy, 262–284
  automatic brightness control in, 265, 265b
  brightness gain in, 265, 265b
  continuous, 278–279, 278f, 278b
  conversion factor in, 265, 265b
  digital, 275–278, 276f, 278b
  equipment inspection checklist, 267, 268b
  image intensification, 263–265, 263b, 264f
  magnification mode in, 266–267, 266f–268f
    patient dose and, 266b
  pulsed, 278–279, 278f, 279b
  quality control for, 280–281, 281b
  radiation safety with, 279–280, 280t
  recording systems in, 273–274, 273f, 274b
  viewing systems for, 267–273
    coupling of devices in, 270, 271b
    liquid crystal display (LCD) monitors in, 271–272,
        272f
    plasma monitors in, 272–273, 273f
    television cameras in, 267–270, 269f–270f
    television monitor in, 270–271, 271f, 271b
  vignetting in, 267
Flux gain, in fluoroscopy, 265
Focal distance, 192–193
Focal range, 192–193
Focal spot, 18, 19f
Focal spot size
  actual, 32, 32f
  anode angle and, 33f, 33b
  effective, 32, 32f
  as exposure technique factors, 158, 158b, 159f
  in image receptors
    digital, 245t
    film-screen, 246t
Focal track, 18, 19f
Focused grid, 190–193, 192b
  convergent point and convergent line with, 192–193,
      192f
  focal distance of, 192–193
  focal range of, 192–193, 192f
  transmitted photons passing through, 190–191, 191f
Focusing cup, 16, 16f, 18f
  during x-ray exposure, 26f
Fog
  in image artifacts, 243
  from scatter, 61, 61f
Foreign bodies, image artifacts due to, 62
Foreshortening, 59, 60f
FOV. see Field of view (FOV)
Frequency, of x-rays, 6
  wavelength and, 6f–7f, 6b
Front screen, of intensifying screen, 116

G

GCF. *see* Grid conversion factor (GCF)
Generator factor, 37, 37t
Generator output, 169
Geriatric patients, in exposure technique, 229
Glass envelope x-ray tube, 19–20, 19f
Gonadal shielding, 9–10
Gray scale, 55, 239
Grayscale Standard Display Function
    (GSDF), 96
Green sensitive film, 114–115
Grid(s), 188–202, 188f
    addition of, 194, 194b
    adjusting mAs for, 168, 168b
    construction of, 189–190
    crossed or cross-hatched, 190, 190f
    decreasing grid ratio of, 195b
    as exposure technique factors, 167–168
    focused, 190–193, 192b
        convergent point and convergent line with,
            192–193, 192f
        focal distance of, 192–193
        focal range of, 192–193, 192f
        transmitted photons passing through, 190–191,
            191f
    grid conversion chart for, 168, 169t
    and image receptor exposure, 167, 167b
    in image receptors
        digital, 245t
        film-screen, 246t
    increasing grid ratio of, 196b
    interspace material in, 189
    linear, 190, 190f
        long-dimension *versus* short-dimension, 193–194,
            193f
    Moiré effect with, 200, 201f
    parallel (nonfocused), 190–191, 191f
        transmitted photons passing through, 190–191,
            191f
    performance of, 194–196
    and radiographic contrast, 167, 167b, 168f
    reciprocating, 193
    removing of, 195b
    and scatter absorption, 167, 167f, 167b
    selection of, 168b
    stationary, 193
    types of, 193–194
    typical, 201, 202b
    usage of, 200–201
    wafer, 193
Grid alignment, 201, 202b
Grid cap, 193
Grid cassette, 193
Grid conversion chart, 168, 169t

Grid conversion factor (GCF), 194, 195t
    when adding grid, 194, 194b
    when decreasing grid ratio, 195b
    when increasing grid ratio, 196b
    when removing grid, 195b
Grid conversions, in image quality calculations,
    249–250, 249t
Grid cutoff, 196–200
    defined, 196
    errors in, 196–200, 199b, 202b
    off-center, 198, 198b, 199f
    off-focus, 198–200, 198b, 200f
    off-level, 197, 197b, 198f
    upside-down focused, 197, 197f, 197b
Grid focus, 190–193
Grid frequency, 189
    and lead content, 189
Grid pattern, 190, 190f
Grid radius, 192–193
Grid ratio, 189, 189f
    calculation of, 189b
    decreasing, 195b
    and exposure to image receptor, 194, 194b
    and grid conversion factor, 194, 195t
    increasing, 196b, 200t
    and lead content, 189
    and patient dose, 196b
    and radiographic contrast, 189, 189b
    range of, 189
    selection of, 196b
Grid uniformity, quality-control check for, 201, 202b
GSDF. *see* Grayscale Standard Display Function (GSDF)
Gurney-Mott theory, 113

H

Half-value layer (HVL), 36b
Health Level Seven standard (HL7), 105
Heat dissipation, in anode tube, 18, 18b
Heat loads, of rotating anode tube, 18
Heat units, 37–38, 37b
Helium-neon laser beam, in computed radiography,
    77, 78f
High-contrast film, 114
High-contrast image, 55, 56f–57f, 239, 239f–240f
High-frequency generators, 28, 28f–29f
HIS. *see* Hospital information systems (HIS)
Histogram analysis, 87–90, 87f–88f, 88b
HL7. *see* Health Level Seven standard (HL7)
Hospital information systems (HIS), 104
HVL. *see* Half-value layer (HVL)
Hydroquinone, in film developing, 119
Hypersthenic body habitus, 170, 171f
Hypo, as fixing agent, 121
Hyposthenic body habitus, 170, 171f

I

Illuminators, 142–143, 143f
Image analysis, 253
    activities on, 254–255
        computed radiography image evaluation, 257–258, 257f–258f
        film image evaluation, 254–257, 254f, 256f
Image artifacts, 62–63, 63f
    in image evaluation, 243–244, 244f
Image brightness, 52–53, 53f–54f, 53b, 238, 238f
    diagnostic, 53
    excessive, 53, 54f
    and image contrast, 53–55
    in image evaluation, 238, 238f
    insufficient, 53, 54f
    milliamperage and, 150, 150b
    postprocessing for, 98–103
    and quantity of radiation, 53
    and tissue density, 51, 51f, 52b
    window level and, 98
Image characteristics, in digital imaging, 68–75
    contrast resolution in, 71b, 73f
    dynamic range as, 83–84, 84b–85b
    field of view as, 68, 69f, 70b
    matrix and pixels in, 68, 69f, 70b
    pixel bit depth in, 70b–71b, 79–81
    pixel density and pixel pitch in, 72, 72f, 72b
    pixel values, 71f, 87f
Image contrast, 53–55, 99–103, 100f–101f, 238–239
    in abdomen, 54, 56f
    and contrast resolution, 55
    and density and brightness, 53–54
    desired level in, 55
    for differentiating among anatomic tissues, 54b
    in digital imaging, 55
    in film-screen imaging, 55
    grids and, 167, 167b, 168f
    high (short-scale), 55, 56f–57f, 239, 239f–240f
    of homogeneous object, 53–54, 55f
    kilovoltage peak and, 155–158, 155b
    low (long-scale), 55, 56f–57f, 239, 239f–240f
    of object with different absorption characteristics, 53–54, 55f
    and sharpness, 58, 59f
    subject, 54
    in thorax, 54, 56f
    window width and, 99, 100b
Image density, 238, 238f
    and image contrast, 53–54, 55f
    milliamperage and, 151, 152f, 152b
    and quantity of radiation, 53
Image display
    digital, 93–104
        display monitors, 94–103

Image display *(Continued)*
        cathode ray tube (CRT), 94, 95f
        contrast resolution of, 99
        landscape, 94
        liquid crystal display, 94, 96f
        luminance of, 96
        performance criteria for, 96
        portrait, 94, 95f
        primary, 96
        types of, 94–95, 95f
        viewing conditions for, 95–96
    laser printers for, 104
    postprocessing, 98–103
        black/white reversal in, 102, 103f
        brightness, 98–99
        contrast enhancement in, 101
        contrast resolution, 99
        edge enhancement in, 102, 102f
        electronic masking, 98
        equalization, 102, 104f
        smoothing, 102
        window level, 98
        window width in, 99, 100b
    for film-screen imaging, 142–143
    illuminators for, 142–143, 143f
Image evaluation, 237–261
    activities on, 251–253, 252t–253t
    analysis of, 253
        activities in, 254–258, 254f, 256f–258f
    criteria for, 237–244
        brightness or density as, 238, 238f
        contrast as, 238–239, 239f–240f
        distortion as, 240–241, 241f
        exposure indicator as, 242–243, 242b
        image artifacts as, 243–244, 244f
        quantum noise as, 241–242, 242f
        spatial resolution or recorded detail as, 240, 241f
    exposure technique factors in, 244–246
        for digital image receptors, 245t
        for film-screen image receptors, 246t
        for image quality, 245–246
Image formation, 42–66
    and differential absorption, 43–51, 44f
        beam attenuation in, 43–46
            defined, 43
            factors affecting, 47–49, 49b, 50t
            and photoelectric effect, 44, 45f
            and photon absorption, 44, 44b
            and scattering, 44–46, 45b
            and tissue density, 48–49, 50t
            and tissue thickness, 47, 47f, 50t
            and tissue type, 47–49, 48f, 50t
            and x-ray beam quality, 49, 49f, 50t
        and image brightness, 51, 51f, 52b

Image formation *(Continued)*
  and image brightness, 52–53, 52b, 53f–54f
  transmission in, 49, 50f
    and exit radiation, 49–51, 51f
    and latent image, 51
    and x-ray interaction with matter, 50b
Image intensification, in fluoroscopy, 263–265, 263b, 264f
Image noise. *see* Quantum noise
Image processing
  digital, 86–92
    automatic rescaling in, 88
    exposure indicator in, 88–90, 89f
    histogram analysis in, 87–90, 87f–88f, 88b
    lookup tables in, 90–92, 91f, 92b, 93f
      with change in pixel values, 91f
      with no change in pixel values, 91f
  film, 119–128
    automatic, 119–124
      automatic film processor for, 119, 120f
      developing in, 119–121, 120t
      drying in, 120t, 122
      fixing in, 121
      stages of, 119, 120t
      washing in, 120t, 121–122
    inadequate processing in, 124, 124t
    processor systems for, 122–124, 123f
      feed tray in, 122, 123f
      immersion heater in, 124
      recirculation system in, 123
      replenishment in, 122, 123b
      solution performance in, 123b
      standby control in, 122
      temperature control in, 123
    silver recovery in, 125–128, 128b
  quality control for, 125, 126f–127f, 128b
Image quality
  activities on
    digital, 246–247, 247f, 247t
    exposure conversions, 250, 250t–251t
    film-screen, 247–248, 247t, 248f
  criteria for, 237–244
    brightness or density as, 238, 238f
    contrast as, 238–239, 239f–240f
    distortion as, 240–241, 241f
    exposure indicator as, 242–243, 242b
    image artifacts as, 243–244, 244f
    quantum noise as, 241–242, 242f
    spatial resolution or recorded detail as, 240, 241f
  exposure technique factors in, 244–246
    for digital image receptors, 245t
    for film-screen image receptors, 246t
  and scatter, 60–61, 61f
  scatter radiation and, 188, 188b

Image quality *(Continued)*
  spatial resolution and recorded detail in, 57, 57b
    and image contrast, 58, 59f
    and patient motion, 58, 58f
Image quality calculations, 248–250, 248t–250t
Image receptor (IR), 43
  computed radiography, 76f, 76b
    analog-to-digital converter of, 77, 78f
    helium-neon laser beam or solid state laser diode in, 77, 78f
    imaging plate of, 75, 75f–77f
    matrix size in, 79b, 80f
    photomultiplier tube of, 77, 78f
    photostimulable phosphor, 75, 76f
    pixel pitch of, 77–79, 79f
    reader unit of, 77, 77f
    sampling frequency of, 77–79, 79f
    sampling pitch of, 77–79
    trapped electrons in, 77
  contrast-to-noise ratio of, 86, 86b, 87f
  detective quantum efficiency with, 85, 85b
  digital, 75–86
    dynamic range with, 83–84, 85f, 85b
    signal-to-noise ratio with, 85–86, 86b
  direct radiography, 81–83
    direct conversion, 83, 84f
    flat-panel detectors as, 81–82, 81f–82f
      indirect conversion, 82–83, 83f
  exposure technique factors for
    digital, 245t
    film-screen, 246t
  exposure to
    beam restriction and, 182, 182b
    grid ratio and, 194, 194b
  kilovoltage peak and exposure to, 152–155, 152b
    in digital imaging, 152, 153b
    in film-screen imaging, 153, 153f, 153b
Image receptor (IR) variations, in automatic exposure control, 219, 219b
Imaging artifacts, digital, 93, 94f
Imaging plate (IP), 75, 75f–77f
  and matrix size, 79b, 80f
Immersion heater, in processor systems, 124
Important relationships
  anode angle and effective focal spot size, 33b
  anode heel effect, 33b
  archival quality of radiographs, 121b–122b
  beam restriction and image receptor exposure, 169b
  Bremsstrahlung interactions, 21b
  brightness and radiographic quality, 53b
  brightness gain, 265b
  cassette spot filming, 274b
  characteristic interactions, 22b
  clearing the unexposed crystals, 121b

Important relationships *(Continued)*
  continuous fluoroscopy, 278b
  coupling systems and the television monitor, 271b
  creating latent image, 52b
  developer temperature and radiographic quality, 124b
  developing or reducing agents, 120b
  differential absorption and image formation, 43b
  differentiating among anatomic tissues, 54b
  digital fluoroscopic systems, 278b
  dissipating heat, 18b
  dual nature of x-ray energy, 6b
  dynamic range and film-screen imaging, 63b, 112b
  energy conversion in x-ray tube, 25b
  exposure errors and film-screen imaging, 153b
  exposure errors in digital imaging, 153b
  exposure indicator value, 151b
  exposure time, tube current, and x-ray quantity, 30b
  factors affecting beam attenuation, 49b
  filament, 16b
  film-screen system speed and mAs, 118b
  focal spot size and spatial resolution, 158b
  grids, scatter, and contrast, 167b
  grids and image receptor exposure, 167b
  image brightness, 52b
  image-intensified fluoroscopy, 263b
  interactions that produce x-ray photons, 20b
  kilovoltage, scatter radiation, and radiographic contrast, 157b
  kilovoltage and digital image quality, 157b
  kilovoltage and speed of electrons, 26b
  kVp and 15% rule, 154b
  kVp and beam penetrability, 27b
  kVp and the radiographic image, 152b
  line-focus principle, 32b
  low-energy photons, patient dose, and image formation, 34b
  magnification mode and patient dose, 266b
  mAs and digital image brightness, 150b
  mAs and film-screen density, 152b
  mAs and quantity of radiation, 149b
  milliamperage, tube current, and x-ray quantity, 30b
  milliamperage and exposure time, 150b
  number of photons and quantum noise, 61b
  OID, size distortion, and spatial resolution, 163b
  production of x-rays, 20b
  pulsed fluoroscopy, 279b
  quantity of electrons, x-rays, and mAs, 31b
  replenishment and solution performance, 123b
  rotating anodes, 19b
  screen speed, light emission, and patient dose, 117b
  screen speed and recorded detail, 116b
  sensitivity specks and latent image centers, 114b

Important relationships *(Continued)*
  shape distortion, 60b
  sharpness of anatomic detail, 57b
  SID, size distortion, and spatial resolution, 161b
  SID and mAs, 160b
  SID and x-ray beam intensity, 159b
  silver halide and film sensitivity, 114b
  silver recovery, 128b
  size distortion, 59b
  speed of electrons and quality of x-rays, 27b
  target, 17b
  thermionic emission, 23b
  tube current, 24b
  tube filtration, radiation quantity and energy, 170b
  tungsten, 18b
  wavelength and frequency, 6b
  x-ray beam scattering, 45b
  x-ray interaction with matter, 50b
  x-ray photon absorption, 44b
Indirect conversion detectors, for direct digital radiography, 83
Inherent filtration, 35, 35f
Input phosphor, 264f
  in magnification mode, 266–267, 266f, 268f
Instantaneous-load tube-rating chart, 38f, 38b
Insulating oil, 20
Intensifying screens, 115–119, 115f
  absorption efficiency of, 117
  composition of, 115–116, 115b
  conversion efficiency of, 117
  fluorescence of, 116
  luminescence of, 116
  purpose of, 115
  quality-control check for, 119b
  speed of, 116–119
    for detail or extremity, 117–118
    factors affecting, 117, 117t
    and light emission, 117b
    and milliamperage, 118, 118b
    and patient dose, 117b
    and recorded detail, 116, 116b, 117t
    relative, 117–118
Intensity, of radiation exposure. *see* Exposure intensity
Interspace material, in grid, 189
Inverse-square law, for source-to-image receptor distance, 158–159, 159b
Invisible image, 51
Ion chambers, in automatic exposure control, 210–212, 211f, 212b
Ionization, 44
Ionization chamber systems, in automatic exposure control, 210–212, 211f, 212b
IP. *see* Imaging plate (IP)
IR. *see* Image receptor (IR)

K

Kilovoltage, 26–28
   and beam penetrability, 27b
   quality-control check for accuracy of, 28b
   and speed of electrons, 26b
   and x-ray quality, 27b
   and x-ray quantity, 27f
Kilovoltage peak (kVp)
   and 15% rule, 154, 154b–155b
   and density, 153, 154f
   and digital image quality, 157, 157b
   and exit-beam intensities, 155, 156f
   in exposure technique charts
      fixed, 227–228, 227t, 227b
      variable, 225–226, 226t, 226b
   as exposure technique factors, 152–158
   and exposure to image receptor, 152–155, 152b
      in digital imaging, 152, 153b
      in film-screen imaging, 153, 153f, 153b
   in image receptors
      digital, 245t
      film-screen, 246t
   optimal, 227
   and radiographic contrast, 155–158, 155b, 157b
   and scatter, 179b
   and scatter radiation, 157, 157b, 179, 179b
   selections, in automatic exposure control, 212–213,
      212b–213b
   of x-ray beams, 11
K-shell electrons, in characteristic interactions,
   21, 22f
kVp. *see* Kilovoltage peak (kVp)

L

Landscape, display monitors, 94
Laser printers, 104
Latent image, 51, 52b
   in computed radiography, 68
Latent image centers
   on film, 113–114
   and sensitivity specks, 114b
Latent image formation, on film, 113–114, 113f
Lateral decentering, 198, 198b, 199f
Lead, for radiation protection, 9–10
Leaded curtains, 9–10
Leakage radiation, 20
Light emission, and screen speed, 117b
Line pair, digital imaging and, 73f
Linear grid, 190, 190f
   long-dimension, 193–194, 193f
   short-dimension, 193–194, 193f
Line-focus principle, 32–33, 32b
   and actual and effective focal spot size, 32, 32f
   and target angle, 32, 32f, 33b

Liquid crystal display (LCD) monitor, 94, 96f
   in viewing systems, of fluoroscopy, 271–272, 272f
Log median (lgM) numbers, on exposure indicator, 89,
   89t
Long-dimension grids, 193–194, 193f
Long-scale contrast, 55, 56f–57f, 239, 239f–240f
Lookup tables (LUT), 90–92, 91f, 92b, 93f
   with altered pixel values to increase contrast, 92f
   with change in pixel values, 91f
   with no change in pixel values, 91f
Low spatial frequency, 74
Low-vacuum tube, 1–2, 3f
Low-contrast image, 55, 56f–57f, 239, 239f–240f
Low-energy photons, and beam filtration, 34, 34b
Luminance, of display monitor, 96
Luminescence
   in computed radiography, 75
   of intensifying screens, 116
LUT. *see* Lookup tables (LUT)

M

mA. *see* Milliamperage (mA)
Magnification, 58–59
   calculating, 163–165
      determining object size in, 164, 165b
      magnification factor in, 163, 164b
      object % of magnification in, 165, 165b
      source-to-object distance in, 163, 164f
Magnification factor (MF), 163, 164b
   in fluoroscopy, 266
Magnification mode, in fluoroscopy, 266–267,
   266f–267f
   patient dose and, 266b
   spatial resolution and, 267
Manifest image, 51
mAs. *see* Milliamperes per second (mAs)
Mathematical application
   adjusting mAs for changes in film-screen system
      speed, 118b
   adjusting mAs for changes in the grid, 168b
   adjusting milliamperage and exposure time to
      maintain mAs, 150b
   adjusting milliamperage or exposure time, 149b
   calculating heat units, 37b
   calculating mAs, 31b
   determining object % of magnification, 165b
   determining object size, 165b
   inverse square law formula, 159b
   magnification factor, 164, 164b
   mAs-distance compensation formula, 160b
   using 15% rule, 155b
Matrix, 68, 69f, 70b
Matrix size, 70b
   in computed radiography, 79b, 80f

Measurement, with exposure technique charts, 224, 225f
Metal envelope x-ray tube, 19–20
Metallic replacement, silver recovery by, 126
MF. *see* Magnification factor (MF)
Milliamperage (mA), 28–29
    and density, 151, 152f, 152b
    and digital image brightness, 150, 150b
    and exposure time, 30–31, 150b
        adjustment of, 149, 149b
        exposure indicator for, 150–151, 151b
        linearity of, 31b
        maintaining mAs with, 149, 150b
    and film-screen speed, 118, 118b
    in fluoroscopy, 263
    and quantum noise, 150, 151f
    source-to-image-receptor distance and, 160, 160b
    and tube current, 28–29, 29b–30b
    of x-ray beams, 11
    and x-ray quality, in exposure time, 148–149, 149f, 149b
    and x-ray quantity, 29f, 29b–30b
Milliampere (mA) selections, in automatic exposure control, 212–213, 212b–213b
Milliamperes per second (mAs), 30
    adjusting milliamperage and exposure time to maintain, 149, 149b
    calculation of, 31b
    and digital image brightness, 150, 150b
    distance conversions, 249, 249t
    in exposure technique charts
        fixed, 227–228, 227t, 227b
        variable, 225–226, 226t, 226b
    and film-screen density, 151, 152f, 152b
    in image quality calculations, 249, 249t
    in image receptors
        digital, 245t
        film-screen, 246t
    readout, in automatic exposure control, 212, 212b
    reciprocity, 31b
    and x-ray quality, and exposure time, 148–149, 149f, 149b
    and x-ray quantity, 31b
Milliamperes per second (mAs)-distance compensation formula, 160, 160b
Minification gain, in fluoroscopy, 265
Minimum response time, in automatic exposure control, 213
Minus-density artifacts, 243
Mobile C-arm units, 274–275, 275f
Modulation transfer function (MTF), 74–75, 75b
Moiré effect, 200, 201f
Monitor brightness, in fluoroscopic equipment inspection, 268b

Motion unsharpness, 58, 58f, 240, 241f
MTF. *see* Modulation transfer function (MTF)

N
Negative contrast agents, 232, 233f
Noise. *see* Quantum noise
Nonfocused grid, 190–191, 191f, 192b
    transmitted photons passing through, 190–191, 191f

O
Object % of magnification, 165, 165b
Object size, determining, 164, 165b
Object-to-image-receptor distance (OID), 58–59
    and air gap, 162, 162f
    defined, 163
    as exposure technique factors, 162–163
    in image receptors
        digital, 245t
        film-screen, 246t
    and size distortion, 162, 163f, 163b
    and spatial resolution, 162, 163b
Off-center grid cutoff, 198, 198b, 199f
Off-focus grid cutoff, 198–200, 198b, 200f
Off-focus radiation, 19–20
Off-level grid cutoff, 197, 197b, 198f
OID. *see* Object-to-image-receptor distance (OID)
Optical density, 131
    diagnostic range of, 131
    formula for, 132b
    and transmittance, 131
Optimal density, 140–141, 140f
Orthochromatic film, 114–115
Output phosphor, 263, 264f
    in magnification mode, 266–267, 266f, 268f

P
Parallel grid, 190–191, 191f, 192b
    transmitted photons passing through, 190–191, 191f
Part thickness
    as exposure technique factors, 172
    and scatter radiation, 180b
Pathological conditions, in exposure technique, 230–231, 231t
Patient centering, in automatic exposure control, 215–217, 216b, 217f
Patient considerations, in automatic exposure control, 218, 218b
Patient dose
    beam restriction and, 180b
    grid ratio and, 196b
    magnification and, 266, 266b
    and screen speed, 117b

Patient motion, in image receptors
　digital, 245t
　film-screen, 246t
Patient thickness, in image receptors
　digital, 245t
　film-screen, 246t
Pediatric patients, in exposure technique, 229
Penetrometer, 129, 129f–130f
Phenidone, in film developing, 119
Phosphor crystal, size of, and screen speed, 117, 117t
Phosphor layer
　of imaging plate, 75
　of intensifying screen, 115–116
　　and screen speed, 117, 117t
Phosphorescence, of intensifying screens, 116
Photocathode, 263, 264f
　in magnification mode, 266f, 267, 268f
Photoelectric effect, 44, 45f
　and Compton effect, 47b
Photoelectron, 44
Photoemission. *see* Photocathode
Photomultiplier tube (PMT)
　in automatic exposure control, 210
　in computed radiography, 77, 78f
Photons, 7
　absorption of, 44, 44b
Photo-spot cameras, in fluoroscopy, 273f, 274
Photostimulable luminescence, 75
Photostimulable phosphor (PSP), 75, 76f
Phototimers, in automatic exposure control, 210, 211f
Phototiming, 209. *see also* Automatic exposure control (AEC)
Pincushion distortion, in fluoroscopy, 267, 267f
Pixel(s), 68, 69f, 70b
Pixel bit depth, 70b–71b, 79–81
　and binary number system, 72b
Pixel density, 72, 72f, 72b
Pixel location, 68, 69f
Pixel pitch, 72, 72f, 72b
　in computed radiography, 77–79, 79f
Pixel size, 70b
Pixel values, 87–88
　changed, 92f
　on lookup tables, 91f
Plasma monitors, in viewing systems, of fluoroscopy, 272–273, 273f
Plus-density artifacts, 243
Portrait, display monitors, 94, 95f
Positioning considerations, in automatic exposure control, 215–218
Positions, in exposure technique, 230
Positive beam-limiting device, 187–188, 187b
Positive contrast agents, 233f

Postprocessing, 98–103
　black/white reversal in, 102, 103f
　brightness, 98–99, 99f
　　window level, 99f, 99b
　contrast enhancement in, 101, 102f
　contrast resolution in, 99
　edge enhancement in, 102, 102f
　electronic masking, 98
　smoothing in, 102, 103f
　subtraction in, 101, 101f
　window width in, 99, 100b
Potter-Bucky diaphragm, 193
Pregnancy, screening for, x-ray and, 11, 12b
Prep button, 23
Processor systems, 122–124, 123f
　feed tray in, 122, 123f
　immersion heater in, 124
　inadequate processing in, 124, 124t
　recirculation system in, 123
　replenishment in, 122, 123b
　solution performance in, 123b
　standby control in, 122
　temperature control in, 123
Projections, in exposure technique, 230
Protective curtain, in fluoroscopic equipment inspection, 268b
PSP. *see* Photostimulable phosphor (PSP)
Pulsed fluoroscopy, 278–279, 278f, 279b

Q
Quality control
　in automatic exposure control, 219, 219b
　for beam filtration, 36b
　for collimator and beam alignment, 187b
　for computed tomography, 96
　for exposure timer accuracy, 30b
　for film processing, 125, 126f–127f, 128b
　for fluoroscopy, 280–281, 281b
　for grid uniformity and alignment, 201, 202b
　for intensifying screens, 119b
　for kilovoltage, 28b
　for radiation output, 31b
Quantization, in computed radiography, 79–81
Quantum, 7
Quantum mottle, 61, 241
Quantum noise, 61–62, 62f
　in fluoroscopy, 268f
　in image evaluation, 241–242, 242f
　and number of photons, 61b

R
Radiation
　discovery of, 1–14
　electromagnetic, 1, 5

Radiation (*Continued*)
  exit, 49–51, 51f
  fundamentals of protection from, 9–13, 12b
    ALARA principle, 9b
    avoiding duplicate exams, 11b
    beam restriction, 11b
    minimizing radiation dose, 10b
    primary exposure factors, 11b
    screening for pregnancy, 12b
  leakage, 20
  off-focus, 19–20
  units of measurement for, 7–8
Radiation detectors, in automatic exposure control,
    209–212, 210f, 210b
  ionization chamber systems as, 210–212, 211f, 212b
  phototimers as, 210, 211f
  selection of, 215, 215b, 216f
  size of, 217–218
Radiation protection, 202
Radiation protection alert
  beam filtration and, 36b
  beam restriction, 169b
  excessive radiation exposure and digital imaging,
    153b
  grid selection, 168b
  kVp/mAs, 155b
Radiation safety, during fluoroscopic imaging,
    279–280, 280t
Radioactivity, 8
Radiographic quality, 52–64, 52f
  distortion in, 58–60
    shape, 59–60, 60f, 60b
    size, 58–59, 59b
  exposure technique charts and, 224b
  image artifacts in, 62–63, 63f
  image brightness in, 52–53, 53f–54f, 53b
    diagnostic, 53
    excessive, 53, 54f
    insufficient, 53, 54f
  image contrast in, 53–55
    in abdomen, 54, 56f
    and contrast resolution, 55
    desired level in, 55
    for differentiating among anatomic tissues, 54b
    in digital imaging, 55
    in film-screen imaging, 55
    of homogeneous object, 53–54, 55f
    of object with different absorption characteristics,
      53–54, 55f
    and sharpness, 58, 59f
    subject, 54
    in thorax, 54, 56f
  quantum noise in, 61–62, 62f
  and scatter, 60–61, 61f

Radiographs
  archival quality of, 121b–122b
  first, 3, 4f
Radiology information systems (RIS), 104
Rare earth elements, in intensifying screen, 115–116
Reader unit, in computed radiography, 77, 77f
Reciprocating grids, 193
Recirculation system, in film processor, 123
Recorded detail, 58
  and image contrast, 58, 59f
  in image evaluation, 240, 241f
  and patient motion, 58, 58f
  and screen speed, 116, 116b, 117t
Recording systems, in fluoroscopy, 273–274, 273f, 274b
Reducing agents, 119, 120b
Reflecting layer, of intensifying screen, and screen
    speed, 117, 117t
Relative exposure, log of, 133, 134f
Relative speed (RS), 117–118
Remnant radiation, 49–50
Replenishment, in processor systems, 122
Reproducibility, of exposure, 31b
Rescaling, automatic, 88
Resolution test pattern, 73f
RIS. *see* Radiology information systems (RIS)
Roentgen, Wilhelm Conrad, 1–2, 2f
Roentgen rays, 4
Roentgenology, 4
Rotating anode tube, 17, 17f–18f, 19b
  focal track and focal spot of, 18, 19f
  heat loads of, 18
  rotor of, 17, 18f
  stator of, 17, 18f
  tungsten of, 17, 17f–18f, 18b
Rotor, of rotating anode tube, 17, 18f
Rotor button, 23
Row gates, in viewing systems, of fluoroscopy, 269–270,
    270f
RS. *see* Relative speed (RS)

S
Safelights, in darkroom, 125
Safety, radiation, during fluoroscopic imaging,
    279–280, 280t
Sampling frequency, in computed radiography, 77–79
  fixed, 80f
  and matrix size, 79b
  and spatial resolution, 79b
Sampling pitch, in computed radiography, 77–79
Scale of contrast, 55
Scatter, and image quality, 60–61, 61f
Scatter control, 178–207
  air gap technique for, 203, 203f, 203b
  beam restriction for, 180

Scatter control (Continued)
  digital imaging and, 204
  radiographic grids for, 188–202
Scatter radiation, 179–180
  beam restriction and, 180–182, 181b, 182f
  in image artifacts, 243
  and image quality, 188, 188b
  kilovoltage peak and, 157, 157b, 179, 179b
  part thickness and, 180b
  x-ray-beam field size and, 179, 180b
Scattering, 44–46, 45b
  coherent, 46
  and Compton effect, 44–45, 46f
    and photoelectric effect, 47b
Screen speed, 116–119
  for detail or extremity, 117–118
  factors affecting, 117, 117t
  in image receptors
    digital, 245t
    film-screen, 246t
  and light emission, 117b
  and milliamperage, 118, 118b
  and patient dose, 117b
  and recorded detail, 116, 116b, 117t
  relative, 117–118
Secondary electron, 44–45
Secondary radiation, 9, 9b
Sensitivity (S) numbers, on exposure indicator, 89, 89t
Sensitivity specks
  on film, 113–114
  and latent image centers, 114b
Sensitometer, 129
Sensitometric curve, in film-screen imaging, 132–135, 133f
  log of relative exposure and, 133, 134f
  other terms for, 133b
  regions of, 133–135, 134f
    shoulder, 135
    straight-line, 135
    toe, 135
Sensitometry, of film, 128–129
  equipment for, 129
    densitometer as, 129, 130f–131f
    penetrometer as, 129, 129f–130f
    sensitometer as, 129
Shape distortion, 59–60, 60f, 60b, 165–167, 166f
  in image evaluation, 241, 241f
Sharpness
  in image evaluation, 237–238, 240
  of recorded detail, 57b, 58
    and image contrast, 58, 59f
    and patient motion, 58, 58f
Shielding
  accessories, 204–205, 204f
  during fluoroscopy, 280
  from radiation, 9–10

Short-dimension grids, 193–194, 193f
Short-scale contrast, 55, 56f–57f, 239, 239f–240f
SID. see Source-to-image-receptor distance (SID)
Signal-to-noise ratio (SNR), of digital imaging system, 85–86, 86b
Silver halide, 112–113
  and film sensitivity, 114b
Silver recovery, 125–128, 128b
Silver-recovery units, 126
Sine waves, of wavelength and frequency, 6, 6f–7f
Single-exposure rating charts, 38b
Single-phase generators, 28, 28f–29f
Size distortion, 58–59, 59b
  in image evaluation, 240
  object-to-image-receptor distance (OID) and, 162, 163f, 163b
  source-to-image-receptor distance and, 161, 161f, 161b
Slope of line, determining, 137b
Smoothing, postprocessing, 102, 103f
SOD. see Source-to-object distance (SOD)
Soft copy viewing, 93–94, 94f
Soft tissue, in exposure technique, 231–232, 232f
Solid state laser diode, in computed radiography, 77
Solution performance, in processor system, 123b
Source-to-image-receptor distance (SID), 58–59
  as exposure technique factors, 158–161
  in image receptors
    digital, 245t
    film-screen, 246t
  inverse-square law for, 158–159, 159b
  mAs-distance compensation formula for, 160, 160b
  and size distortion, 161, 161f, 161b
  and x-ray beam intensity, 159, 159b, 160f
Source-to-object distance (SOD), 163, 164f
Source-to-skin distance (SSD), in fluoroscopy, 280
Space charge, 24
Space charge effect, 24
Spatial frequency, pixel density and pixel pitch and, 72–74, 74b
Spatial resolution, 57–58, 57b
  and focal spot size, 158, 158b, 159f
  and image contrast, 58, 59f
  in image evaluation, 240, 241f
  magnification mode and, 267
  object-to-image-receptor distance (OID) and, 162, 163b
  and patient motion, 58, 58f
  pixel density and pixel pitch and, 72–74, 72f–74f, 72b
  sampling frequency and, in computed radiography, 77–79
  and source-to-image-receptor distance, 161, 161b
Spectral emission, of film, 114–115
Spectral matching, of film, 114–115

Spectral sensitivity, of film, 114–115
Speed exposure point, 135, 136f–137f
Speed point, 135, 136f
Splints, in exposure technique, 230
Spot-film camera, in fluoroscopy, 263, 264f
Standby control, of processor system, 122
Stationary anode tube, 17, 17f, 19f
Stationary grids, 193
Stator, of rotating anode tube, 17, 18f
Steel wool metallic replacement unit, 126
Subject contrast, 54
Subtraction, postprocessing, 101, 101f

T
Table tilt motion, in fluoroscopic equipment
    inspection, 268b
Target, of anode, 17, 17b
Target angle, 32, 32f
    and effective focal spot size, 33f, 33b
Target interactions, 20–22
    Bremsstrahlung, 20, 21f, 21b
    characteristic, 21–22, 22f, 22b
Technique charts. see Exposure technique charts
Television cameras, in viewing systems, of fluoroscopy,
    267–270, 269f–270f
Television monitor, in viewing systems, of fluoroscopy,
    270–271, 271f, 271b
Temperature control, in processor system, 123
Thermionic emission, 23, 23b
Thickness
    in image receptors
        digital, 245t
        film-screen, 246t
    and scatter radiation, 180b
    tissue, and beam attenuation, 47, 47f–48f, 50t
Thin-film transistor (TFT) array, in flat-panel
    detectors, 81
    direct conversion, 83
    indirect conversion, 82
Thiosulfate, as fixing agent, 121
Thorax, image contrast in, 54, 56f
Three-phase generators, 28, 28f–29f
Thyroid shields, 9–10
Time, radiation protection and, 10
Tissue atomic number, and beam attenuation, 47–48,
    50t
Tissue composition, and image contrast, 56f
Tissue density
    and beam attenuation, 48–49, 50t
    and image brightness, 51–53, 51f, 52b, 53f–54f
Tissue thickness
    and beam attenuation, 47, 47f–48f, 50t
    and scatter radiation, 180b
Tissue type, and beam attenuation, 47–49, 48f, 50t
Tissue volume, and scatter radiation, 180b

Total filtration, 35
Tower, in fluoroscopic equipment inspection, 268b
Transmission, 49, 50f
    and exit radiation, 49–51, 51f
    and latent image, 51
    and x-ray interaction with matter, 50b
Transmittance, and optical density, 131
    formula for, 132b
    percent, 132t
Trapped electrons, in computed radiography, 75–76
Trough filter, 36, 37f
Tube current, 24, 24b
    milliamperage and, 28–29, 30b
    during x-ray exposure, 26f
Tube filtration, 169–170, 170b
Tungsten, in anode tubes, 17, 17f–18f, 18b

U
Unrestricted primary beam, 180, 181f
Upside-down focused grid cutoff, 197, 197f, 197b

V
Values of interest (VOI), in histogram analysis, 87–88
Variable kVp/fixed mAs technique chart, 225–226,
    226t, 226b
Videotape, in recording systems, of fluoroscopy, 274
Vidicon-type camera tube, in viewing systems, of
    fluoroscopy, 267–269, 269f
Viewing systems, for fluoroscopy, 267–273
    charge-coupled device in, 269–270, 270f
    coupling of devices in, 270, 271b
    liquid crystal display (LCD) monitors in, 271–272,
        272f
    plasma monitors in, 272–273, 273f
    television cameras in, 267–270, 269f
    television monitor in, 270–271, 271f, 271b
Vignetting, in fluoroscopy, 267
Visibility, of recorded detail, 58, 237–238
    and image contrast, 58, 59f
    and patient motion, 58, 58f
Visible image, 51
VOI. see Values of interest (VOI)
Voltage ripple, 28

W
Wafer grid, 193
Washing, of film, 120t, 121–122
Wavelength, of x-rays, 6
    frequency and, 6f–7f, 6b
Wedge filter, 36, 37f
Wide-latitude film, 114
Window level
    and brightness, 98
    and contrast, 99
Window width, 99, 100b

X

X-ray(s)
Bremsstrahlung, 23f
characteristic, 21, 22f–23f
discovery of, 1–5, 3f
dual nature of, 6, 6b
as energy, 5–8, 5f–7f
frequency of, 6
wavelength and, 6f–7f, 6b
properties of, 8–9, 9b
radiographic unit for, 12f
wavelength of, 6
frequency and, 6f–7f, 6b
X-ray beam, 15–41
X-ray-beam field size
result of increasing, 182t
and scatter radiation, 179, 180b
X-ray beam intensity, source-to-image-receptor
distance and, 159, 159b, 160f
X-ray beam quality, and beam attenuation, 49, 49f, 50t
X-ray button, 23
X-ray emission spectrum, 22–23, 23f
X-ray exposure, 23–24
deadman switches in, 23
energy conversion in x-ray tube in, 24, 25b
exposure or x-ray button in, 23
filament current in, 23
making, 25b
preparing tube for, 24, 24b, 25f
rotor or prep button for, 23
space charge effect in, 24
space charge in, 24
thermionic emission in, 23, 23b
tube current in, 24, 24b, 26f
X-ray generators, 28, 28f–29f
X-ray production, 16–20, 20b

X-ray quality, 26–31
beam filtration and, 36f
defined, 26
kilovoltage and, 26–28, 26b–27b
quality-control check for, 28b
radiation output and, 31b
speed of electrons and, 27b
X-ray quantity
beam filtration and, 36f
defined, 26–31
exposure time and, 30b
generators for, 28, 28f–29f
and image brightness and density, 53
kilovoltage and, 26–28, 26b, 27f
mAs and, 31b
milliamperage and, 28–29, 29f, 29b–30b
voltage ripple and, 28
X-ray table, 12f
X-ray tube, 16
anode of, 17–18, 17f–18f
cathode of, 16, 16f, 18f
dual-focus, 16
energy conversion in, 24, 25b
extending life of, 39, 39f
filament of, 16, 16f, 16b, 18f
large and small, 16, 16f
during x-ray exposure, 25f
focusing cup of, 16, 16f, 18f, 26f
glass envelope, 19–20, 19f
metal envelope, 19–20
X-ray tube current, 24, 24b
X-ray tube housing, 19–20, 19f
X-ray tube-rating charts, 38f, 38b

Z

Zebra pattern, 200, 201f